Joint Repair and Replacement:
Clinical Updates and Perspectives

Joint Repair and Replacement: Clinical Updates and Perspectives

Editors

Massimiliano Mosca
Silvio Caravelli
Alberto Grassi

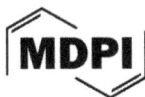

Basel • Beijing • Wuhan • Barcelona • Belgrade • Novi Sad • Cluj • Manchester

Editors

Massimiliano Mosca
U.O. Ortopedia Bentivoglio,
IRCCS Istituto Ortopedico
Rizzoli
Bologna
Italy

Silvio Caravelli
U.O. Ortopedia Bentivoglio,
IRCCS Istituto Ortopedico
Rizzoli
Bologna
Italy

Alberto Grassi
II Clinic of Orthoapedics and
Traumatology, IRCCS Istituto
Ortopedico Rizzoli
Bologna
Italy

Editorial Office
MDPI
St. Alban-Anlage 66
4052 Basel, Switzerland

This is a reprint of articles from the Special Issue published online in the open access journal *Journal of Clinical Medicine* (ISSN 2077-0383) (available at: https://www.mdpi.com/journal/jcm/special_issues/bone_loss).

For citation purposes, cite each article independently as indicated on the article page online and as indicated below:

Lastname, A.A.; Lastname, B.B. Article Title. *Journal Name* **Year**, *Volume Number*, Page Range.

ISBN 978-3-7258-0491-7 (Hbk)
ISBN 978-3-7258-0492-4 (PDF)
doi.org/10.3390/books978-3-7258-0492-4

Cover image courtesy of Silvio Caravelli

© 2024 by the authors. Articles in this book are Open Access and distributed under the Creative Commons Attribution (CC BY) license. The book as a whole is distributed by MDPI under the terms and conditions of the Creative Commons Attribution-NonCommercial-NoDerivs (CC BY-NC-ND) license.

Contents

About the Editors vii

Silvio Caravelli, Giulia Puccetti, Emanuele Vocale, Marco Di Ponte, Camilla Pungetti, Annalisa Baiardi, Alberto Grassi, et al.
Reconstructive Surgery and Joint-Sparing Surgery in Valgus and Varus Ankle Deformities: A Comprehensive Review
Reprinted from: *J. Clin. Med.* 2022, 11, 5288, doi:10.3390/jcm11185288 1

Jaime Oraa, Maider Beitia, Nicolás Fiz, Sergio González, Xabier Sánchez, Diego Delgado and Mikel Sánchez
Custom 3D-Printed Cutting Guides for Femoral Osteotomy in Rotational Malalignment Due to Diaphyseal Fractures: Surgical Technique and Case Series
Reprinted from: *J. Clin. Med.* 2021, 10, 3366, doi:10.3390/jcm10153366 12

Alessandro Bruschi, Luca Cevolani, Benedetta Spazzoli, Marco Focaccia, Stefano Pasini, Tommaso Frisoni and Davide Maria Donati
Periacetabular Tumour Resection under Anterosuperior Iliac Spine Allows Better Alloprosthetic Reconstruction than Above: Bone Contact Matters
Reprinted from: *J. Clin. Med.* 2022, 11, 4499, doi:10.3390/jcm11154499 21

Michele Fiore, Andrea Sambri, Matteo Filippini, Lorenzo Morante, Claudio Giannini, Azzurra Paolucci, Claudia Rondinella, et al.
Are Static Spacers Superior to Articulated Spacers in the Staged Treatment of Infected Primary Knee Arthroplasty? A Systematic Review and Meta-Analysis
Reprinted from: *J. Clin. Med.* 2022, 11, 4854, doi:10.3390/jcm11164854 33

Massimiliano Mosca, Alberto Grassi and Silvio Caravelli
Osteochondral Lesions of Ankle and Knee. Will Future Treatments Really Be Represented by Custom-Made Metal Implants?
Reprinted from: *J. Clin. Med.* 2022, 11, 3817, doi:10.3390/jcm11133817 57

Giuseppe Anzillotti, Alberto Iacomella, Matteo Grancagnolo, Enrico Maria Bertolino, Maurilio Marcacci, Cristiano Sconza, Elizaveta Kon, et al.
Conservative vs. Surgical Management for Femoro-Acetabular Impingement: A Systematic Review of Clinical Evidence
Reprinted from: *J. Clin. Med.* 2022, 11, 5852, doi:10.3390/jcm11195852 59

Marco Girolami, Cristiana Griffoni, Emanuela Asunis, Luigi Falzetti, Stefano Bandiera, Giovanni Barbanti Brodano, Riccardo Ghermandi, et al.
Custom-Made 3D-Printed Implants for Anterior Column Reconstruction in the Upper Cervical Spine after Intralesional Extracapsular Excision—Report of 2 Cases and Literature Review
Reprinted from: *J. Clin. Med.* 2022, 11, 6058, doi:10.3390/jcm11206058 69

Eugenio Cammisa, Iacopo Sassoli, Matteo La Verde, Stefano Fratini, Vito Gaetano Rinaldi, Giada Lullini, Vittorio Vaccari, et al.
Bilateral Knee Arthroplasty in Patients Affected by Windswept Deformity: A Systematic Review
Reprinted from: *J. Clin. Med.* 2022, 11, 6580, doi:10.3390/jcm11216580 81

Andrea Fidanza, Irene Schettini, Gabriele Palozzi, Vasileios Mitrousias, Giandomenico Logroscino, Emilio Romanini and Vittorio Calvisi
What Is the Inpatient Cost of Hip Replacement? A Time-Driven Activity Based Costing Pilot Study in an Italian Public Hospital
Reprinted from: *J. Clin. Med.* 2022, *11*, 6928, doi:10.3390/jcm11236928 90

Michela Saracco, Andrea Fidanza, Stefano Necozione, Giulio Maccauro and Giandomenico Logroscino
Could Short Stems THA Be a Good Bone-Saving Option Even in Obese Patients?
Reprinted from: *J. Clin. Med.* 2022, *11*, 7114, doi:10.3390/jcm11237114 100

Giovanni Trisolino, Alessandro Depaoli, Giovanni Gallone, Marco Ramella, Eleonora Olivotto, Paola Zarantonello, Stefano Stallone, et al.
A 20-Year Retrospective Study of Children and Adolescents Treated by the Three-in-One Procedure for Patellar Realignment
Reprinted from: *J. Clin. Med.* 2023, *12*, 702, doi:10.3390/jcm12020702 111

Patrick Reinbacher, Andrzej Hecker, Joerg Friesenbichler, Maria Smolle, Lukas Leitner, Sebastian Klim, Alexander Draschl, et al.
Simultaneous Bilateral Total Hip Arthroplasty with Straight-Stems and Short-Stems: Does the Short One Do a Better Job?
Reprinted from: *J. Clin. Med.* 2023, *12*, 1028, doi:10.3390/jcm12031028 125

Enrico Guerra, Alessandro Marinelli, Fabio Tortorella, Michelle Dos Santos Flöter, Alice Ritali, Andrea Sessa, Giuseppe Carbone, et al.
Elbow Arthroscopy for the Treatment of Radial Head Fractures: Surgical Technique and 10 Years of Follow Up Results Compared to Open Surgery
Reprinted from: *J. Clin. Med.* 2023, *12*, 1558, doi:10.3390/jcm12041558 133

Luca De Marziani, Angelo Boffa, Lucia Angelelli, Luca Andriolo, Alessandro Di Martino, Stefano Zaffagnini and Giuseppe Filardo
Infrared Thermography in Symptomatic Knee Osteoarthritis: Joint Temperature Differs Based on Patient and Pain Characteristics
Reprinted from: *J. Clin. Med.* 2023, *12*, 2319, doi:10.3390/jcm12062319 143

Sebastian Martin Klim, Patrick Reinbacher, Maria Anna Smolle, Andrzej Hecker, Michael Maier, Joerg Friesenbichler, Andreas Leithner, et al.
Femoral Anteversion in Total Hip Arthroplasty: Retrospective Comparison of Short- and Straight-Stem Models Using CT Scans
Reprinted from: *J. Clin. Med.* 2023, *12*, 2391, doi:10.3390/jcm12062391 154

Luca De Marziani, Angelo Boffa, Simone Orazi, Luca Andriolo, Alessandro Di Martino, Stefano Zaffagnini and Giuseppe Filardo
Joint Response to Exercise Is Affected by Knee Osteoarthritis: An Infrared Thermography Analysis
Reprinted from: *J. Clin. Med.* 2023, *12*, 3399, doi:10.3390/jcm12103399 164

About the Editors

Massimiliano Mosca

Massimiliano Mosca is an Orthopaedic surgeon and complex unit chief at the IRCCS Istituto Ortopedico Rizzoli in Bologna (Italy). He graduated and specialized at the University of Bologna, always fascinated in the pathology and surgery of the foot and ankle. He carries out teaching and clinical activities for UNIBO degree courses. He authored numerous scientific articles dealing mainly with the articular and extrarticular pathology of the tibio-podalic complex. He is also a volunteer orthopedic surgeon in developing countries; he went to Camerum and helped adult and young patients suffering from serious deformities, such as congenital clubfoot, varus or valgus knees, and outcomes of childhood cerebral palsy or poliomyelitis.

Silvio Caravelli

Silvio Caravelli graduated in Medicine and Surgery from the University of L'Aquila; he specialized in Orthopaedics and Traumatology with honors at the University of Bologna. He discussed his PhD dissertation thesis in Biomedical and Neuromotor Sciences in 2019, shifting his research activity to the Laboratory of Biomechanics and the Technological Innovation of the IRCCS Istituto Ortopedico Rizzoli. He carries out his research in the field of articular and extra-articular pathology of the lower limb and biomechanics of the foot and ankle. His areas of interest are mainly, but not exclusively, aimed at researching and understanding the field of kinematics in in vivo ankle prosthetic components, as well as the treatment of degenerative arthropathy, regenerative surgery and complex deformities of the ankle and foot. He has carried out part of his scientific and clinical activity at the FIFA Excellence Center—Sports Medicine Aspetar Hospital in Doha (Qatar), under the guide of Prof. Pieter D'Hooghe. He participated in national and international conferences as a speaker, presenting the results of his research activities carried out at the IRCCS Istituto Ortopedico Rizzoli. His scientific output covers various fields of interest and is published in nationally and internationally indexed journals. He has collaborated in the drafting of several volumes and international books of orthopedic and traumatological interest as author, co-author and editorial collaborator. He also carries out continuous reviewer activities for international scientific journals. He is an active member of the Italian Society of Orthopaedic and Traumatology (SIOT) and Italian Society of Foot and Ankle Study (SISPEC).

Alberto Grassi

Alberto Grassi is an orthopaedic surgeon, with expertise in the fields of the knee, ligament and meniscus, and sports traumatology. He completed his MD at the University of Bologna, Italy, in 2010, and his medical school thesis was published in 2012. He completed his residency in Orthopaedics and Traumatology at Rizzoli Orthopaedic Institute of Bologna, Italy, in 2016, and he completed a PhD in Biomedical Sciences at the University of Bologna. Since 2009, he collaborated with Prof. Stefano Zaffagnini and Prof. Maurilio Marcacci in clinical and research settings, which allowed him to publish over 90 papers in peer-reviewed and indexed journals, over 30 book chapters, surgical videos and abstracts for international congresses. His major research interests are meniscal allograft and scaffold replacement, biomechanics of knee ligament reconstructions, non-invasive assessment of knee laxities, and evidence-based medicine and the meta-analysis of sports trauma conditions. He was a fellow of Dr Annunziato "Ned" Amendola at Duke University, North Carolina, USA, in 2016, and winner of the European Arthroscopy Fellowship in 2018, visiting European centres of arthroscopic surgery in Germany, France, Denmark, Italy, Spain and Portugal. He is an active member of the Italian Society of Knee surgery and Arthroscopy (SIGASCOT), where he has a relevant role in the Sports Committee (2014-2016) and Arthroscopy Committee (2016–2018 and 2018–2020). He is also an active member of ESSKA and ESMA, and a member of the ESSKA Arthroscopy Committee (2018–2020). In 2018, he received the National Qualification for his role as Associate Professor in Orthopaedics.

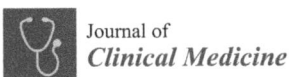

Review

Reconstructive Surgery and Joint-Sparing Surgery in Valgus and Varus Ankle Deformities: A Comprehensive Review

Silvio Caravelli [1,*], Giulia Puccetti [1], Emanuele Vocale [1], Marco Di Ponte [1], Camilla Pungetti [2], Annalisa Baiardi [1], Alberto Grassi [1] and Massimiliano Mosca [1]

1 II Clinic of Orthopaedics and Traumatology, IRCCS Istituto Ortopedico Rizzoli, 40136 Bologna, Italy
2 Department Orthopaedics and Traumatology, Ospedale Maggiore "Pizzardi", 40133 Bologna, Italy
* Correspondence: doct.car@gmail.com

Abstract: Osteoarthritis (OA) of the ankle affects about 1% of the world's adult population, causing an important impact on patient lives and health systems. Most patients with ankle OA can show an asymmetrical wear pattern with a predominant degeneration of the medial or the lateral portion of the joint. To avoid more invasive ankle joint sacrificing procedures, joint realignment surgery has been developed to restore the anatomy of the joints with asymmetric early OA and to improve the joint biomechanics and symptoms of the patients. This narrative, comprehensive, all-embracing review of the literature has the aim to describe the current concepts of joint preserving and reconstructive surgery in the treatment of the valgus and varus ankle early OA, through an original iconography and clear indications and technical notes.

Keywords: ankle deformity; early osteoarthritis; reconstruction; joint-sparing; surgery; review

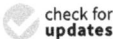

Citation: Caravelli, S.; Puccetti, G.; Vocale, E.; Di Ponte, M.; Pungetti, C.; Baiardi, A.; Grassi, A.; Mosca, M. Reconstructive Surgery and Joint-Sparing Surgery in Valgus and Varus Ankle Deformities: A Comprehensive Review. *J. Clin. Med.* 2022, *11*, 5288. https://doi.org/10.3390/jcm11185288

Academic Editor: Christian Carulli

Received: 24 June 2022
Accepted: 2 September 2022
Published: 8 September 2022

Publisher's Note: MDPI stays neutral with regard to jurisdictional claims in published maps and institutional affiliations.

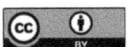

Copyright: © 2022 by the authors. Licensee MDPI, Basel, Switzerland. This article is an open access article distributed under the terms and conditions of the Creative Commons Attribution (CC BY) license (https:// creativecommons.org/licenses/by/ 4.0/).

1. Introduction

Ankle osteoarthritis (OA) affects about 1% of the world's adult population [1], causing an important socioeconomic impact on patients and health systems [2,3]. Unlike the hip and the knee, ankle OA is reported in about 80% of the cases related to trauma [4,5], and a part of the population involved is represented by active and high-performance-demanding patients, with a large part younger than 50 years [1].

Most patients with ankle OA show an asymmetrical wear pattern [6] with a predominant degeneration of the medial or the lateral portion of the joint. If left untreated, these patients will have a progression of the disease up to end-stage global osteoarthritis [7].

To avoid more invasive ankle joint sacrificing procedures, joint realignment surgery has been developed to restore the anatomy of the joints with asymmetric early osteoarthritis and improve the biomechanics of the joints and symptoms of the patients [6–8]. This narrative, comprehensive, all-embracing review of the literature has the aim to describe the current joint preserving and reconstructive surgery in the treatment of the valgus and varus ankle early osteoarthritis.

2. Etiology

About 80% of ankle OA has a post-traumatic origin, such as articular fractures or repeated trauma [9,10]. The fractures that can lead to an asymmetric *valgus* ankle are represented by the distal diaphysis of the tibia, tibial plafond, and distal fibular fractures [3]. Another frequent cause of *valgus* ankle osteoarthritis is repeated ankle sprains with associated insufficiency of the deltoid ligament complex [11].

The deltoid ligament complex has a fundamental role in preventing the lateral translation and valgus inclination of the talus [12]. It has been demonstrated that lesions of the deep portion of the deltoid ligament can lead to a lateral translation of the talus and cause valgus ankle osteoarthritis [11–13]. Moreover, the adult flatfoot deformity associated with tibialis posterior (TP) dysfunction and hindfoot abnormalities can be recognized as a cause of ankle OA [14,15].

Varus deformities can also be related to previous fractures (mostly lower-leg fractures [16,17] and/or repetitive ankle sprains [18]), as well as bone deformities, chronic lateral capsulo-ligamentous insufficiency or muscle imbalance, or neurologic diseases such as cerebral palsy or nerve disorders. As with valgus deformities, the *varus* ones can be associated with a concomitant deformity that may be seen at the supramalleolar, intraarticular, and/or inframalleolar level [18–20].

3. Management of *Valgus* Ankle Early Osteoarthritis
3.1. Diagnosis
3.1.1. Clinical Assessment

It is necessary to obtain a full clinical history of the patient, including comorbidities, previous surgeries, trauma, and fractures. Both the lower limbs need to be fully exposed; it is necessary to evaluate the alignment of the entire limb during weight-bearing and the posture during standing and walking [11].

The painful areas of the ankle and foot have to be evaluated, as well as the motion of the joints. The instability of the medial or lateral ligamentous complex should be clinically tested. Tightness of the Achilles tendon has to be studied with the knee in extension and flexion.

Tiptoe position and the function of the tibialis posterior tendon should be assessed; the hindfoot alignment, plantar arch, and midfoot are then considered. The mobility of the hindfoot and midfoot and any deformity should be highlighted and defined if mobile or rigid [11]. The position of the forefoot, in particular of the first ray, should be determined, as well as the eventual supination or pronation of the forefoot and toe deformities [21].

3.1.2. Radiographic Assessment

In the literature, authors routinely reported weight-bearing standardized radiographs for radiographic evaluation. These require anteroposterior and lateral views of the ankle and lateral and dorsoplantar views of the foot [3,22]. Besides, it is also useful to perform a *mortise view* of the tibiotalar joint [14]. A Saltzman view is included for the evaluation of the hindfoot alignment.

Patients with a deformity involving the ipsilateral hip or knee should be assessed with a panoramic weight-bearing radiograph of the entire limb.

One of the most important parameters for the analysis of the valgus deformity of the tibiotalar joint is the medial distal tibial angle (MDTA, Figure 1), which measures the angle between the longitudinal axis of the tibia and the transverse axis of the tibial plafond. The mean value reported in the literature differs between measurements on radiographs and studies on cadavers. In vivo radiographic measurements reported a mean value of $92.4 \pm 3.1°$ (84–100°) and studies on cadavers a mean value of $93.3 \pm 3.2°$ [3,23]. Moreover, the measures could differ between radiographs in standard and mortise views of the ankle; it is recommended to perform the angle measurements on standardized radiographs.

Another fundamental measurement for the preoperative evaluation of a valgus ankle is the medial tibiotalar angle (MTTA). The MTTA measure the position of the articular surface of the talus concerning the main axis of the tibia, with a mean value of $9.5° \pm 1.2°$ [14]. The difference between the MDTA and the MTTA gives the talar tilt and measures the incongruence of the tibiotalar joint [4]. The talar tilt in a normal aligned ankle has a value of less than 4° [24]. As reported by Krähenbühl et al. [25], the MDTA and talar tilt are useful measurements to distinguish between a supramalleolar and an intraarticular deformity. An MDTA value greater than 92° indicates a supramalleolar valgus deformity. A talar tilt greater than 4° is related to an incongruent tibiotalar joint and an intraarticular deformity.

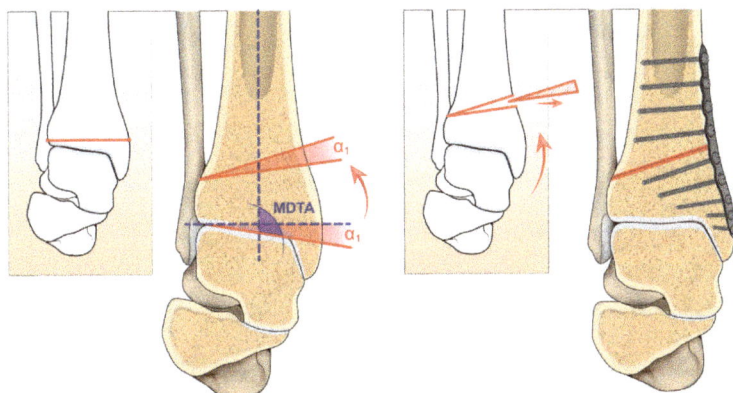

Figure 1. Visual artwork showing α angle of correction and MDTA (medial distal tibial angle). α: angular correction desired.

In selected cases with degenerative alterations of the ankle and other adjacent joints, it is recommended to use single-photon emission computed tomography (SPECT/CT) to evaluate the exact location of the degenerative joint changes and their biological activity [21,26].

Eventually, magnetic resonance imaging (MRI) will be useful in the evaluation of the amount of residual cartilage layer, the grade of joint degeneration, eventual osteochondral lesions, and the quality of the ankle ligaments and tendons [22,27].

4. Indications and Contraindications

The main indication for a realignment surgery procedure is represented by an asymmetric OA with a valgus deformity associated with a lateral articular surface preserved [7,28]. Some authors reported that at least 50% of the articular surface should be preserved for this surgery [4,29]. In selected patients, another indication is isolated lateral osteochondral lesions of the ankle [30]. In some cases, a realignment procedure represents the first surgical step in ankle replacement surgery [31], making it easier and faster. It reduces the time of surgery and complications and improving the final alignment of the definitive components [3].

The contraindications to a realignment surgery can be found in an end-stage OA with less than 50% of cartilage preserved, patients in poor general health or not able to follow the postoperative protocol [28], vascular or neurological diseases, poor bone quality [4], acute or chronic infections of the ankle, unmanageable hindfoot instability [3], or neuropathic disorders.

Relative contraindications are represented by advanced age (older than 70 years) [3], smoking, diabetes mellitus, soft tissue or skin disorders, or abnormalities [4,32].

5. Supramalleolar Osteotomy

A supramalleolar osteotomy is a surgical procedure introduced by Takakura et al. [14,33] in 1995. In a *supramalleolar valgus deformity*, the most indicated surgical procedure is a medial closing wedge osteotomy.

5.1. Preoperative Planning

To determine the height of the wedge of the osteotomy, the width of the distal tibia (W) is measured on an anteroposterior weight-bearing radiograph. The height of the wedge to remove from the tibia is the result of the formula: $H = \tan \alpha_1 \times W$, with α_1 as the desired angular correction [3,34] (Figure 1). The osteotomy distal plane should be perpendicular to the medial cortex of the tibia. The proximal plane is inclined based on the angle of correction desired and the height of the wedge to remove (as a general rule, it is suggested there be an overcorrection of 2–4°) [4]. For anomalous MDTA, the center of rotation of angular (CORA) is measured. It is represented by the intersection of the mid-diaphyseal line and the line from the center of the joint and perpendicular to the abnormal MDTA. CORA may be at the level of the joint line (usually due to misalignment or degeneration of the anatomical joint line) or proximal (usually due to tibial defects/fractures) [34–36].

5.2. Clinical Results

Hintermann et al. [37] reported 48 cases of ankle malunited fracture sequaele, treated by supramalleolar osteotomy, finding a correction of malalignment in all patients at the follow-up. At the follow-up of 7.1 years, good–excellent results were found in 42 patients. Pagenstert et al. [7] reported 35 cases of realignment surgery for valgus or varus osteoarthritis. At a mean follow-up of 5 years, the authors found a significant improvement in pain and functionality.

Knupp et al. [8] reported 92 patients with valgus or varus malalignment treated with realignment surgery. At a mean follow-up of 43 months, they reported clinical and radiological improvements, with a subsequent ankle arthrodesis or arthroplasty in 10 patients.

6. Distal Fibular Lengthening Osteotomy

The unsatisfactory reduction of a distal fibular fracture, or the loss of the reduction obtained with the surgery, could lead to an alteration of the anatomical axis and distribution of the loads on the articular surfaces, with a consequent deformity in the valgus of the tibiotalar joint [38,39]. The incidence of malunion after ankle fractures is reported as between 5% and 68% [40,41].

The fibula represents the tibiotalar joint lateral buttress and contributes to maintain the normal anatomy and position of the talus in the mortise. The most frequent malunion of the fibula is shortening and external rotation and can lead to a widening of the mortise and lateralization and instability of the talus [42,43]. Typically, an ankle with a malunion of the fibula is characterized by a widened medial joint space due to the external rotation and lateral translation of the talus [43–45]. As described, the translation and instability of the talus have important implications for the function of the tibiotalar joint: a translation of 1 mm of the talus can lead to a reduction of the joint contact surface by up to 40% [38,39,44].

Speed et al. [41] first described the corrective osteotomy of a malunited fibula in 1936. Since then, several authors have reported encouraging results with this type of surgical procedure. Weber et al. [46] described a Z-lengthening osteotomy, Roberts et al. [47] described an oblique osteotomy at the level of the initial fracture, and Yablon and Leach [48] used a transverse fibular osteotomy with or without the use of bone graft (Figure 2).

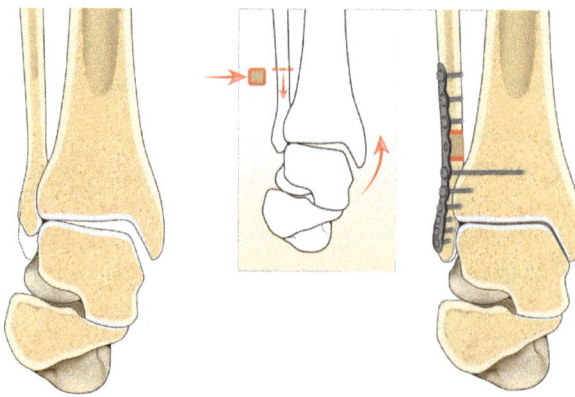

Figure 2. Visual artwork showing fibular lengthening osteotomy technique.

The oblique or Z-lengthening osteotomy is indicated only for shortening of minimum entity and malrotations of less than 10°. In cases of important deformities, a transverse osteotomy must be preferred [49]. It is important to note that in this procedure the debridement of the syndesmotic scar tissue is mandatory to enable lengthening the fibula, otherwise, the fibula cannot be pushed downwards to the tibiofibular joint [46]. Due to the altered anatomy of the fibula and also due to instability of the syndesmosis, it is common to detect a high talar tilt value on the radiograph. Most authors measured radiographic parameters on weight-bearing radiographs internally rotated at 20° [43].

Three main alterations of the normal anatomy of the ankle are common on an anteroposterior 20° internally rotated radiograph: unequal joint space, a broken Shenton's line, and a broken curve between the lateral part of the talar articular surface and fibular recess [38,43,50]. Other parameters important for the evaluation and planning are the talar tilt, the talocrural angle, and the bimalleolar angle.

Leaving out the already explained talar tilt, the talocrural angle represents the angle between the line of the tibial plafond and a line connecting the tips of the lateral and medial malleolus [43]. If this measurement is greater than 3° compared to the contralateral side, a fibular shortening is present. The bimalleolar angle is formed by a line connecting the tips of the two malleoli and a vertical line that follows the fibular intramedullary space (Figure 3). A difference greater than 2.5° compared to the contralateral side indicates a fibular shortening [43,51].

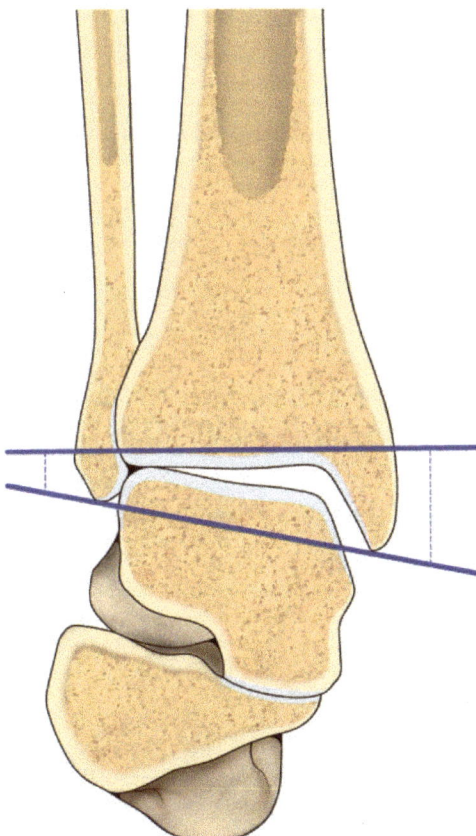

Figure 3. Visual artwork highlighting the bimalleolar angle.

To assess the amount of fibular shortening on the affected side, it can be useful to compare the relationship between the medial and lateral malleolus to those on the normal contralateral ankle [42].

Computerized tomography (CT) is useful for the evaluation of malrotation and to detect the incongruence of the lateral malleolus in the fibularis tibiae notch [42,46].

Clinical Results

Weber et al. reported 23 cases of fibular malunion treated with lengthening osteotomy, with 73% good–excellent results [50]. El-Rosasy et al. [42] described 17 cases, with 12 good or excellent and 5 unsatisfactory results. Van Wensen et al. [43] found, in their case series, 75% good or excellent results. Mosca et al. [38] reported the outcomes of 23 patients treated with ankle joint rebalancing through fibular lengthening, with an improvement of the AOFAS score from a preoperative 32.6 ± 7.6 points to a postoperative score of 74.0 ± 8.9 points and all cases treated with radiographic evidence of good alignment.

7. Ligament Reconstructions

The deltoid ligament complex has a fundamental role in the medial stability of the ankle. Besides, it contributes to preventing the lateral translation and the valgus angulation of the talus [11,12]. In case of concomitant insufficiency of the deltoid ligament, its reconstruction is indicated.

As reported by Hogan et al. [11], the reconstruction of the deltoid ligament complex represents a valid additional treatment when ligamentous stability and balancing are required. Instead, an isolated reconstruction of the deltoid ligament is not an effective treatment of the valgus ankle OA and cannot have satisfactory outcomes as an isolated procedure.

Various techniques have been described for the repair or reconstruction of the deltoid ligament. It is possible to repair the deltoid ligament anatomically by reattachment and retensioning it to its origin on the medial malleolus with anchors or trans-osseous sutures [14]. Wiltberger and Mallory described a technique using a tendinous autograft, splitting the posterior tibial tendon (PTT). The PTT was left attached to its insertion and the split proximal end passed through a bone tunnel in the medial malleolus [11,52].

8. Associated Procedures (Calcaneal Osteotomy, Evans Osteotomy, Subtalar and Midfoot Arthrodesis, Cotton Osteotomy, Posterior Tibial Tendon Repair or Reconstruction)

In cases of associated valgus deformity of the hindfoot or of the mid- or forefoot, or posterior tibial tendon dysfunction, additional procedures could be considered.

9. Management of Varus Ankle Early Osteoarthritis

9.1. Diagnosis

9.1.1. Clinical Assessment

The patient's examination has a central role in the evaluation work-up: during the clinical examination, it is important to expose not only the foot but the entire lower limb because the varus malalignment can be related not only to the ankle but also to the entire lower limb. The patient must be examined barefoot, during walking and standing, and the position of the ankle, the foot, and the hindfoot should be assessed. It is not rare to point out heel varus, cavus foot, and/or a first ray plantarflexion while examining the foot during weight-bearing. Using the Coleman Block test, it is possible to assess the role of the first ray on the varus hindfoot position. Clinical evaluation should also take into consideration the compensatory valgus position of the hindfoot. After visual examination, palpation must be performed; it is important to focus on the search for a tender spot on the course of the medial and lateral ligament complexes and tendons; the joint lines of the ankle, subtalar, and Chopart joints should be always palpated to highlight painful points.

The functionality of muscles should be evaluated and particular attention must be paid to possible tightness of the heel cord and function of plantar flexors. The stability of the ankle and the hindfoot should be manually assessed. It is also important to measure the tibiotalar range of motion both in plantarflexion/dorsiflexion and in eversion/inversion.

The last part of the clinical examination should include a neurovascular status examination and in particular tibial nerve function.

9.1.2. Radiographic Assessment

The radiographic examination is performed through weight-bearing X-rays: dorsoplantar and lateral plain radiographs of the foot, ankle mortise, and hindfoot alignment view (Saltzman view).

Panoramic lower limb radiographs should also be included allowing the surgeon to assess the bony deformities of the entire lower extremity. Preoperative CT scans, SPECT-CT [26], or a weight-bearing CT (WBCT) could be useful to better comprehend the case, assess the quality of the bone, and identify cysts preoperatively [53]. Magnetic resonance imaging (MRI) may be helpful to evaluate possible tendon and muscle pathologies [54].

9.1.3. Surgical Treatment

If conservative treatment has given no benefit to the patient, surgical treatment should be taken into consideration. The surgical options are joint-sparing techniques, arthrodesis, and arthroplasty. Regardless of the technique, the goal is to reach a plantigrade, fully functional, and stable foot. To obtain an optimal treatment, associated deformities, forefoot malalignment, lesser toe deformities, Achilles tendon tightness, knee deformities, and contralateral lower limb malalignment, lateral chronic ankle instability, and hindfoot OA must be recognized.

10. Supramalleolar Osteotomy

The aims of supramalleolar osteotomy (SMOT) are both restoration of the lower-leg axis (to improve intra-articular load distribution) and to slow down or to stop the degeneration of the tibiotalar joint [3,55,56] (Figure 4).

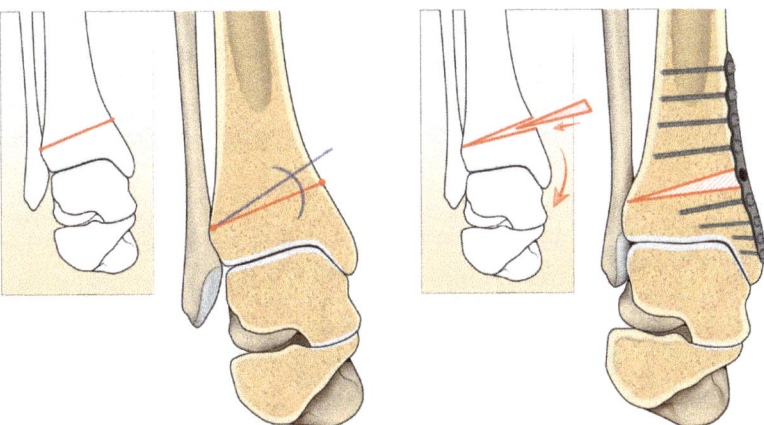

Figure 4. Visual artwork showing supramalleolar osteotomy in varus ankle deformity.

Before performing a SMOT it is important to assess different parameters preoperatively, such as the medial distal tibial angle to quantify the supramalleolar varus deformity, the tibiotalar tilt to evaluate intra-articular deformity in the coronal plane, and the calcaneal moment arm to quantify inframalleolar deformity in the coronal plane. Based on leg length, the osteotomy can be performed either in a medial opening-wedge or lateral closing-wedge fashion when the varus deformity is larger than 10° and/or a previously fused distal tibiofibular joint is present [16]. It may (in most cases) or may not be associated with a fibular osteotomy in case of an overlong fibula. Knupp and colleagues [34] modified a classification of varus ankle providing a treatment algorithm for the joint sparing procedure. It is extremely useful if an isolated supramalleolar osteotomy may not be sufficient to correct the deformity.

Depending on the case, different procedures could be associated, such as an intra-articular distal tibia osteotomy, if varus talar tilt persists due to asymmetric joint wear (it could be done simultaneously with medial opening wedge osteotomy as described by Hintermann and colleagues [57]). Other concomitant procedures could be done if ligamentous instability or fixed hindfoot deformity is present [7].

Indications and Contraindications

The common indications for SMOT are represented by supramalleolar varus deformity with a partially preserved tibiotalar joint, end-stage ankle OA requiring total ankle replacement, or ankle arthrodesis (as a staged procedure to improve the overall leg axis).

Contraindications to SMOT are end-stage varus OA with degeneration of the entire tibiotalar joint.

11. Discussion

Ankle OA results from mainly post-traumatic causes. The typical patient is relatively young and active and because of that, their expectations are higher than those of the patient affected by hip or knee OA. In the early stages of varus ankle OA, the best option is represented by an osteotomy to shift the weight load from medial to lateral [3,55,56]. Through surgery, it is possible to resume normal biomechanics and to achieve pain relief, functional improvement, and also slow down the degeneration process [7,33,58–62].

On the other hand, it is important to underline that 25% of patients who undergo a SMOT procedure need a secondary procedure [63]. Krähenbühl and colleagues [6], in a prospective study showed the need of a secondary ankle replacement or an ankle arthrodesis at long-term follow-up.

Risk factors associated with failure of an early OA treatment are young age at the time of the surgery and a Takakura preoperative score 3B. Additionally, a preoperative tibiotalar varus tilt greater than $7°$ can be considered a risk factor [6], as well as a varus ankle with the talus tilted within the mortise, and degenerative changes located in the medial gutter as described by Tanaka [64].

On the other hand, Kim and colleagues [55] in their retrospective study showed significant pain relief in most of the 31 patients who underwent supramalleolar medial wedge OT (Visual Analog Scale (VAS) 7.1 + 0.8/3.4 + 1.3); they also showed a functional improvement (American Orthopedic Foot and Ankle Society (AOFAS) hindfoot score 62.9 + 4.0/83.1 + 7.5) at a mean of 13.2 + 1.4 months after surgery. In another series of 35 patients who had undergone supramalleolar osteotomies by Pagenstert and colleagues [7], 91% postponed total ankle replacement.

Today, computer tomography-based 3D planning allows the operators to make a precise prediction of the correction and the possibility of performing the surgical procedure using patient-specific cutting guides, increasing its accuracy [65].

However, it is important to underline the fact that complete pain relief cannot be achieved by SMOT because of preexisting irreversible degenerative changes of the tibiotalar joint.

12. Complications and Pitfalls

The intraoperative complications of these procedures include neurovascular or tendon lesions. An accurate surgery is necessary to minimize this risk [3].

Wound healing problems are frequent, above all in patients with risk factors such as smokers, diabetes, or poor quality of soft tissues.

Over- or under-correction of the deformity can be linked to inaccurate preoperative planning or technical errors [48] and could lead to an impingement syndrome, deformity of the ankle, or faster cartilage wear.

A malunion or nonunion can occur at the site of the osteotomy. Among the possible causes of this complication, inappropriate surgical technique, violation of the lateral cortex of the tibia [3], and a non-anatomic reduction or a secondary displacement are included.

A loss of correction is possible in case of non-compliance of the patient regarding the early postoperative period or case of inadequate fixation [14].

The bone graft used in the procedure of fibular lengthening could be reabsorbed or collapse. An appropriate surgical technique with a stable fixation could prevent this complication [48].

Moreover, pain or discomfort at the level of the hardware is possible, and in some cases, a subsequent hardware removal procedure after the consolidation of the osteotomy is necessary.

Months after the procedure, a progression of osteoarthritis of the tibiotalar joint can occur [6].

One of the most feared complications is infection, which can be superficial or deep [66]. A superficial infection can appear as delayed or poor healing of the wound, necrosis of the wound, or hematoma. In contrast, deep infection can involve hardware, soft tissues, or reach the bone.

13. Summary

Patients with osteoarthritis of the ankle in most cases present a varus or valgus malalignment.

When osteoarthritis has not reached its final stage, a joint realignment surgical procedure can slow down the cartilage wear and relieve symptoms. Realignment surgery of the ankle has to be carefully planned, evaluating the origin of the deformity and associated pathological conditions of the ankle and the foot.

The literature has shown promising results for the various techniques available for the correction of ankle malalignment.

Author Contributions: Conceptualization, S.C. and C.P.; Methodology, E.V. and A.G.; writing—original draft preparation, M.D.P. and G.P.; writing—review and editing, S.C.; Software, A.B.; Supervision, M.M. All authors have read and agreed to the published version of the manuscript.

Funding: This research received no external funding.

Institutional Review Board Statement: Not applicable.

Informed Consent Statement: Not applicable.

Conflicts of Interest: The authors declare no conflict of interest.

References

1. Glazebrook, M.; Daniels, T.; Younger, A.; Foote, C.; Penner, M.; Wing, K.; Lau, J.; Leighton, R.; Dunbar, M. Comparison of Health-Related Quality of Life Between Patients with End-Stage Ankle and Hip Arthrosis. *J. Bone Jt. Surg.* **2008**, *90*, 499–505. [CrossRef]
2. Buckwalter, J.A.; Saltzman, C.; Brown, T. The impact of osteoarthritis: Implications for research. *Clin. Orthop. Relat. Res.* **2004**, *427*, S6–S15. [CrossRef]
3. Barg, A.; Pagenstert, G.I.; Horisberger, M.; Paul, J.; Gloyer, M.; Henninger, H.B.; Valderrabano, V. Supramalleolar osteotomies for degenerative joint disease of the ankle joint: Indication, technique and results. *Int. Orthop.* **2013**, *37*, 1683–1695. [CrossRef]
4. Hintermann, B.; Knupp, M.; Barg, A. Supramalleolar Osteotomies for the Treatment of Ankle Arthritis. *J. Am. Acad. Orthop. Surg.* **2016**, *24*, 424–432. [CrossRef]
5. Saltzman, C.L.; Salamon, M.L.; Blanchard, G.M.; Huff, T.; Hayes, A.; Buckwalter, J.A.; Amendola, A. Epidemiology of ankle arthritis: Report of a consecutive series of 639 patients from a tertiary orthopaedic center. *Iowa Orthop. J.* **2005**, *25*, 44–46.
6. Krähenbühl, N.; Zwicky, L.; Bolliger, L.; Schädelin, S.; Hintermann, B.; Knupp, M. Mid-to long-term results of supramalleolar osteotomy. *Foot Ankle Int.* **2017**, *38*, 124–132. [CrossRef]
7. Pagenstert, G.I.; Hintermann, B.; Barg, A.; Leumann, A.; Valderrabano, V. Realignment Surgery as Alternative Treatment of Varus and Valgus Ankle Osteoarthritis. *Clin. Orthop. Relat. Res.* **2007**, *462*, 156–168. [CrossRef]
8. Knupp, M.; Stufkens, S.A.S.; Bolliger, L.; Barg, A.; Hintermann, B. Classification and Treatment of Supramalleolar Deformities. *Foot Ankle Int.* **2011**, *32*, 1023–1031. [CrossRef]

9. Valderrabano, V.; Horisberger, M.; Russell, I.; Dougall, H.; Hintermann, B. Etiology of Ankle Osteoarthritis. *Clin. Orthop. Relat. Res.* **2009**, *467*, 1800–1806. [CrossRef]
10. Egloff, C.; Hügle, T.; Valderrabano, V. Biomechanics and pathomechanisms of osteoarthritis. *Swiss Med. Wkly.* **2012**, *142*, w13583. [CrossRef] [PubMed]
11. Hogan, M.V.; Dare, D.M.; Deland, J.T. Is deltoid and lateral ligament reconstruction necessary in varus and valgus ankle osteoarthritis, and how should these procedures be performed? *Foot Ankle Clin.* **2013**, *18*, 517–527. [CrossRef]
12. Savage-Elliott, I.; Murawski, C.D.; Smyth, N.A.; Golanó, P.; Kennedy, J.G. The deltoid ligament: An in-depth review of anatomy, function, and treatment strategies. *Knee Surg. Sports Traumatol. Arthrosc.* **2013**, *21*, 1316–1327. [CrossRef]
13. Deland, J.T.; de Asla, R.J.; Segal, A. Reconstruction of the Chronically Failed Deltoid Ligament: A New Technique. *Foot Ankle Int.* **2004**, *25*, 795–799. [CrossRef]
14. Valderrabano, V.; Paul, J.; Monika, H.; Pagenstert, G.I.; Henninger, H.B.; Barg, A. Joint-preserving surgery of valgus ankle osteoarthritis. *Foot Ankle Clin.* **2013**, *18*, 481–502. [CrossRef]
15. Bluman, E.M.; Chiodo, C.P. Valgus Ankle Deformity and Arthritis. *Foot Ankle Clin.* **2008**, *13*, 443–470. [CrossRef]
16. Horisberger, M.; Valderrabano, V.; Hintermann, B. Posttraumatic Ankle Osteoarthritis After Ankle-Related Fractures. *J. Orthop. Trauma* **2009**, *23*, 60–67. [CrossRef]
17. Valderrabano, V.; Hintermann, B.; Horisberger, M.; Fung, T.S. Ligamentous Posttraumatic Ankle Osteoarthritis. *Am. J. Sports Med.* **2006**, *34*, 612–620. [CrossRef]
18. Barg, A.; Saltzman, C.L. Joint-preserving procedures in patients with varus deformity: Role of supramalleolar osteotomies. *Foot Ankle Clin.* **2019**, *24*, 239–264. [CrossRef]
19. Stufkens, S.A.; Van Bergen, C.J.; Blankevoort, L.; Van Dijk, C.N.; Hintermann, B.; Knupp, M. The role of the fibula in varus and valgus deformity of the tibia: A biomechanical study. *J. Bone Jt. Surg.* **2011**, *93*, 1232–1239. [CrossRef]
20. Horn, D.M.; Fragomen, A.T.; Rozbruch, S.R. Supramalleolar Osteotomy Using Circular External Fixation with Six-Axis Deformity Correction of the Distal Tibia. *Foot Ankle Int.* **2011**, *32*, 986–993. [CrossRef]
21. Hintermann, B.; Knupp, M.; Barg, A. Joint-Preserving Surgery of Asymmetric Ankle Osteoarthritis with Peritalar Instability. *Foot Ankle Clin.* **2013**, *18*, 503–516. [CrossRef] [PubMed]
22. Saltzman, C.L.; El-Khoury, G.Y. The Hindfoot Alignment View. *Foot Ankle Int.* **1995**, *16*, 572–576. [CrossRef]
23. Knupp, M.; Ledermann, H.; Magerkurth, O.; Hinterman, B. The Surgical Tibiotalar Angle: A Radiologic Study. *Foot Ankle Int.* **2005**, *26*, 713–716. [CrossRef] [PubMed]
24. Tanaka, Y.; Takakura, Y.; Fujii, T.; Kumai, T.; Sugimoto, K. Hindfoot alignment of hallux valgus evaluated by a weightbearing subtalar x-ray view. *Foot Ankle Int.* **1999**, *20*, 640–645. [CrossRef]
25. Krähenbühl, N.; Susdorf, R.; Barg, A.; Hintermann, B. Supramalleolar osteotomy in post-traumatic valgus ankle osteoarthritis. *Int. Orthop.* **2020**, *44*, 535–543. [CrossRef] [PubMed]
26. Knupp, M.; Pagenstert, G.I.; Barg, A.; Bolliger, L.; Easley, M.E.; Hintermann, B. SPECT-CT compared with conventional imaging modalities for the assessment of the varus and valgus malaligned hindfoot. *J. Orthop. Res.* **2009**, *27*, 1461–1466. [CrossRef]
27. Gyftopoulos, S.; Bencardino, J.T. Normal Variants and Pitfalls in MR Imaging of the Ankle and Foot. *Magn. Reson. Imaging Clin. N. Am.* **2010**, *18*, 691–705. [CrossRef]
28. Barg, A.; Pagenstert, G.I.; Leumann, A.G.; Müller, A.M.; Henninger, H.B.; Valderrabano, V. Treatment of the Arthritic Valgus Ankle. *Foot Ankle Clin.* **2012**, *17*, 647–663. [CrossRef]
29. Scholten, P.E.; Sierevelt, I.N.; Van Dijk, C.N. Hindfoot endoscopy for posterior ankle impingement. *J. Bone Jt. Surg.* **2018**, *90*, 2665–2672. [CrossRef]
30. Valderrabano, V.; Miska, M.; Leumann, A.; Wiewiorski, M. Reconstruction of osteochondral lesions of the talus with autologous spongiosa grafts and autologous matrix-induced chondrogenesis. *Am. J. Sports Med.* **2013**, *41*, 519–527. [CrossRef]
31. Barg, A.; Elsner, A.; Anderson, A.E.; Hintermann, B. The Effect of Three-Component Total Ankle Replacement Malalignment on Clinical Outcome: Pain Relief and Functional Outcome in 317 Consecutive Patients. *J. Bone Jt. Surg.* **2011**, *93*, 1969–1978. [CrossRef] [PubMed]
32. Gougoulias, N.; Khanna, A.; Maffulli, N. How successful are current ankle replacements?: A systematic review of the literature. *Clin. Orthop. Relat. Res.* **2010**, *468*, 199–208. [CrossRef]
33. Takakura, Y.; Tanaka, Y.; Kumai, T.; Tamai, S. Low tibial osteotomy for osteoarthritis of the ankle. Results of a new operation in 18 patients. *J. Bone Jt. Surg.* **1995**, *77*, 50–54. [CrossRef]
34. Knupp, M.; Barg, A.; Bolliger, L.; Hintermann, B. Reconstructive Surgery for Overcorrected Clubfoot in Adults. *J. Bone Jt. Surg.* **2012**, *94*, e1101-7. [CrossRef]
35. Mulhern, J.L.; Protzman, N.M.; Brigido, S.A.; Deol, P.P.S. Supramalleolar osteotomy: Indications and surgical techniques. *Clin. Podiatr. Med. Surg.* **2015**, *32*, 445–461. [CrossRef]
36. Bonasia, D.E.; Dettoni, F.; Femino, J.E.; Phisitkul, P.; Germano, M.; Amendola, A. Total ankle replacement: Why, when and how? *Iowa Orthop. J.* **2010**, *30*, 119.
37. Hintermann, B.; Barg, A.; Knupp, M. Corrective supramalleolar osteotomy for malunited pronation-external rotation fractures of the ankle. *J. Bone Jt. Surg.* **2011**, *93*, 1367–1372. [CrossRef]

38. Mosca, M.; Buda, R.; Ceccarelli, F.; Fuiano, M.; Vocale, E.; Massimi, S.; Benedetti, M.G.; Grassi, A.; Caravelli, S.; Zaffagnini, S. Ankle joint re-balancing in the management of ankle fracture malunion using fibular lengthening: Prospective clinical-radiological results at mid-term follow-up. *Int. Orthop.* **2020**, *45*, 411–417. [CrossRef]
39. Giannini, S.; Faldini, C.; Acri, F.; Leonetti, D.; Luciani, D.; Nanni, M. Surgical treatment of post-traumatic malalignment of the ankle. *Injury* **2010**, *41*, 1208–1211. [CrossRef]
40. Tarr, R.R.; Resnick, C.T.; Wagner, K.S.; Sarmiento, A. Changes in Tibiotalar Joint Contact Areas Following Experimentally Induced Tibial Angular Deformities. *Clin. Orthop. Relat. Res.* **1985**, *199*, 72–80. [CrossRef]
41. Ng, A.; Barnes, E.S. Management of Complications of Open Reduction and Internal Fixation of Ankle Fractures. *Clin. Podiatr. Med. Surg.* **2009**, *26*, 105–125. [CrossRef] [PubMed]
42. El-Rosasy, M.; Ali, T. Realignment-lengthening osteotomy for malunited distal fibular fracture. *Int. Orthop.* **2013**, *37*, 1285–1290. [CrossRef] [PubMed]
43. van Wensen, R.J.; van den Bekerom, M.P.; Marti, R.K.; van Heerwaarden, R.J. Reconstructive osteotomy of fibular malunion: Review of the literature. *Strateg. Trauma Limb Reconstr.* **2011**, *6*, 51–57. [CrossRef] [PubMed]
44. Egger, A.C.; Berkowitz, M.J. Operative Treatment of the Malunited Fibula Fracture. *Foot Ankle Int.* **2018**, *39*, 1242–1252. [CrossRef] [PubMed]
45. Yablon, I.G.; Heller, F.G.; Shouse, L.E.R.O.Y. The key role of the lateral malleolus in displaced fractures of the ankle. *J. Bone Jt. Surg.* **1977**, *59*, 169–173. [CrossRef]
46. Weber, D.; Friederich, N.F.; Müller, W. Lengthening osteotomy of the fibula for post-traumatic malunion. *Int. Orthop.* **1998**, *22*, 149–152. [CrossRef]
47. Roberts, C.; Sherman, O.; Bauer, D.; Lusskin, R. Ankle Reconstruction for Malunion by Fibular Osteotomy and Lengthening with Direct Control of the Distal Fragment: A Report of Three Cases and Review of the Literature. *Foot Ankle* **1992**, *13*, 7–13. [CrossRef]
48. Yablon, I.G.; Leach, R.E. Reconstruction of malunited fractures of the lateral malleolus. *J. Bone Jt. Surg.* **1989**, *71*, 521–527. [CrossRef]
49. Speed, J.S.; Boyd, H.B. Operative reconstruction of malunited fractures about the ankle joint. *J. Bone Jt. Surg.* **1936**, *18*, 270–286.
50. Weber, B.G.; Simpson, L.A. Corrective Lengthening Osteotomy of the Fibula. *Clin. Orthop. Relat. Res.* **1985**, *199*, 61–67. [CrossRef]
51. Davis, J.L.; Giacopelli, J.A. Transfibular osteotomy in the correction of ankle joint incongruity. *J. Foot Ankle Surg.* **1995**, *34*, 389–399. [CrossRef]
52. Wiltberger, B.R.; Mallory, T.H. A new method for the reconstruction of the deltoid ligament of the ankle. *Orthop. Rev.* **1972**, *1*, 37–41.
53. Kim, J.-B.; Yi, Y.; Kim, J.-Y.; Cho, J.-H.; Kwon, M.-S.; Choi, S.-H.; Lee, W.-C. Weight-bearing computed tomography findings in varus ankle osteoarthritis: Abnormal internal rotation of the talus in the axial plane. *Skelet. Radiol.* **2017**, *46*, 1071–1080. [CrossRef] [PubMed]
54. Hintermann, B. What the Orthopaedic Foot and Ankle Surgeon Wants to Know from MR Imaging. *Semin. Musculoskelet. Radiol.* **2005**, *9*, 260–271. [CrossRef]
55. Easley, M.E. Surgical Treatment of the Arthritic Varus Ankle. *Foot Ankle Clin.* **2012**, *17*, 665–686. [CrossRef]
56. Tanaka, Y. The concept of ankle joint preserving surgery: Why does supramalleolar osteotomy work and how to decide when to do an osteotomy or joint replacement. *Foot Ankle Clin.* **2012**, *17*, 545–553. [CrossRef]
57. Knupp, M.; Pagenstert, G.; Valderrabano, V.; Hintermann, B. Osteotomien zur Entlastung der Varusarthrose im oberen Sprunggelenk [Osteotomies in varus malalignment of the ankle]. *Oper Orthop Traumatol.* **2008**, *20*, 262–273. (In German) [CrossRef]
58. Hintermann, B.; Ruiz, R.; Barg, A. Novel Double Osteotomy Technique of Distal Tibia for Correction of Asymmetric Varus Osteoarthritic Ankle. *Foot Ankle Int.* **2017**, *38*, 970–998. [CrossRef]
59. Takakura, Y.; Takaoka, T.; Tanaka, Y.; Yajima, H.; Tamai, S. Results of Opening-Wedge Osteotomy for the Treatment of a Post-Traumatic Varus Deformity of the Ankle*. *J. Bone Jt. Surg.* **1998**, *80*, 213–218. [CrossRef]
60. Beijk, I.; Johannes, B.; de Vries Astrid, J.; van Raaij Tom, M. Is there an optimal degree of correction for ankle varus deformity after supramalleolar osteotomy? A systematic review. *Foot Ankle Surg.* **2022**. [CrossRef]
61. Li, X.; Xu, X. Joint Preservation for Posttraumatic Ankle Arthritis After Tibial Plafond Fracture. *Foot Ankle Clin.* **2022**, *27*, 73–90. [CrossRef] [PubMed]
62. Wagner, E.; Wagner, P. Correction of Sagittal Plane Deformity of the Distal Tibia. *Foot Ankle Clin.* **2022**, *27*, 129–144. [CrossRef]
63. Barg, A.; Saltzman, C.L. Single-Stage Supramalleolar Osteotomy for Coronal Plane Deformity. *Curr. Rev. Musculoskelet. Med.* **2014**, *7*, 277–291. [CrossRef]
64. Tanaka, Y.; Takakura, Y.; Hayashi, K.; Taniguchi, A.; Kumai, T.; Sugimoto, K. Low tibial osteotomy for varus-type osteoarthritis of the ankle. *J. Bone Jt. Surg. Br. Vol.* **2006**, *88*, 909–913. [CrossRef] [PubMed]
65. van Raaij, T.; van der Wel, H.; Beldman, M.; de Vries, A.; Kraeima, J. Two-Step 3D-Guided Supramalleolar Osteotomy to Treat Varus Ankle osteoarthritis. *Foot Ankle Int.* **2022**, *43*, 937–941. [CrossRef] [PubMed]
66. Espinosa, N. What Leads to Failure of Joint-preserving Surgery for Ankle Osteoarthritis? When This Surgery Fails, What Next? *Foot Ankle Clin.* **2013**, *18*, 555–569. [CrossRef]

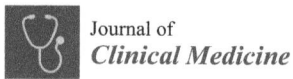

Article

Custom 3D-Printed Cutting Guides for Femoral Osteotomy in Rotational Malalignment Due to Diaphyseal Fractures: Surgical Technique and Case Series

Jaime Oraa [1], Maider Beitia [2], Nicolás Fiz [1], Sergio González [1], Xabier Sánchez [3], Diego Delgado [2] and Mikel Sánchez [1,2,*]

[1] Arthroscopic Surgery Unit, Hospital Vithas Vitoria, 01008 Vitoria-Gasteiz, Spain; jaime.oraa@ucatrauma.com (J.O.); nicolas.fiz@ucatrauma.com (N.F.); sergio.gonzalez@ucatrauma.com (S.G.)
[2] Advanced Biological Therapy Unit, Hospital Vithas Vitoria, 01008 Vitoria-Gasteiz, Spain; maider.beitia@ucatrauma.com (M.B.); diego.delgado@ucatrauma.com (D.D.)
[3] Osteomodel, 20018 San Sebastian, Spain; xabier.sanchez@osteomodel.com
* Correspondence: mikel.sanchez@ucatrauma.com; Tel.: +34-945-252077

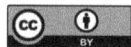

Citation: Oraa, J.; Beitia, M.; Fiz, N.; González, S.; Sánchez, X.; Delgado, D.; Sánchez, M. Custom 3D-Printed Cutting Guides for Femoral Osteotomy in Rotational Malalignment Due to Diaphyseal Fractures: Surgical Technique and Case Series. *J. Clin. Med.* 2021, 10, 3366. https://doi.org/10.3390/jcm10153366

Academic Editors: Silvio Caravelli, Alberto Grassi and Massimiliano Mosca

Received: 19 May 2021
Accepted: 28 July 2021
Published: 29 July 2021

Publisher's Note: MDPI stays neutral with regard to jurisdictional claims in published maps and institutional affiliations.

Copyright: © 2021 by the authors. Licensee MDPI, Basel, Switzerland. This article is an open access article distributed under the terms and conditions of the Creative Commons Attribution (CC BY) license (https://creativecommons.org/licenses/by/4.0/).

Abstract: Femoral shaft fractures are one of the most common injuries in trauma patients. The gold standard treatment consists of closed reduction and intramedullary nailing, providing a high fracture healing rate and allowing early mobilization. However, rotational malalignment is a well-known complication following this procedure, and excessive femoral anteversion or femoral retroversion can trigger functional complaints. In order to achieve the ideal degree of femoral rotation, a 3D planning and printing cutting guides procedure was developed to correct femoral malrotation. A patient series with malalignment after a femoral diaphyseal fracture was operated on with the customized guides and evaluated in this study. Computed tomography scans were performed to accurately determine the number of degrees of malrotation, allowing the design of specific and personalized surgical guides to correct these accurately. Once designed, they were produced by 3D printing. After surgery with the customized guides to correct femoral malrotation, all patients presented a normalized anteversion angle of the femur (average −10.3°, range from −5° to −15°), according to their contralateral limb. These data suggest that the use of customized cutting guides for femoral osteotomy is a safe and reproducible surgical technique that offers precise results when correcting femoral malrotation.

Keywords: 3D printing; 3D technology; femoral osteotomy; femoral malrotation; femoral anteversion; femoral shaft fractures

1. Introduction

Femoral shaft fractures (FSF) are one of the most common injuries in trauma patients, with an incidence of between 10 and 21 per 100,000 people per year [1,2]. Their causes are often related to high energy mechanisms such as traffic accidents and are commonly associated with multiple injuries, life-threatening complications, sequelae and limb deformities, namely shortening and malrotation, if not treated appropriately [3].

The gold standard treatment for FSF consists of closed reduction and intramedullary nailing. This technique provides a high fracture healing rate and allows early mobilization [4,5]. However, a rotational malalignment is a well-known complication following this procedure, and a difference in rotation greater than 15° compared with the healthy side can be responsible for functional complaints [6,7]. This complication may occur in 28% of the patients [8], although other studies showed that the incidence of malrotation after intramedullary nailing for femur fractures ranges from 19% to 56% [9–11]. Femoral malrotation is calculated by measuring the femoral version, which is defined according to the technique described by Jeanmart et al., determining the angle between a line tangential to the dorsal bony contours of the femoral condyles and a line drawn through the axis of the femoral neck [12,13].

The average values of femoral anteversion range from 10° to 15°, and exceeding these values on both sides can lead to pathological conditions [14]. On the one hand, excessive femoral anteversion can imply anterior knee pain and patellofemoral instability, anterior hip pain and labral tears in patients with concomitant femoro-acetabular impingement, posterior extra-articular hip impingement and ischiofemoral impingement. It is also a frequent reason for an internally rotated gait, which can cause discomfort when walking, with tripping, and difficulties with running and doing sports. On the other hand, a lack of femoral anteversion (or femoral retroversion) can cause damage to the labrum and articular cartilage of the hip and early osteoarthritis, and an externally rotated gait [7,15–26].

By means of derotation osteotomies, surgeons seek to resolve the malrotation resulting from the initial surgery for FSF. However, achieving the ideal degree of femoral version is difficult and challenging. One of the reasons is that current surgical techniques for correcting malrotation are observer-dependent, based on measurements of intraoperative clinical and radiological parameters [27–31].

Therefore, new techniques need to be developed to allow for more accurate correction. In this regard, the use of custom 3D planning and printing cutting guides is a novel tool in surgical interventions to correct femoral malrotation. Advances in 3D technology in recent years have led to an exponential increase in its use in medicine, and especially in orthopedic surgery [32–35].

3D printing is an additive manufacturing technique that allows us to transform a digital model into a three-dimensional object. Three-dimensional models are obtained by processing digital radiological studies of patients, such as computed tomography (CT) scans, and when the virtual model has been obtained, it can be printed. Objects are built layer by layer, using different technologies and materials depending on the final application for which they are intended. 3D printing allows manufacturing by successively adding material to the object, so as to create complex structures that could not be obtained with other technologies [36].

CT scans can accurately determine the degree of malrotation, enabling the design of a specific and personalized surgical guide. Its design and 3D printing according to the surgical plan would improve the predictability of osteotomy procedures [37,38]. Another option to solve this problem could be the use of navigated surgery, but, to our knowledge, there are so far no publications on this technique.

In the present study, we describe in detail a new surgical technique based on the design and 3D printing of customized cutting guides for femoral osteotomies with rotational malalignment after a diaphyseal fracture, and the clinical outcomes in a case series.

2. Materials and Methods

2.1. Patients

Six patients with a medical history of closed FSF after a traffic accident are described in Table 1. Five of them had undergone surgery at other centers, and were brought into our clinic for a second opinion; the other patient did not have any previous surgery.

Table 1. Clinical and surgical data of the patients.

	Patient 1	Patient 2	Patient 3	Patient 4	Patient 5	Patient 6
Age (years)	23	72	40	30	59	35
Sex	Female	Male	Male	Male	Female	Male
Side	Left	Left	Left	Right	Right	Left
Previous distal femur deformity	Internal rotation	External rotation	External rotation	Internal rotation	External rotation	Internal rotation
Pre-angulation (°)	−60	40	43	−44	1	−24
Correction (°)	45	50	50	33	15	19
Post-angulation (°)	−15	−10	−7	−11	−14	−5

Clinical examination showed groin and/or knee pain, with an in-toe or out-toe gait. On the initial telemetry all the patients presented signs of femoral malrotation, so a CT scan was performed to calculate the degree of femoral torsion.

2.2. Design and 3D Printing

The CT images were treated with 3D reconstruction software (Mimics®, Materialise, Belgium), obtaining a 3D composition of the femoral head, proximal metaphysis and condyles of both lower extremities (Figure 1A). The rotational malalignment was accurately measured by the software according to Jeanmart's technique, as described above [12], and compared with the contralateral limb (Figure 1B).

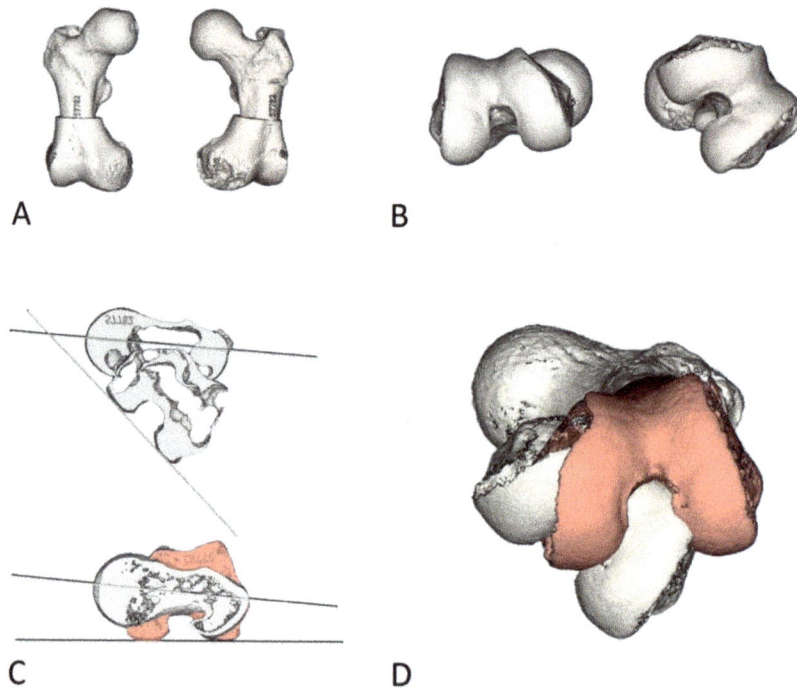

Figure 1. Calculation of correction degrees (Patient 3). A 3D composition of the femoral head, proximal metaphysis and condyles of both lower extremities are obtained from CT images (**A**), and the rotational malalignment of both limbs is evaluated (**B**). The degrees of malrotation are calculated by software according to Jeanmart's technique (top, (**C**)), as well as the degrees needed for correction (red) (bottom, (**C**)). Once the position of the distal femur is established before and after (red) rotation correction (**D**), the guides are designed to correct the necessary number of degrees and to fit the patient's bone surface.

After quantifying the required degree of correction, preoperative planning was performed (Figure 1C,D). A diaphyseal derotational osteotomy with intramedullary fixation was considered for all the patients. A segmentation process was performed, in which 3D volume is generated from a CT scan, and custom surgical guides were made for the correction of the femoral rotation.

The planning, design and manufacturing process is divided into different phases. Initially, the desired anatomical area, in this case the femur, is segmented. The Mimics Innovation Suite from Materialise is used for this purpose. Subsequently, using Nx Unigraphics from Siemens and Magics (Materialise, Materialise, Belgium; NX Unigraphics, Munich, Germany), the surgery is planned and simulated. During this phase we compare different strategies and results in order to obtain an optimal outcome.

Once the correction is defined, customized guides are designed with Nx Unigraphics and Magics. Depending on the bone deformity, these can be placed separated or joined together as required to facilitate placement during the surgical procedure. After defining the design, all components are manufactured in biocompatible ABS M30i with a Stratasys F380mc printer and after undergoing a validated cleaning process, they are sent to the hospital for sterilization by a Low Temperature Hydrogen Peroxide and Plasma sterilizer (Matachana 130 HPO®) and subsequent surgical use.

2.3. Surgical Technique

The femoral diaphysis was exposed through a postero-lateral approach, between the vastus lateralis and lateral intermuscular septum (Figure 2A). The two initial surgical guides were pinned to the bone surface with two monocortical Kisrchner wires and two monocortical screws for each piece (Figure 2B). The 3D-printed guides adapted accurately to osteophytes and fracture lips, ensuring perfect rotational positioning and precision in placement.

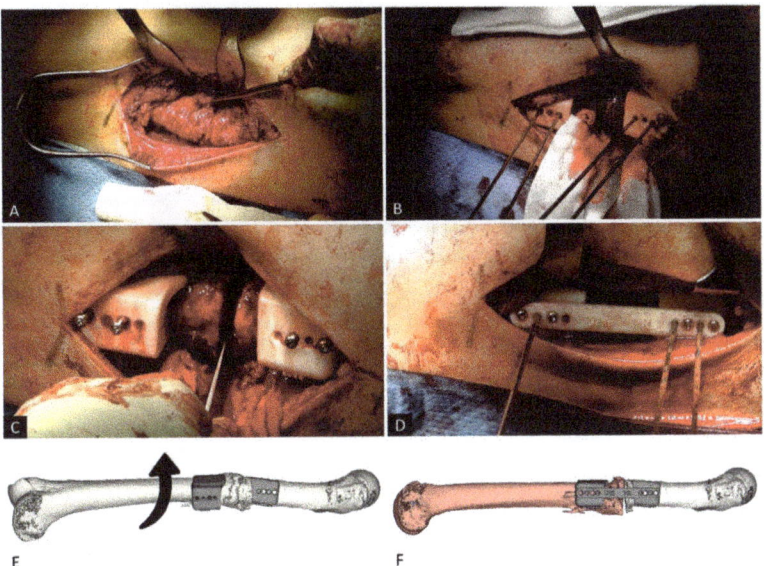

Figure 2. Surgical technique (Patient 3). After exposing the femoral diaphysis through a postero-lateral approach (**A**), the two initial surgical guides are pinned to the bone surface (**B**). Subsequently, the osteotomy is carried out by removing all previous osteosynthesis material (**C**). The correction is performed with an external or internal rotation of the distal femoral fragment and the third 3D- printed guide is used to connect the other two, providing the correct femoral rotation degree (**D**). The degrees of rotation of the distal femoral fragment are defined by the alignment of the two guides (**E**). Once the two guides are aligned and connected by the third piece, the distal fragment is already correctly rotated according to the surgical planning (**F**). Finally, the osteotomy is completed by inserting the intramedullary nail and removing the surgical guides.

The next step was to remove previous osteosynthesis material (T2 femoral nail, Kuntscher nail or Russell-Taylor nail). After conducting a femur osteotomy through the previous fracture site, correction of internal or external femoral torsion was performed with an external or internal rotation of the distal femoral fragment, respectively (Figure 2C–E). Then, the third 3D-printed guide was used to connect the other two, and provide the correct femoral rotation degree (Figure 2D–F). Finally, a new T2 nail (Stryker) was introduced, with both proximal and distal locking. As the screws in the guides were monocortical, it was not necessary to remove the guides to place the new nail, which maintained the correction and provided stability for the derotation femoral osteotomy. Once the nail was placed, the surgical guides were removed, and correct positioning was checked under fluoroscopy.

In cases of fracture sequelae, it may be easier to apply the guides separately to better adapt each part of the guide to the deformed relief of the bone. Furthermore, in cases of idiopathic anteversion without fracture and in cases with poorly exuberant callus bone, the different parts of the guide are first joined together and then separated before correcting the rotation (Figure 3).

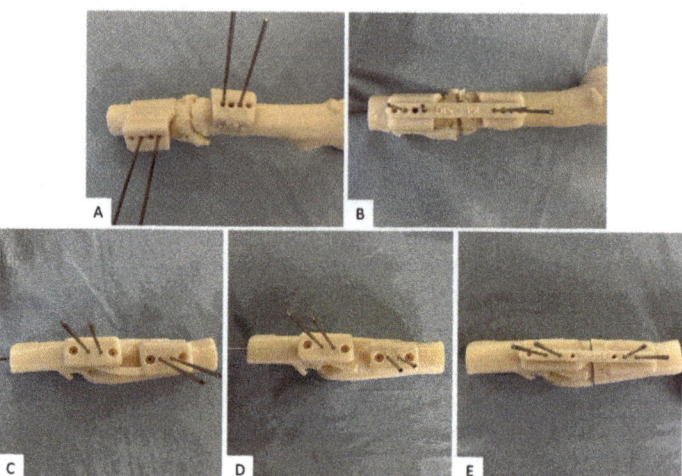

Figure 3. Surgical procedure. Guides are fixed separately in cases of fracture sequelae to correctly adapt them to the relief of the bone (**A**) and then the rotation is performed until the wires are aligned (**B**). In cases of idiopathic anteversion without fracture and in cases with poorly exuberant callus bone, the guide is first fixed with the pieces joined together (**C**), and then separated (**D**) and rotated until the alignment of the wires is achieved (**E**).

The success of the surgery is assessed both clinically and radiologically. Thus, X-rays are employed to see the consolidation status of the osteotomy and, additionally, teleradiography is performed to confirm the rotation. This rotation is then compared with the initial one. As for the physical examination, the hip is explored for internal and external rotation and to assess the symmetry between both hips (Figure 4).

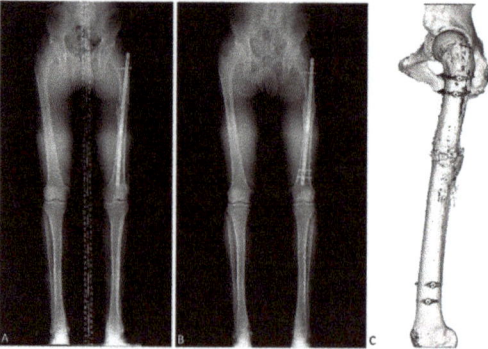

Figure 4. Pre- and postoperative image study (Patient 3). Teleradiographs are conducted to observe rotation before (**A**) and after surgery (**B**). It also indicates callus formation over time. The CT scan also indicates whether the alignment of the femur is correct after surgery (**C**).

3. Results

Results are shown in Table 1. A total of six derotation osteotomies were performed in six patients: two female and four male. The average age was 43 years (range 23–72 years). Three of the patients presented a femoral external rotation deformity (average +28°, range from +1° to +43°), while the other three patients displayed an internal rotation deformity of the femur (average −43°, range from −24° to −60°). After surgery, all patients presented a normalized anteversion angle of the femur (average −10.3°, range from −5° to −15°), with respect to their contralateral limb.

As explained before, the etiology was post-traumatic in all the patients, in each case due to a traffic accident, and five of the six patients had previously undergone surgery. The mean time elapsed from the first surgery to the surgery performed by our medical team was 179.2 months (range 10–600 months). Three of the patients had a T2 nail (Stryker) implanted at the first operation, another patient had a Russell-Taylor nail (Smith & Nephew), while the remaining patient had a Küntscher nail. No major complications had occurred in this time (after first surgery), nor any deep or superficial infections.

4. Discussion

This study describes a new surgical technique to correct femoral malrotation using custom 3D-printed cutting guides. In addition, we present a series of six patients who consulted for femoral malalignment after an FSF, in which a femoral derotation osteotomy was performed using the customized guides. The results suggest this is a safe process with great precision to establish the proper rotation of the femur. Using 3D-printed guides makes the surgery shorter and technically easier, with less radiation inside the operating room. Furthermore, this procedure is inexpensive.

Customized osteotomy guides solve one of the major difficulties when correcting malrotations by providing a highly accurate calculation and correction of the degrees of malrotation. Several methods of calculating intraoperative femoral rotation were published in the literature. A work by Krettek et al. described simple and useful techniques used to analyze limb alignment after initial fixation of femoral and tibial fractures [39]. Jagernauth et al. used a protractor to correct the femoral internal rotation after intramedullary nailing, performing a derotation osteotomy leaving the previous nail in situ [40]. A method carried out by Espinoza et al. set femoral rotation in acute fractures using the inherent anteversion of the intramedullary nail [41]. Stambough et al. determined femoral anteversion measuring the trochanteric prominence angle in adolescents with symptomatic excessive femoral anteversion [42]. Although all these techniques offer a variety of possibilities for solving the proposed challenge, they present some limitations, such as the requirement of a high dose of radiation in the operating room, or the help of an experienced radiology technician to achieve the correct visualization of the necessary projections. However, the major drawback of these techniques is that the correction to be performed is observer-dependent and, therefore, it should be taken into consideration that these techniques are somewhat susceptible to error.

On the other hand, the technique described in the present study calculates the degrees to be corrected by means of virtual planning prior to surgery based on the patient's imaging studies, from which the guides are designed to accurately correct the degrees of rotation as well as fitting the patient's bone tissue with exactitude. Consequently, the surgeon only needs to follow the indications provided by the custom 3D-printed guide, thus avoiding a subjective estimation of the number of degrees to be corrected during the surgical intervention, and the resulting error. This was confirmed by the fact that patients who underwent this surgical technique achieved a normalized anteversion within the recommended range (from −5° to −15°).

The major disadvantage of this procedure is that it requires open surgery. As a consequence, there is an increased risk of blood loss during the operation as well as a possible risk of delay in the union or nonunion at the level of the osteotomy. This was resolved by Buly et al. by performing 55 femoral derotation osteotomies in 43 patients for version abnormalities using an intramedullary hand saw, with the advantage of not requiring exposure of the osteotomy site [43]. Rotational control was achieved by placing 1/8-inch smooth Steinmann pins into the femur, proximal and distal to the osteotomy to the desired amount of rotational correction. However, the angular correction was again observer-dependent, controlled visually using flat, triangular guides from a blade plate instrument set. Other authors also carried out rotational femoral osteotomies using an intramedullary saw [44,45].

It should be noted that the positioning of the 3D-printed guides is a critical step in this type of surgery [46]. Thus, the detailed and meticulous fabrication of the guides is mandatory, as well as correct positioning in the bone, taking into account the fracture ends and reference bone reliefs used in the design of the guides. Suboptimal intraoperative guide positioning could lead to incomplete or excessive correction.

In the case of bilateral femur malrotation due to bilateral FSF, it is not possible to compare with a healthy limb, and the desired femoral anteversion should be estimated based on the mean values of the population.

In recent years, the techniques of designing and manufacturing surgical guides have been improved, as well as the printing material. This is a modern and personalized technique, in constant evolution, in which different custom guides are manufactured for each case. Its versatility makes it a promising alternative for other types of surgical intervention. It might be a valid surgical treatment of acute fractures with severe comminution of the fracture site, since only a CT scan of both lower extremities is needed, and the preparation time of the guides is relatively short; around 5–6 h. It may even be an option for treatment with osteosynthesis plates or external fixation, when needed, in other pathologies such as hypophosphatemic osteomalacia, osteogenesis imperfecta, polyostotic fibrous dysplasia, vitamin D-resistant hypophosphatemic rickets and other lower extremity bone deformities.

This study has several limitations, including the small sample size, and further studies are needed to evaluate the technique more in greater depth. In addition, it presents the usual shortcomings associated with retrospective studies of this kind.

5. Conclusions

The design and 3D printing of customized cutting guides for femoral osteotomies with rotational malalignment after a diaphyseal fracture is a reproducible surgical technique that offers precise results when correcting femoral malrotation. Following surgery, all patients presented a normalized anteversion angle of the femur. The use of patient-tailored surgical guides could be implemented in different types of surgical interventions, improving aspects such as accuracy and surgery times.

Author Contributions: Conceptualization, J.O., N.F., D.D. and M.S.; methodology, J.O., M.B. and M.S.; software, X.S.; investigation, J.O., N.F. and S.G.; writing—original draft preparation, J.O. and M.B.; writing—review and editing, D.D. and M.S.; supervision, M.S. All authors have read and agreed to the published version of the manuscript.

Funding: This research received no external funding.

Institutional Review Board Statement: The study was conducted according to the guidelines of the Declaration of Helsinki, and approved by the Ethics Committee CEIm-E (protocol code UCA-PLA-2016-01 and 10/2018).

Informed Consent Statement: Informed consent was obtained from all subjects involved in the study.

Data Availability Statement: The data presented in this study are available within the article.

Conflicts of Interest: The authors declare no conflict of interest.

References

1. Weiss, R.J.; Montgomery, S.M.; Al Dabbagh, Z.; Jansson, K.-A. National Data of 6409 Swedish Inpatients with Femoral Shaft Fractures: Stable Incidence between 1998 and 2004. *Injury* **2009**, *40*, 304–308. [CrossRef] [PubMed]
2. Enninghorst, N.; McDougall, D.; Evans, J.A.; Sisak, K.; Balogh, Z.J. Population-Based Epidemiology of Femur Shaft Fractures. *J. Trauma Acute Care Surg.* **2013**, *74*, 1516–1520. [CrossRef] [PubMed]

3. Denisiuk, M.; Afsari, A. Femoral Shaft Fractures. In *StatPearls*; StatPearls Publishing: Treasure Island, FL, USA, 2021.
4. Winquist, R.A.; Hansen, S.T.; Clawson, D.K. Closed Intramedullary Nailing of Femoral Fractures. A Report of Five Hundred and Twenty Cases. 1984. *J. Bone Joint Surg. Am.* **2001**, *83*, 1912. [CrossRef] [PubMed]
5. Bucholz, R.W.; Jones, A. Fractures of the Shaft of the Femur. *J. Bone Joint Surg. Am.* **1991**, *73*, 1561–1566. [CrossRef]
6. Bråten, M.; Terjesen, T.; Rossvoll, I. Femoral Shaft Fractures Treated by Intramedullary Nailing. A Follow-up Study Focusing on Problems Related to the Method. *Injury* **1995**, *26*, 379–383. [CrossRef]
7. Karaman, O.; Ayhan, E.; Kesmezacar, H.; Seker, A.; Unlu, M.C.; Aydingoz, O. Rotational Malalignment after Closed Intramedullary Nailing of Femoral Shaft Fractures and Its Influence on Daily Life. *Eur. J. Orthop. Surg. Traumatol.* **2014**, *24*, 1243–1247. [CrossRef]
8. Jaarsma, R.L.; Pakvis, D.F.M.; Verdonschot, N.; Biert, J.; van Kampen, A. Rotational Malalignment after Intramedullary Nailing of Femoral Fractures. *J. Orthop. Trauma* **2004**, *18*, 403–409. [CrossRef]
9. Hüfner, T.; Citak, M.; Suero, E.M.; Miller, B.; Kendoff, D.; Krettek, C.; Citak, M. Femoral Malrotation after Unreamed Intramedullary Nailing: An Evaluation of Influencing Operative Factors. *J. Orthop. Trauma* **2011**, *25*, 224–227. [CrossRef]
10. Kenawey, M.; Krettek, C.; Ettinger, M.; Hankemeier, S.; Breitmeier, D.; Liodakis, E. The Greater Trochanter-Head Contact Method: A Cadaveric Study with a New Technique for the Intraoperative Control of Rotation of Femoral Fractures. *J. Orthop. Trauma* **2011**, *25*, 549–555. [CrossRef]
11. Stephen, D.J.G.; Kreder, H.J.; Schemitsch, E.H.; Conlan, L.B.; Wild, L.; McKee, M.D. Femoral Intramedullary Nailing: Comparison of Fracture-Table and Manual Traction. A Prospective, Randomized Study. *J. Bone Joint Surg. Am.* **2002**, *84*, 1514–1521. [CrossRef]
12. Jeanmart, L.; Baert, A.L.; Wackenheim, A. *Atlas of Pathological Computer Tomography: Volume 3: Computer Tomography of Neck, Chest, Spine and Limbs*; Springer: Berlin/Heidelberg, Germany, 1983; ISBN 978-3-642-68538-5.
13. Wissing, H.; Buddenbrock, B. Determining rotational errors of the femur by axial computerized tomography in comparison with clinical and conventional radiologic determination. *Unfallchirurgie* **1993**, *19*, 145–157. [CrossRef]
14. Fabry, G.; MacEwen, G.D.; Shands, A.R. Torsion of the Femur. A Follow-up Study in Normal and Abnormal Conditions. *J. Bone Joint Surg. Am.* **1973**, *55*, 1726–1738. [CrossRef]
15. Parikh, S.; Noyes, F.R. Patellofemoral Disorders: Role of Computed Tomography and Magnetic Resonance Imaging in Defining Abnormal Rotational Lower Limb Alignment. *Sports Health* **2011**, *3*, 158–169. [CrossRef]
16. Steensen, R.N.; Bentley, J.C.; Trinh, T.Q.; Backes, J.R.; Wiltfong, R.E. The Prevalence and Combined Prevalences of Anatomic Factors Associated with Recurrent Patellar Dislocation: A Magnetic Resonance Imaging Study. *Am. J. Sports Med.* **2015**, *43*, 921–927. [CrossRef]
17. Kitaoka, H.B.; Weiner, D.S.; Cook, A.J.; Hoyt, W.A.; Askew, M.J. Relationship between Femoral Anteversion and Osteoarthritis of the Hip. *J. Pediatr. Orthop.* **1989**, *9*, 396–404. [CrossRef]
18. Tönnis, D.; Heinecke, A. Acetabular and Femoral Anteversion: Relationship with Osteoarthritis of the Hip. *J. Bone Joint Surg. Am.* **1999**, *81*, 1747–1770. [CrossRef]
19. Eckhoff, D.G. Effect of Limb Malrotation on Malalignment and Osteoarthritis. *Orthop. Clin. N. Am.* **1994**, *25*, 405–414. [CrossRef]
20. Terjesen, T.; Benum, P.; Anda, S.; Svenningsen, S. Increased Femoral Anteversion and Osteoarthritis of the Hip Joint. *Acta Orthop. Scand.* **1982**, *53*, 571–575. [CrossRef] [PubMed]
21. Siebenrock, K.A.; Steppacher, S.D.; Haefeli, P.C.; Schwab, J.M.; Tannast, M. Valgus Hip with High Antetorsion Causes Pain Through Posterior Extraarticular FAI. *Clin. Orthop. Relat. Res.* **2013**, *471*, 3774–3780. [CrossRef] [PubMed]
22. Gómez-Hoyos, J.; Schröder, R.; Reddy, M.; Palmer, I.J.; Martin, H.D. Femoral Neck Anteversion and Lesser Trochanteric Retroversion in Patients With Ischiofemoral Impingement: A Case-Control Magnetic Resonance Imaging Study. *Arthroscopy* **2016**, *32*, 13–18. [CrossRef]
23. Eckhoff, D.G.; Montgomery, W.K.; Kilcoyne, R.F.; Stamm, E.R. Femoral Morphometry and Anterior Knee Pain. *Clin. Orthop. Relat. Res.* **1994**, 64–68. [CrossRef]
24. Bruce, W.D.; Stevens, P.M. Surgical Correction of Miserable Malalignment Syndrome. *J. Pediatr. Orthop.* **2004**, *24*, 392–396. [CrossRef]
25. MacWilliams, B.A.; McMulkin, M.L.; Davis, R.B.; Westberry, D.E.; Baird, G.O.; Stevens, P.M. Biomechanical Changes Associated with Femoral Derotational Osteotomy. *Gait Posture* **2016**, *49*, 202–206. [CrossRef] [PubMed]
26. Moya, L.; Buly, R.; Henn, F.; Kelly, B.; Ma, Y.; Molisani, D. Femoral Retroversion in Patients with Femoroacetabular Impingement: A Cofactor in the Development of Hip Osteoarthritis. *Orthop. Proc.* **2010**, *92-B*, 526. [CrossRef]
27. Ramme, A.J.; Egol, J.; Chang, G.; Davidovitch, R.I.; Konda, S. Evaluation of Malrotation Following Intramedullary Nailing in a Femoral Shaft Fracture Model: Can a 3D c-Arm Improve Accuracy? *Injury* **2017**, *48*, 1603–1608. [CrossRef] [PubMed]
28. Deshmukh, R.G.; Lou, K.K.; Neo, C.B.; Yew, K.S.; Rozman, I.; George, J. A Technique to Obtain Correct Rotational Alignment during Closed Locked Intramedullary Nailing of the Femur. *Injury* **1998**, *29*, 207–210. [CrossRef]
29. Hawi, N.; Kabbani, A.-R.; O'Loughlin, P.; Krettek, C.; Citak, M.; Liodakis, E. Intraoperative Measurement of Femoral Antetorsion Using the Anterior Cortical Angle Method: A Novel Use for Smartphones. *Int. J. Med. Robot.* **2013**, *9*, 29–35. [CrossRef]
30. Jaarsma, R.L.; Verdonschot, N.; van der Venne, R.; van Kampen, A. Avoiding Rotational Malalignment after Fractures of the Femur by Using the Profile of the Lesser Trochanter: An in Vitro Study. *Arch. Orthop. Trauma Surg.* **2005**, *125*, 184–187. [CrossRef]
31. Hawi, N.; Liodakis, E.; Suero, E.M.; Stuebig, T.; Citak, M.; Krettek, C. Radiological Outcome and Intraoperative Evaluation of a Computer-Navigation System for Femoral Nailing: A Retrospective Cohort Study. *Injury* **2014**, *45*, 1632–1636. [CrossRef]

32. Lal, H.; Patralekh, M.K. 3D Printing and Its Applications in Orthopaedic Trauma: A Technological Marvel. *J. Clin. Orthop. Trauma* **2018**, *9*, 260–268. [CrossRef]
33. Wong, K.C. 3D-Printed Patient-Specific Applications in Orthopedics. *Orthop. Res. Rev.* **2016**, *8*, 57–66. [CrossRef]
34. Chai, W.; Xu, M.; Zhang, G.; Zhang, L.; Gou, W.; Ni, M.; Chen, J. Computer-Aided Design and Custom-Made Guide in Corrective Osteotomy for Complex Femoral Deformity. *J. Huazhong Univ. Sci. Technol. Med. Sci.* **2013**, *33*, 398–405. [CrossRef] [PubMed]
35. Krettek, C.; Bruns, N. Aktueller Stand und neue Entwicklungen des 3D-Drucks in der Unfallchirurgie. *Unfallchirurg* **2019**, *122*, 256–269. [CrossRef] [PubMed]
36. Andrés-Cano, P.; Calvo-Haro, J.A.; Fillat-Gomà, F.; Andrés-Cano, I.; Perez-Mañanes, R. Papel del cirujano ortopédico y traumatólogo en la impresión 3D: Aplicaciones actuales y aspectos legales para una medicina personalizada. *Rev. Esp. Cir. Ortop. Traumatol.* **2021**, *65*, 138–151. [CrossRef]
37. Fiz, N.; Delgado, D.; Sánchez, X.; Sánchez, P.; Bilbao, A.M.; Oraa, J.; Sánchez, M. Application of 3D Technology and Printing for Femoral Derotation Osteotomy: Case and Technical Report. *Ann. Transl Med.* **2017**, *5*, 400. [CrossRef]
38. Victor, J.; Premanathan, A. Virtual 3D Planning and Patient Specific Surgical Guides for Osteotomies around the Knee: A Feasibility and Proof-of-Concept Study. Bone Joint J. *Bone Joint J.* **2013**, *95-B*, 153–158. [CrossRef]
39. Krettek, C.; Miclau, T.; Grün, O.; Schandelmaier, P.; Tscherne, H. Intraoperative Control of Axes, Rotation and Length in Femoral and Tibial Fractures. Technical Note. *Injury* **1998**, *29* (Suppl. 3), C29–C39. [CrossRef]
40. Jagernauth, S.; Tindall, A.J.; Kohli, S.; Allen, P. New Technique: A Novel Femoral Derotation Osteotomy for Malrotation Following Intramedullary Nailing. *Case Rep. Orthop.* **2012**, *2012*, 1–2. [CrossRef] [PubMed]
41. Espinoza, C.; Sathy, A.K.; Moore, D.S.; Starr, A.J.; Reinert, C.M. Use of Inherent Anteversion of an Intramedullary Nail to Avoid Malrotation in Femur Fractures. *J. Orthop. Trauma* **2014**, *28*, e34–e38. [CrossRef]
42. Stambough, J.B.; Davis, L.; Szymanski, D.A.; Smith, J.C.; Schoenecker, P.L.; Gordon, J.E. Knee Pain and Activity Outcomes After Femoral Derotation Osteotomy for Excessive Femoral Anteversion. *J. Pediatr. Orthop.* **2018**, *38*, 503–509. [CrossRef]
43. Buly, R.L.; Sosa, B.R.; Poultsides, L.A.; Caldwell, E.; Rozbruch, S.R. Femoral Derotation Osteotomy in Adults for Version Abnormalities. *J. Am. Acad. Orthop. Surg.* **2018**, *26*, e416–e425. [CrossRef]
44. Stahl, J.-P.; Alt, V.; Kraus, R.; Hoerbelt, R.; Itoman, M.; Schnettler, R. Derotation of Post-Traumatic Femoral Deformities by Closed Intramedullary Sawing. *Injury* **2006**, *37*, 145–151. [CrossRef] [PubMed]
45. Gérard, R.; Stindel, E.; Moineau, G.; Le Nen, D.; Lefèvre, C. Rotational Femoral Osteotomies Using an Endomedullary Saw. *Orthop. Traumatol. Surg. Res.* **2009**, *95*, 414–419. [CrossRef] [PubMed]
46. Rosseels, W.; Herteleer, M.; Sermon, A.; Nijs, S.; Hoekstra, H. Corrective Osteotomies Using Patient-Specific 3D-Printed Guides: A Critical Appraisal. *Eur. J. Trauma Emerg Surg.* **2019**, *45*, 299–307. [CrossRef] [PubMed]

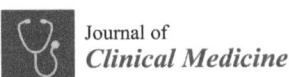

Article

Periacetabular Tumour Resection under Anterosuperior Iliac Spine Allows Better Alloprosthetic Reconstruction than Above: Bone Contact Matters

Alessandro Bruschi *, Luca Cevolani, Benedetta Spazzoli, Marco Focaccia, Stefano Pasini Tommaso Frisoni and Davide Maria Donati

Unit of 3rd Orthopaedic and traumatologic Clinic Prevalently Oncologic, IRCCS Istituto Ortopedico Rizzoli, Via Pupilli 1, 40136 Bologna, Italy; luca.cevolani@ior.it (L.C.); benedetta.spazzoli@ior.it (B.S.); marco.focaccia@ior.it (M.F.); stefano.pasini@ior.it (S.P.); tommaso.frisoni@ior.it (T.F.); davidemaria.donati@ior.it (D.M.D.)
* Correspondence: alessandro.bruschi@ior.it

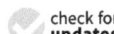

Citation: Bruschi, A.; Cevolani, L.; Spazzoli, B.; Focaccia, M.; Pasini, S.; Frisoni, T.; Donati, D.M. Periacetabular Tumour Resection under Anterosuperior Iliac Spine Allows Better Alloprosthetic Reconstruction than Above: Bone Contact Matters. *J. Clin. Med.* 2022, 11, 4499. https://doi.org/10.3390/jcm11154499

Academic Editors: Massimiliano Mosca, Alberto Grassi and Silvio Caravelli

Received: 29 June 2022
Accepted: 30 July 2022
Published: 2 August 2022

Publisher's Note: MDPI stays neutral with regard to jurisdictional claims in published maps and institutional affiliations.

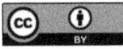

Copyright: © 2022 by the authors. Licensee MDPI, Basel, Switzerland. This article is an open access article distributed under the terms and conditions of the Creative Commons Attribution (CC BY) license (https://creativecommons.org/licenses/by/4.0/).

Abstract: Background: Periacetabular resections are more affected by late complications than other pelvic resections. Reconstruction using bone allograft is considered a suitable solution. However, it is still not clear how the bone-allograft contact surface impacts on mechanical and functional outcome. Materials and methods: This paper presents the results of a retrospective analysis of 33 patients with resection of the entire acetabulum and reconstruction with an allograft-prosthetic composite for the period 1999 to 2010. Patients were divided in two groups, based on type of resection. In Group 1. patients had resections under anterosuperior iliac spine allowing the highest bone-allograft surface contact in reconstruction, while in Group 2 patients had resections over it. Results: Mechanical survival of the implant and Musculoskeletal Tumor Society functional score were calculated. Impact of age and artificial ligament were investigated as well. Patients in Group 1 had 38% mechanical failure rate of the implant while patients in Group 2 had 88%. Average functional score was higher in Group 1 compared with patients in Group 2. An artificial ligament was shown to have non-significant impact on survival of the reconstruction in Group 1, while significantly improving survival of reconstruction in Group 2. Conclusion: Bone-allograft contact matters: resection under anterosuperior iliac spine allows better mechanical survival and offers better reconstruction functional scores.

Keywords: pelvic resection; alloprosthetic composite; bone sparing; multiplanar osteotomies; surgical navigation; 3D custom made prosthesis

1. Introduction

Pelvic resections involving acetabulum are more affected by late complications than other pelvic resections, and, hence, the worst functional prognosis should be expected [1]. The resulting large bone and soft tissue defects, the perioperative complications and the post-operative tumour treatment frequently result in complications threatening the implant survival. Factors majorly determining complications are post-operative chemotherapy, the long surgical intraoperative time and the type of reconstruction [2–6]. Indeed, reaching a suitable reconstruction following this type of resection is a major challenge for the orthopaedic oncologist [3]. Different reconstructive techniques have been proposed over the years: Harrington reconstruction, iliofemoral coaptation or pseudoarthrosis, ischiofemoral arthrodesis, saddle prosthesis, alloprosthetics composite and 3D custom made prostheses [3,7,8]. When reconstruction is not a suitable option, flail hip can be performed [9]. Among all these techniques, alloprosthetics composite reconstruction consists of a bone allograft customized on the operative table to restore pelvic bone defect combined with a total hip arthroplasty. In most cases, it is a reliable solution after periacetabular tumour resection in terms of durability and function [3,6]. However mechanical, infective and local tumour relapse complications range from 30% to 90% [2,6,10–12]. Infection and dislocation are the most common complications in the early stages [2,3,6], while, loosening and mechanical failure are later complications [6,10]. However, type II pelvic resections can involve much more than the periacetabular area, and, thus, it is unclear if extension of the resection due to tumour location impacts on the functional outcome of the reconstruction over time [1]. The extension of resection is reported with no effect on outcome of a periacetabular reconstruction in [5,6], while other reports [5,11,13,14] showed better outcome in cases with limited bone excision. We, therefore, decided to retrospectively review our series of patients who experienced pelvic resection and reconstruction with allograft prosthetic composite to investigate if the extension of bone-allograft interface in the reconstruction impacts on survival of reconstruction, thus, pivoting the choice of the type of resection when this is possible.

2. Materials and Methods

2.1. Criteria of Data Collection

We retrospectively reviewed 69 patients treated with internal hemipelvectomy for a bone tumour involving the periacetabular area between November 1990 and August 2010. According to the Enneking and Dunham classification, all the patients had a type II alone or a combined type II resection; i.e., extending to ilium, ischium, pubis or sacrum, depending on tumour location [15]. Inclusion criteria: (a) patients with locally aggressive benign (Stage III) or malignant bone tumour of the periacetabular area; (b) diagnosis performed with either needle or incisional biopsy confirmed by an expert pathologist; (c) type II resection alone or combined type II resection of the pelvis; (d) follow up longer than 24 months; (e) no infection or local tumour relapse. Exclusion criteria: follow up less than 24 months; infective or local tumour relapse complications. According to the inclusion and exclusion criteria, 33 patients were considered for the retrospective analysis.

2.2. Classification System of Pelvic Resections Used

The 33 patients were divided into 2 groups following the classification system here suggested: Group 1 (resection under anterosuperior iliac spine allowing high bone-allograft contact in the reconstruction: 1A type resection) and Group 2 (resection above anterosuperior iliac spine allowing low bone-allograft contact in the reconstruction: all other resections) (Figure 1) (Table 1).

Table 1. Classification System.

Region of Proximal Osteotomy Line:	Region of Distal Osteotomy Line:
1 Osteotomy inside an area comprised between the roof of the acetabulum and a line that connects the apex of the ischiatic notch and the anterosuperior iliac spine	A Osteotomy involving the ipsilateral pubic ramus
2 Osteotomy inside an area comprised between the anterosuperior iliac spine and the lateral margin of posterosuperior iliac spine bone bulk	B Osteotomy involving the pubic symphysis
3 Osteotomy inside an area comprised between the lateral margin of posterosuperior iliac spine bone bulk and the sacro-iliac joint (excluded)	C Osteotomy involving the contralateral pubic ramus
4 Osteotomy medial to the sacro-iliac joint (included)	

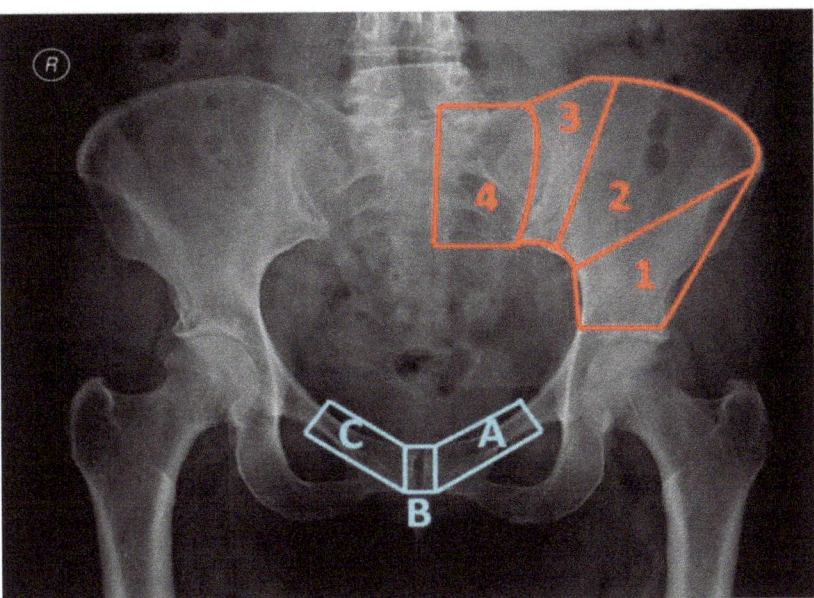

Figure 1. Classification system based on the amount of bone resected. Numbers are related to the four different regions in which the proximal osteotomy (super acetabular) can be made. Letters define the distal osteotomy (medial) location.

The classification system was based on where the proximal osteotomy and the distal osteotomy were made at the time of surgery to achieve wide margins resection. We defined 4 regions in the super acetabular area (Figure 1) in which the proximal osteotomy had been performed in the different cases. Region 1 was contained between the roof of the acetabulum and a line that connects the apex of the greater sciatic notch and the anterosuperior iliac spine. Region 2 was comprised of the area between the anterosuperior iliac spine and the lateral margin of posterosuperior iliac spine. Region 3 was the area in between the lateral margin of the posterosuperior iliac spine bone and the sacroiliac joint. Region 4 included the sacroiliac joint, and thus, it was placed in the sacral wing. For the distal (medial) osteotomy, we identified three osteotomy locations: type A osteotomy involved the ipsilateral pubic ramus, type B osteotomy was in the pubic symphysis and type C involved the contralateral pubic ramus.

The Senior Author (DD) participated in all procedures and more than 5 senior surgeons have been involved in the procedures during the considered period of time. In 4 patients only the extended iliofemoral (lateral) approach was used. In all other patients, inguinal extension was performed in order to better expose iliac vessels and nerves, including the obturator bundle. To improve the exposure of the posterior column of the acetabulum, in 7 patients a trochanteric osteotomy was performed and repaired using a cable grip device or a tension band wire. An extra-articular resection, removing the entire hip en bloc. during tumour excision was used in 9 patients. All procedures were performed using a frozen, non-irradiated, pelvic allograft shaped to match the bone excised. Grafts were thawed in Rifampin solution (Lepetit, Milan, Italy) for 60 min before use. Cultures for aerobic and anaerobic bacteria were performed after thawing. The first 9 patients received a reconstruction using a bipolar cup or a metal-backed cup cemented in the acetabular allograft. The other 14 patients were reconstructed with different acetabular cups. In all these cases, the acetabulum was cemented, and bone screws supplemented fixation of the cup to the allograft. To protect the allograft from possible fracture of the medial acetabular, a contoured neutralization plate along the innominate bone was used in 6 of these patients. The remaining 10 patients were treated with a McMinn acetabular prosthesis (Waldemar

Link, Hamburg, Germany), which incorporated a large central stem, from 45 mm to 85 mm in length. We did not use additional screws for fixation, nor a contoured neutralization plate, in this type of reconstruction. In all procedures involving the iliac wing, we used three or four large cancellous screws fitted with washers (Synthes, Paoli, PA, USA) passing through the graft, into the sacrum (Figure 2). In allograft-host junctions at the symphysis pubis, an anterior plate was fixed onto the contralateral pubic bone with screws and locking nuts, or the symphysis was fixed with screws and cerclage wires. In 21 patients, to avoid early hip prosthetic dislocation, we decided to use one or two artificial ligaments. They were fixed to the proximal femur (inter trochanteric area) with a screw, after having passed the screw into the allograft ileopubic branch through drilled holes and twisting it around the prosthetic neck. A Ligament Advanced Repair System (LARS) artificial ligament was used in the reconstruction (Corin Group, Cirencester, UK) in Figure 2.

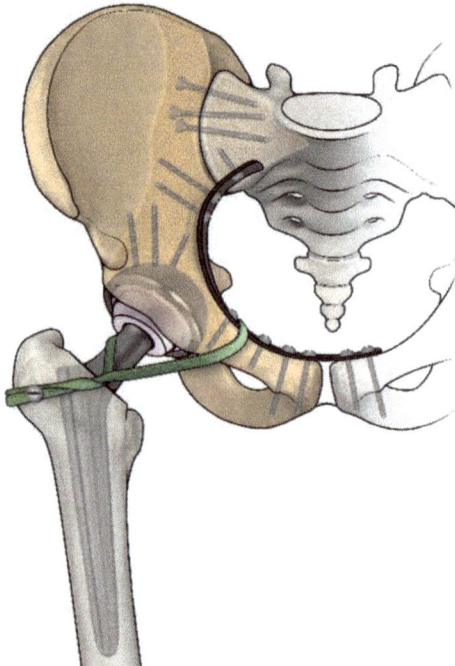

Figure 2. Ileo-femoral artificial ligament used for immediate stabilization of the hip joint.

2.3. Data Collection

According with the described classification, Group 1 included 16 patients who had received 1A resection, while Group 2 included 17 patients who had received other resections (two 1B, one 2A, two 2B, one 3B, seven 4A and four 4B). Characteristics of patients are recorded in Table 2. Resection margin results were wide in all patients.

In Group 1 (16 cases), six patients were younger than 40 years old at the time of the surgical procedure, while ten were older. Ten patients were treated with a hip artificial ligament.

In Group 2 (17 cases), eight patients were younger than 40 years old, while nine were older at the time of the surgical procedure. In 11 hip artificial ligaments were used in the reconstruction.

The end point of the analysis was composite revision, with either revision of the acetabular cup or allograft retrieval (including acetabular cup).

Table 2. Data on the 33 patients of the study. Chs c = central chondrosarcoma; Chs dediff = dedifferentiated chondrosarcoma; GCT = giant cells tumour; Os L = low grade osteosarcoma; Os H = high grade osteosarcoma; Spindle cell s = spindle cell sarcoma; Ewimg = Ewing sarcoma; Angios = angiosarcoma; Dod = dead of disease; Ned = no evidence of disease.

Number	Gender	Age	Diagnosis	Stage	Resection Type	Postoperative Chemotherapy	Patient Follow Up (Months)	Status
1	M	40	Chs c	II B	1A	No	194	Ned
2	M	32	Chs c	I B	1A	No	187	Ned
3	F	56	Chs c	I A	2A	No	256	Ned
4	F	69	Chs c	I B	1A	No	168	Ned
5	M	34	GCT	3	1A	No	286	Ned
6	F	59	Chs c	I B	4A	No	255	Ned
7	M	38	Chs c	I A	1A	No	194	Dod
8	M	62	Chs c	IB	1A	No	110	Ned
9	F	49	Chs dediff	II B	4B	Yes	100	Dod
10	F	25	Chs c	I B	3B	No	277	Ned
11	M	22	Os L	I A	2B	No	258	Ned
12	F	17	Os H	II B	4A	Yes	252	Ned
13	F	22	Os H	II B	4A	Yes	252	Ned
14	M	21	Chs c	IIB	4A	No	295	Ned
15	F	33	GCT	3	1A	No	230	Ned
16	M	57	Chs dediff	II B	4B	No	300	Ned
17	M	56	Chs c	IB	1A	No	142	Ned
18	M	60	Chs c	I B	4B	No	146	Ned
19	M	65	Chs c	II B	2B	No	266	Dod
20	F	37	Chs c	II B	4B	No	305	Ned
21	M	51	Chs c	I B	1B	No	138	Ned
22	F	63	Angios	IIB	4A	No	38	Dod
23	M	29	Tcg	III	4A	No	331	Ned
24	F	51	Os H	II B	1A	Yes	65	Dod
25	M	48	Chs c	I B	1A	No	169	Ned
26	M	66	Chs c	I B	1A	No	123	Ned
27	F	24	Chs dediff	II B	1A	No	276	Ned
28	F	43	Os H	I B	1A	No	167	Ned
29	M	59	GCT	3	1A	No	250	Ned
30	F	35	Spindle cell s	II B	4A	Yes	184	Ned
31	M	53	Chs c	I A	1B	No	173	Ned
21	F	59	Chs c	I B	1A	No	51	Ned
33	M	18	Ewing	II	1A	Yes	157	Ned

Patients had regular follow ups, every three months in the first three years, every six months in the fourth and fifth year and once a year thereafter. Functional status was calculated during follow-up through the Musculoskeletal Tumor Society evaluation score (MSTS93) [16].

All follow up radiographs were compared with previous ones: loosening was considered when the cup was displaced, compared to the previous follow-up. Reabsorption was defined when more than 1 cm of the allograft around the cup was eroded over time or when large progressive lucencies were seen around the fixation devices. Fracture of the allograft was considered when a bone interruption inside the body, or in the margins of the allograft, was seen. Dislocation of the hip prosthesis was considered when the femoral head lost articular contact with the acetabular cup. Breakage of plate and screws was evident when these fixation devices lost their integrity as one single element. Non-union was finally defined as failure of union by one year after surgery.

2.4. Statistical Analysis

Statistical analysis was performed using the Statistical Package for the Social Sciences (SPSS) software version 21.0 (SPSS Inc., Chicago, IL, USA). Kaplan-Meier analysis with the log-rank test was used in order to calculate the failure rate and the mean failure time of the 2 groups [17]. In all reconstructions, the endpoint of the analysis was at least one surgical operation for revision of the implant. Functional evaluation of the patients in the two groups was recorded at two and five years, and at the final follow up. The planned functional evaluation was completed in all but eight patients. Two of them lacked the two years follow up, five the five years follow up and one lacked the final follow up. Cox regression multivariate analysis (with Wald's backward method) was used to calculate the impact of age (</>40 years old) and artificial ligament on failure rate in the two groups at 120 months (Table 2).

3. Results

3.1. Impact of Bone-Allograft Contact on the Reconstruction

Patients in Group 1 had a reconstruction with better survival and functional scores compared to patients in Group 2. In Group 1 the implant had a 38% failure rate and a mean failure time of 144 months (+/−69 months). While patients in Group 2 had an 88% failure rate with a mean failure time of 109 months (+/−84 months) (95% CI, $p = 0.021$) (Figure 3). The endpoint of analysis was at least one surgical operation for revision of implant due to mechanical failure (aseptic loosening, fracture or resorption of the allograft, dislocation or breakage of the hardware).

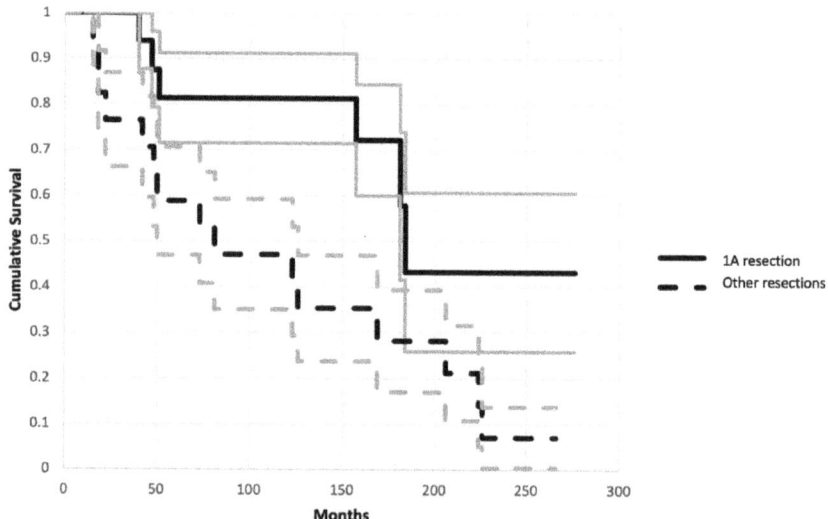

Figure 3. Kaplan-Meier plot shows different cumulative survival in Group 1 (A1 resection) and in Group 2 (Other resections) (CI 95%, $p = 0.02$). Endpoint of analysis was at least one surgical operation for revision of implant due to mechanical failure (aseptic loosening, fracture or resorption of the allograft, dislocation or breakage of the hardware). Grey lines represent standard deviation.

Post-hoc sample size analysis for survival of implant (16 patients in Group 1 and 17 patients in Group 2, with 38% failure rate in Group 1 and 88% in Group 2, $p > 0.05$) showed power of the study to be 88%.

In Group 1, average functional score was 81% at two years follow up, 77% at five years and 68% at final follow up (mean time 145 months). In Group 2 the average functional score at two, five years and at the final follow up (mean time 109 months) were 62%, 70% and 54%, respectively.

In Group 1 (16 patients), failure occurred in 7 patients (%). Six of these patients presented implant failure for loosening of the acetabular cup and were treated with acetabular cup substitution. Another patient failed due to reabsorption of the acetabular wall and was treated with substitution of the acetabular cup with a cemented one. None of these patients underwent allograft removal. Of the six failed patients, in three of them an artificial ligament had been used in the primary reconstruction.

In Group 2 (17 patients), failure occurred in 15 patients (%). Seven patients presented cup loosening and were treated with acetabular cup revision (one 1B, one 2B, one 3B, three 4B and one 4B). Four patients had a fracture of the allograft, treated with acetabular cup revision with an acetabular reinforcement cage in one case (2A), removal of the composite and saddle prosthesis in another case (4B), removal of the implant and flail hip in another patient (1B) and acetabular cup revision with iliac crest bone autograft in the other one (4A). One patient underwent a femoral head revision for dislocation (4A), one patient had a revision of the implant without allograft removal, due to breakage of the neutralization plate (4B). Finally, two more patients presented with non-union of the bone graft. One had the implant and the graft removed and substituted by saddle prosthesis (2B); while, in the other, the implant was revised with an iliac bone crest autograft without allograft removal (4A). In six failures of Group 2 an artificial ligament had not been used, three of them failed with removal of the allograft.

3.2. Impact of Age on the Reconstruction

In both groups, patients older than 40 years old had lower failure rates. In Group 1, patients older than 40 years old had a survival rate of 90%, while patients younger than 40 years old had 67% survival at 120 months (CI 95%, $p = 0.048$). In Group 2, patients older than 40 years old had a survival rate of 56%, while patients younger than 40 years old had a 38% survival rate at 120 months (CI 95%, $p = 0.048$).

3.3. Impact of Artificial Ligament on the Reconstruction

In Group 1 there was no significant difference in implant survival if the artificial ligament was used or not. On the other hand, in Group 2, survival of the reconstruction benefited from the use of the artificial ligament.

Considering patients in Group 1, those in whom an artificial ligament was used in the reconstruction had an 83% survival rate, while those with no artificial ligament used in the reconstruction had an 80% survival rate, at 120 months (CI 95%, $p = 0.02$) (Figure 4).

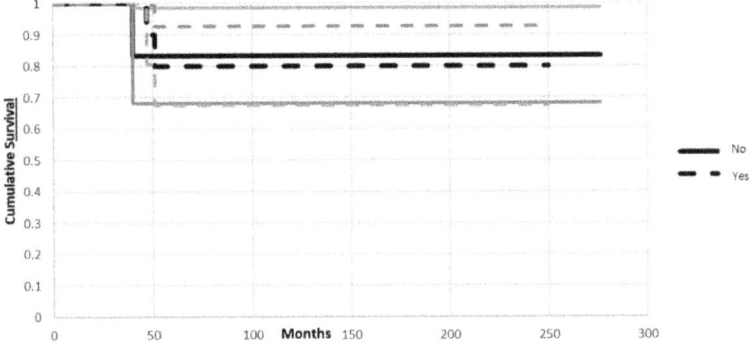

Figure 4. Kaplan-Meier plot shows similar survival rate in Group 1 with ligament in the reconstruction (Yes) or without artificial ligament in the reconstruction (No), at 120 months (CI 95%, $p = 0.02$). The endpoint of analysis was at least one surgical operation for revision of implant due to mechanical failure (aseptic loosening, fracture or resorption of the allograft, dislocation or breakage of the hardware). Grey lines represent standard deviation.

In Group 2, those in whom an artificial ligament was used in the reconstruction had a 64% survival rate, while those with no artificial ligament used in the reconstruction had a 17% survival rate, at 120 months (CI 95%, $p = 0.02$) (Figure 5).

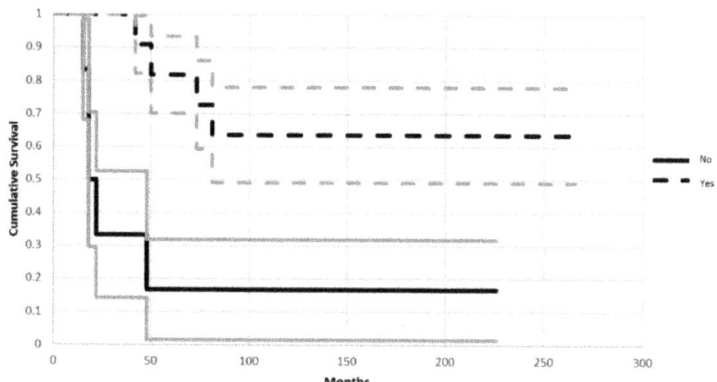

Figure 5. Kaplan-Meier plot shows improved mechanical survival in Group 2 (Yes) using artificial ligament, at 120 months (CI 95%, $p = 0.02$). The endpoint of analysis was at least one surgical operation for revision of implant due to mechanical failure (aseptic loosening, fracture or resorption of the allograft, dislocation or breakage of the hardware). Grey lines represent standard deviation.

4. Discussion

This study was a retrospective analysis on a limited number of patients, but due to rarity of the site of operation and the need for long term follow-ups this case series was larger than others in the literature.

4.1. Impact of Bone-Allograft Contact on the Reconstruction

Reconstruction in Group 1 had a better implant survival if compared to Group 2, scoring a failure rate of 38% vs. 88% (average 144 months +/−69 months vs. 109 +/−84). Concerning functional score, Group 1 scored 81%, 77% and 68% vs. 62%, 70% and 54%, respectively, at two year follow up, five year follow up and final follow up. These results indicate that providing higher bone-allograft contact allows more mechanical durability and higher performance of functional reconstruction. These results are comparable with those of Beadel et al., where type II pelvic resections had a better functional score than type II combined [18]. In our opinion, our results integrate Beadel's conclusion under a mechanical point of view, as in that series deep infection severely impaired the mechanical outcome of larger resections [18]. Other series, considering resection type, also suggest that larger resections are consistently influenced by related deep infection, so, the potential mechanical outcome remains unclear in those series as they appear to be indirectly influenced by infection [4,5,19]. Compared with the MSTS reported in literature (average functional result 70%), in our study Group 1 scored higher and Group 2 lower than 70% [3,4,6]. One of the reasons to explain the better results in Group 1 is related to the direction of the iliac osteotomy. In Group 1, the osteotomy under the anterosuperior iliac spine endures less vertical mechanical shear stress at the bone-allograft interface (Figure 6); therefore, multiplanar osteotomies could be suitable options to tackle this problem in proximal osteotomies over to the anterosuperior iliac spine [20] (Figure 7). On the other hand, the distal osteotomy (pubic area) affects pelvic ring integrity; in type A resections pubic symphysis is spared, while it is not spared in types B and C [21,22]. This factor could contribute to better results in 1A resections.

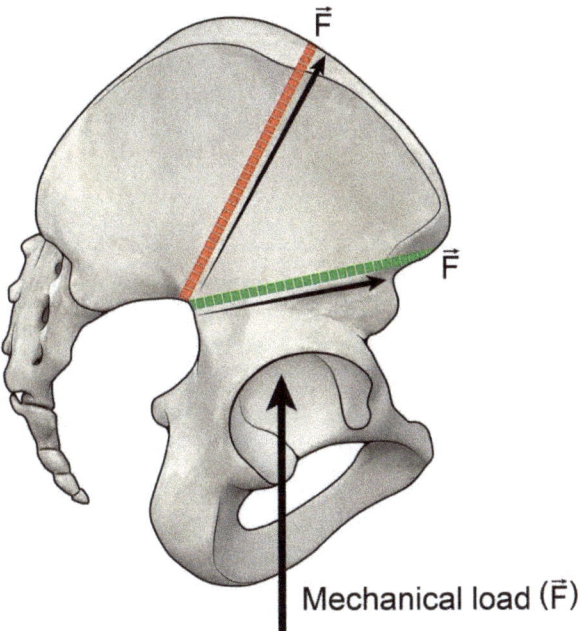

Figure 6. Shear stress vertical forces are less when the osteotomy line is made under the anterosuperior iliac spine.

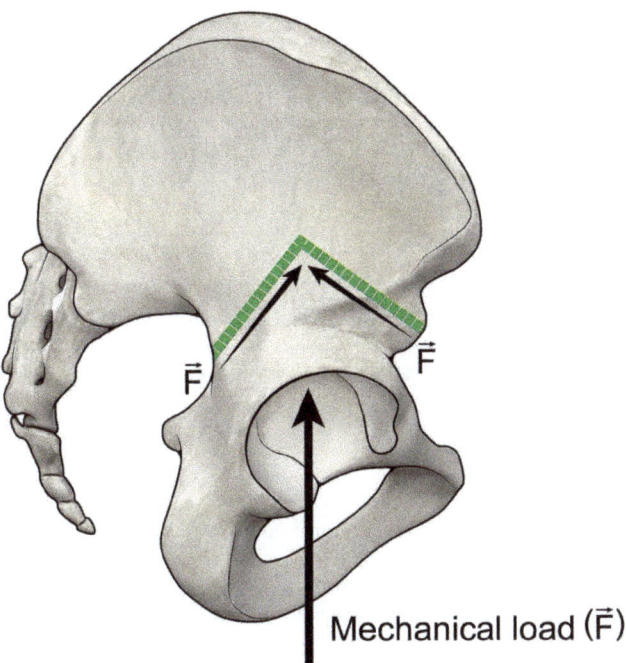

Figure 7. Biomechanics of a multiplanar osteotomy: the mechanical load is distributed along the two osteotomy lines with limited vertical shear stress.

Long-term survival and functional results of alloprosthetic composite reconstruction in this series was fair. However, we believe surgically navigated resections and 3D custom made reconstructions assisted by patient specific instrumentation should provide better results [20,23–27]. Actually, some studies highlight the importance of bone stock sparing resections in order to improve mechanical properties of the reconstruction, such as in the following scenarios, which preserve wide oncological margins while sparing the bone mass needed for a suitable bone-reconstruction contact: iliac multiplanar osteotomies, surgically navigated resections and 3D custom made reconstructions [13,14,20,23,24,28].

4.2. Impact of Age on the Reconstruction

In both groups, patients older than 40 years old had lower failure rates at 120 months. The lifestyle and the higher functional requests of a younger patient could justify mechanical overuse and earlier failure of the implant. Influence of age on cementless fixation is of paramount interest in orthopaedics, as most orthopaedic implants are placed in elderly bone tissues. Despite the fact that it is reported that bone and mineral metabolism decreases with ageing, the impact of age on bone-implant interface remains unclear in humans [29]. Almost all studies investigating this topic have been conducted on animals presenting contrasting results: some studies state ageing decreases bone callus formation and causes lower bone ingrowth in porous implants [29], while in other studies older animals present lower interface shear stress and comparable fixation survival if compared to younger animals [18,22,30,31]. Despite ageing probably having a negative effect on bone-allograft union, these works support the idea that the higher shear stress forces in younger patients can overcome the good performance of a younger bone.

4.3. Impact of Artificial Ligament on the Reconstruction

In Group 1, the use of an artificial ligament to stabilize hip articulation had no significant impact on the mechanics of the reconstruction. On the other hand, in Group 2, the artificial ligament significantly impacted on the mechanics of reconstruction, giving 64% and 17% survival rates, at 120 months. The mechanical role of artificial ligaments in improving mechanics of the reconstruction is well known [6,32,33]. However, due to lower soft tissue excision, a limited resection probably has lower impact on hip stability. The correct indication for the use of artificial ligament is to be defined, as it has been demonstrated to increase the risk of infection and synovitis in some series [34–36]. Therefore, in reconstruction with limited soft tissue sacrifice, this risk could be avoided without any consequence on the stability of the reconstruction.

5. Conclusions

In conclusion, where periacetabular tumour resection is performed can influence reconstruction survival and function. In this study, resections under anterosuperior iliac spine allowed more bone-allograft contact in the reconstruction and were demonstrated to perform better in terms of long-term failure (38% at long term follow up), yielding better functional outcomes (75%), if compared to resections above the anterosuperior iliac spine. Studies comparing functional results after resections inside the iliac wing (low contact reconstruction) and after resections directly in the sacroiliac joint (higher contact reconstruction) should be considered. These studies could demonstrate that pursuing a higher contact reconstruction may provide better functional results, even at the cost of a wider resection. Furthermore, older age and the use of an artificial ligament in selected cases showed better clinical and functional scores. In the future, multiplanar osteotomies, surgical navigation and 3D custom made prostheses could improve the results of all resections, allowing better bone-reconstruction contact.

Author Contributions: Conceptualization, A.B. and D.M.D.; methodology, L.C.; software, L.C.; validation, D.M.D., B.S. and T.F.; formal analysis, D.M.D.; investigation, S.P.; resources, M.F.; data curation, A.B.; writing—original draft preparation, A.B. and D.M.D.; writing—review and editing,

A.B. and D.M.D.; visualization, A.B. and D.M.D.; supervision, D.M.D. and L.C. All authors have read and agreed to the published version of the manuscript.

Funding: This research and APC were funded by the Italian Ministry of Health- 5 × 1000 Year 2018, Income 2017 "Custom made implants produced with additive technology supporting surgical musculoskeletal reconstruction in cancer patients".

Institutional Review Board Statement: The study was conducted in accordance with the Declaration of Helsinki, and approved by the Local Ethics Committee (protocol code *583/2021/Oss/IOR* on the 21 July 2021).

Data Availability Statement: Not applicable.

Acknowledgments: Authors gratefully acknowledge Maria Pia Cumani (Laboratorio di Disegno Anatomico, Dip.Scienze Biomediche e Neuromotorie, Università di Bologna c/o Istituto Ortopedico Rizzoli—Bologna, Italy) for originally created the figures in this paper.

Conflicts of Interest: The authors declare no conflict of interest.

References

1. Mayerson, J.L.; Wooldridge, A.N.; Scharschmidt, T.J. Pelvic Resection: Current Concepts. *J. Am. Acad. Orthop. Surg.* **2014**, *22*, 214–222. [CrossRef]
2. Delloye, C.; Banse, X.; Brichard, B.; Docquier, P.-L.; Cornu, O. Pelvic Reconstruction with a Structural Pelvic Allograft After Resection of a Malignant Bone Tumor. *J. Bone Jt. Surg.* **2007**, *89*, 579–587. [CrossRef]
3. Brown, T.S.; Salib, C.G.; Rose, P.S.; Sim, F.H.; Lewallen, D.G.; Abdel, M.P. Reconstruction of the Hip after Resection of Periacetabular Oncological Lesions: A Systematic Review. *Bone Jt. J.* **2018**, *100-B*, 22–30. [CrossRef]
4. Campanacci, D.; Chacon, S.; Mondanelli, N.; Beltrami, G.; Scoccianti, G.; Caff, G.; Frenos, F.; Capanna, R. Pelvic Massive Allograft Reconstruction after Bone Tumour Resection. *Int. Orthop.* **2012**, *36*, 2529–2536. [CrossRef] [PubMed]
5. Jaiswal, P.K.; Aston, W.J.S.; Grimer, R.J.; Abudu, A.; Carter, S.; Blunn, G.; Briggs, T.W.R.; Cannon, S. Peri-Acetabular Resection and Endoprosthetic Reconstruction for Tumours of the Acetabulum. *J. Bone Jt. Surg. Br.* **2008**, *90-B*, 1222–1227. [CrossRef]
6. Donati, D.; Di Bella, C.; Frisoni, T.; Cevolani, L.; DeGroot, H. Alloprosthetic Composite Is a Suitable Reconstruction After Periacetabular Tumor Resection. *Clin. Orthop.* **2011**, *469*, 1450–1458. [CrossRef]
7. Kiatisevi, P.; Sukunthanak, B.; Pakpianpairoj, C.; Liupolvanish, P. Functional Outcome and Complications Following Reconstruction for Harrington Class II and III Periacetabular Metastasis. *World J. Surg. Oncol.* **2015**, *13*, 4. [CrossRef] [PubMed]
8. Jansen, J.A.; van de Sande, M.A.J.; Dijkstra, P.D.S. Poor Long-Term Clinical Results of Saddle Prosthesis After Resection of Periacetabular Tumors. *Clin. Orthop.* **2013**, *471*, 324–331. [CrossRef]
9. Takami, M.; Ieguchi, M.; Aono, M.; Hoshi, M.; Takada, J.; Oebisu, N.; Iwai, T. Flail Hip Joint Following Periacetabular Tumor Resection of the Pelvis Using Upper Surface of the Femoral Neck as a Saddle: A Case Report. *Oncol. Lett.* **2015**, *10*, 3529–3531. [CrossRef]
10. Langlais, F.; Lambotte, J.C.; Thomazeau, H. Long-Term Results of Hemipelvis Reconstruction with Allografts. *Clin. Orthop.* **2001**, *388*, 178–186. [CrossRef]
11. Ozaki, T.; Hoffmann, C.; Hillmann, A.; Gosheger, G.; Lindner, N.; Winkelmann, W. Implantation of Hemipelvic Prosthesis After Resection of Sarcoma. *Clin. Orthop.* **2002**, *396*, 197–205. [CrossRef]
12. Hillmann, A.; Hoffmann, C.; Gosheger, G.; Rödl, R.; Winkelmann, W.; Ozaki, T. Tumors of the Pelvis: Complications after Reconstruction. *Arch. Orthop. Trauma Surg.* **2003**, *123*, 340–344. [CrossRef]
13. Angelini, A.; Kotrych, D.; Trovarelli, G.; Szafrański, A.; Bohatyrewicz, A.; Ruggieri, P. Analysis of Principles Inspiring Design of Three-Dimensional-Printed Custom-Made Prostheses in Two Referral Centres. *Int. Orthop.* **2020**, *44*, 829–837. [CrossRef]
14. De Paolis, M.; Sambri, A.; Zucchini, R.; Frisoni, T.; Spazzoli, B.; Taddei, F.; Donati, D.M. Custom-Made 3D-Printed Prosthesis in Periacetabular Resections Through a Novel Ileo-Adductor Approach. *Orthopedics* **2022**, *45*, e110–e114. [CrossRef]
15. Enneking, W.F.; Dunham, W.K. Resection and Reconstruction for Primary Neoplasms Involving the Innominate Bone. *J. Bone Jt. Surg.* **1978**, *60*, 731–746. [CrossRef]
16. Enneking, W.F.; Dunham, W.; Gebhardt, M.C.; Malawar, M.; Pritchard, D.J. A System for the Functional Evaluation of Reconstructive Procedures after Surgical Treatment of Tumors of the Musculoskeletal System. In *Classic Papers in Orthopaedics*; Springer: London, UK, 1993; pp. 241–246.
17. Kaplan, E.L.; Meier, P. Nonparametric Estimation from Incomplete Observations. *J. Am. Stat. Assoc.* **1958**, *53*, 457–481. [CrossRef]
18. Beadel, G.P.; McLaughlin, C.E.; Wunder, J.S.; Griffin, A.M.; Ferguson, P.C.; Bell, R.S. Outcome in Two Groups of Patients with Allograft-Prosthetic Reconstruction of Pelvic Tumor Defects. *Clin. Orthop.* **2005**, *438*, 30–35. [CrossRef]
19. Guo, W.; Li, D.; Tang, X.; Yang, Y.; Ji, T. Reconstruction with Modular Hemipelvic Prostheses for Periacetabular Tumor. *Clin. Orthop.* **2007**, *461*, 180–188. [CrossRef]
20. Avedian, R.S.; Haydon, R.C.; Peabody, T.D. Multiplanar Osteotomy with Limited Wide Margins: A Tissue Preserving Surgical Technique for High-Grade Bone Sarcomas. *Clin. Orthop.* **2010**, *468*, 2754–2764. [CrossRef]

21. Coccolini, F.; Stahel, P.F.; Montori, G.; Biffl, W.; Horer, T.M.; Catena, F.; Kluger, Y.; Moore, E.E.; Peitzman, A.B.; Ivatury, R.; et al. Pelvic Trauma: WSES Classification and Guidelines. *World J. Emerg. Surg.* **2017**, *12*, 5. [CrossRef]
22. Pool-Goudzwaard, A.; Hoek van Dijke, G.; van Gurp, M.; Mulder, P.; Snijders, C.; Stoeckart, R. Contribution of Pelvic Floor Muscles to Stiffness of the Pelvic Ring. *Clin. Biomech.* **2004**, *19*, 564–571. [CrossRef] [PubMed]
23. Gerbers, J.G.; Jutte, P.C. Hip-Sparing Approach Using Computer Navigation in Periacetabular Chondrosarcoma. *Comput. Aided Surg.* **2013**, *18*, 27–32. [CrossRef] [PubMed]
24. Yi, C.; Zheng, J.; Li, R.; Lan, Y.; He, M.; Lai, J.; Guan, T.; Pang, F.; Mo, Z.; Chen, P.; et al. Preliminary Proposal: A Classification System for Reconstruction with Autologous Femoral Head after Periacetabular Tumors Resection. *J. Orthop. Surg.* **2021**, *16*, 119. [CrossRef] [PubMed]
25. Xiao, C.; Zhou, Y.; Zhang, W.; Luo, Y.; Tu, C. An Acetabular-Preserving Procedure for Pelvic Giant Cell Tumor Involving Partial Acetabulum. *World J. Surg. Oncol.* **2017**, *15*, 200. [CrossRef] [PubMed]
26. Lam, Y.; Yau, R.; Ho, K.W.Y.; Mak, K.; Fong, S.; So, T.Y.C. Is It Possible and Safe to Perform Acetabular-Preserving Resections for Malignant Neoplasms of the Periacetabular Region? *Clin. Orthop.* **2017**, *475*, 656–665. [CrossRef] [PubMed]
27. Fang, C.; Cai, H.; Kuong, E.; Chui, E.; Siu, Y.C.; Ji, T.; Drstvenšek, I. Surgical Applications of Three-Dimensional Printing in the Pelvis and Acetabulum: From Models and Tools to Implants. *Unfallchirurg* **2019**, *122*, 278–285. [CrossRef]
28. Wong, K.C.; Kumta, S.M.; Geel, N.V.; Demol, J. One-Step Reconstruction with a 3D-Printed, Biomechanically Evaluated Custom Implant after Complex Pelvic Tumor Resection. *Comput. Aided Surg.* **2015**, *20*, 14–23. [CrossRef]
29. Syftestad, G.T.; Urist, M.R. Bone Aging. *Clin. Orthop.* **1982**, *162*, 288–297. [CrossRef]
30. Heck, D.A.; Nakajima, I.; Kelly, P.J.; Chao, E.Y. The Effect of Load Alteration on the Biological and Biomechanical Performance of a Titanium Fiber-Metal Segmental Prosthesis. *J. Bone Jt. Surg.* **1986**, *68*, 118–126. [CrossRef]
31. Eckhoff, D.G.; Turner, A.S.; Aberman, H.M. Effect of Age on Bone Formation around Orthopaedic Implants. *Clin. Orthop.* **1995**, *312*, 253–260.
32. Fujishiro, T.; Nishikawa, T.; Takikawa, S.; Saegusa, Y.; Yoshiya, S.; Kurosaka, M. Reconstruction of the Iliofemoral Ligament with an Artificial Ligament for Recurrent Anterior Dislocation of Total Hip Arthroplasty. *J. Arthroplast.* **2003**, *18*, 524–527. [CrossRef]
33. Aota, S.; Kikuchi, S.; Ohashi, H.; Kitano, N.; Hakozaki, M.; Konno, S. Soft Tissue Reinforcement with a Leeds-Keio Artificial Ligament in Revision Surgery for Dislocated Total Hip Arthroplasty. *HIP Int.* **2018**, *28*, 324–329. [CrossRef] [PubMed]
34. Klein, W.; Jensen, K.-U. Synovitis and Artificial Ligaments. *Arthrosc. J. Arthrosc. Relat. Surg.* **1992**, *8*, 116–124. [CrossRef]
35. Ochen, Y.; Beks, R.B.; Emmink, B.L.; Wittich, P.; van der Velde, D.; Houwert, R.M.; Keizer, J. Surgical Treatment of Acute and Chronic AC Joint Dislocations: Five-Year Experience with Conventional and Modified LARS Fixation by a Single Surgeon. *J. Orthop.* **2020**, *17*, 73–77. [CrossRef] [PubMed]
36. Sinagra, Z.P.; Kop, A.; Pabbruwe, M.; Parry, J.; Clark, G. Foreign Body Reaction Associated with Artificial LARS Ligaments: A Retrieval Study. *Orthop. J. Sports Med.* **2018**, *6*, 232596711881160. [CrossRef] [PubMed]

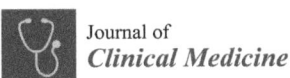

Review

Are Static Spacers Superior to Articulated Spacers in the Staged Treatment of Infected Primary Knee Arthroplasty? A Systematic Review and Meta-Analysis

Michele Fiore [1], Andrea Sambri [1,*], Matteo Filippini [1], Lorenzo Morante [1], Claudio Giannini [1], Azzurra Paolucci [1], Claudia Rondinella [1], Renato Zunarelli [1], Pierluigi Viale [2] and Massimiliano De Paolis [1]

[1] Orthopaedics and Traumatology Unit, IRCCS Azienda Ospedaliera, Universitaria di Bologna, 40138 Bologna, Italy
[2] Infectious Disease Unit, IRCCS Azienda Ospedaliera, Universitaria di Bologna, 40138 Bologna, Italy
* Correspondence: andrea_sambri@libero.it

Abstract: In the treatment of knee periprosthetic joint infection with a two-stage protocol, static spacers allow for the local delivery of high doses of antibiotics and help to preserve soft tissue tension. Articulated spacers were introduced to better preserve flexion after the reimplantation. The aim of this systematic review is to provide a comprehensive data collection of the results of these different spacers. An in-depth search on the main clinical databases was performed concerning the studies reporting data on the topic. A total of 87 studies and 4250 spacers were included. No significant differences were found both in pooling data analysis and meta-analysis of comparative studies about infection recurrences, complications, and clinical scores. Mean active knee flexion at last follow-up after total knee reimplantation was found to be significantly higher using articulated spacers (91.6° ± 7° for static spacers vs. 100.3° ± 9.9° for articulated spacers; $p < 0.001$). Meta-analysis also recognized this strong significant difference ($p < 0.001$). This review has confirmed that articulated spacers do not appear to be inferior to static spacers regarding all clinical outcomes, while they are superior in terms of active flexion. However, the low quality of the studies and the risk for selection bias with complex patients preferentially treated with static spacers need to be accounted for.

Keywords: knee arthroplasty; periprosthetic joint infection; two-stage protocol; static spacer; articulated spacer; knee revision surgery

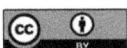

1. Introduction

Periprosthetic joint infection (PJI) is one of the main complications following primary total knee arthroplasty (TKA), with high morbidity and a significant negative impact on the outcome. Because of the increase in the number of arthroplasties, the incidence of PJI has been increasing steadily as well, and it has been reported to range from 0.5% to 1.9%, currently representing a growing social and economic issue for health systems [1,2]. Treatment of PJI represents one of the main challenges of modern orthopedics, requiring a multidisciplinary approach, as it aims for infection control, pain relief, and restoration of joint function [3].

The main treatment options for primary PJIs include debridement and implant retention (DAIR), even with the use of local adjuvants (Debridement, Antibiotic Pearls, and Retention of the Implant—DAPRI) [4], single-stage revision, one-and-half revision with long-lasting spacer, and two-stage revision. Currently, there are well-established guidelines for the management of infections after knee arthroplasty, with DAIR recommended only for early infections with an immature bacterial biofilm and exchange of the prosthesis required for late infection or in case of implant loosening [5,6]. In particular, two-stage treatment has proven to be the most cross-adaptive and the most recommended in cases of infections with highly virulent bacteria and/or bone or soft tissue problems (with possible fistulas) [6–9]. The two-stage procedure consists of the removal of the infected prosthesis and cement, followed by extensive debridement of the non-viable tissue and multiple washes. A temporary spacer impregnated with antibiotic is then implanted and left in place for a variable amount of time. Postoperatively, long-term antibiotic therapy is set up. Empirical intravenous broad-spectrum antibiotic therapy is generally begun immediately after surgery. After culture results, antibiotic therapy is modified, using an oral regimen whenever possible [10].

The reimplantation is performed once the infection has been eradicated, on the basis of clinical and laboratory criteria. However, if there is any suspicion of persistent infection, a repeat debridement with exchange of the spacer should be undertaken.

The use of an antibiotic-loaded cement spacer is an established method to increase knee stability and for local antibiotic administration prior to implantation of the definitive prosthesis [11–14]. Many different types of spacers are regularly used in surgical practice. Static spacers have demonstrated excellent results over the years in terms of eradicating the infection and therefore remain a valid treatment option [8]. However, several risks associated with the use of the static spacer are described in the literature, such as reduced function between the two stages, shortening of the soft tissues, increased bone loss, and an increased risk of spacer displacement [15]. To overcome these problems, articulated spacers are increasingly used, which allow one to avoid the shortening of soft tissues, to reduce bone loss, and to guarantee the patient a better function between the two stages [16]. Several categories of mobile spacers are regularly used, including prefabricated cement-on-cement components, intraoperatively molded cement-on-cement and cement-on-polyethylene components, and autoclaved femoral component on polyethylene [17].

Currently, the scientific evidence to support the use of static or articulated spacers is still not conclusive, both for the functional outcomes and the infection eradication rates. Thus, the choice is often determined by the surgeon's experience.

The aim of this systematic literature review is to provide a comprehensive data collection on two-stage reimplantation using different types of spacers, in terms of infection control, complications, and functional outcomes.

2. Materials and Methods

This systematic review was conducted in accordance with the 2020 PRISMA guidelines (Preferred Reporting Items of Systematic Reviews) [18].

All studies (randomized controlled trials (RCT), prospective (PCCS) and retrospective comparative studies (RCCS), prospective (PCS) and retrospective case series (RCS)) reporting the use of static or articulated cement or hybrid metal/cement/polyethylene spacers in two-stage surgery to treat PJI of a primary knee arthroplasty were included. The two-stage surgical protocol consists of the following: (1) a first surgery with total removal of the infected implant, extended surgical debridement, and placement of a spacer (usually an antibiotic-laden spacer)—this step may be repeated in the case of failure to control the infection; (2) a second surgery for further debridement and reimplantation (regardless of the type of implant used).

No restrictions were made based on the initial indication for knee replacement surgery, as the study focused on the treatment outcome of a complication, namely the PJI. Due to the wide time window of the studies included in this review, the definition of PJI has not been uniformly stated. The criteria adopted by the individual authors for the most recent studies are those which were discussed in the 2018 International Consensus Meeting on Orthopedic Infections [5]. With regard to the remaining articles, the authors of this review unanimously agreed that the criteria adopted by the authors of the individual studies included in this review were always diagnostically appropriate to identify patients with plausible PJI. Otherwise, non-conforming studies were excluded.

Studies reporting the results of PJI treatments other than two-stage protocols (including DAIR with or without partial component replacement, single-stage with partial or total explantation, one-and-half procedure with long-lasting spacer, permanent spacer, megaprosthesis, and resection arthroplasty) were excluded. Studies reporting the results of various treatments of knee PJI were excluded. Cases in which single- or two-stage protocols were used in the treatment of a recurrence of infection were excluded. Only studies with a minimum follow-up of 12 months and a minimum of 5 patients were included. Biomechanical studies, cadaveric studies, "in vitro" studies, and animal model studies were excluded. Only studies in English were included.

Studies eligible for this systematic review were identified through an electronic systematic search of the studies published from 1 January 2000 up to 30 June 2022, published on PubMed (https://pubmed.ncbi.nlm.nih.gov/ (accessed on 30 June 2022)), Scopus (https://www.scopus.com (accessed on 30 June 2022)), and Web of Science (www.webofscience.com (accessed on 30 June 2022)) databases. Terms used for the search included "infection", "prosthesis-related infection", "knee joint", "knee arthroplasty", "knee replacement", "periprosthetic infection", "2-stage", "two-stage", "explant", "re-implantation", "static spacer", "articulated spacer", "mobile spacer", "dynamic spacer". Articles that were considered relevant by electronic search were retrieved in full text, and a cross-referencing search of their bibliographies was performed, to find further related articles. Reviews and meta-analyses were also analyzed, in order to broaden the search to studies that might have been missed through the electronic search. All duplicates were removed, and all the articles retrieved have been analyzed. After the first screening, records without eligibility criteria were excluded (Figure 1). Remnant studies were categorized by type, according to the Oxford Centre for Evidence-Based Medicine (OCEBM). To assess the quality of the articles, the revised Cochrane risk-of-bias tool for randomized trials (RoB2) (Figure 2a) and the Cochrane risk of bias in non-randomized studies of interventions (ROBINS-I) assessment tool (Figure 2b) were utilized [19,20]. Each study was assessed by two reviewers (Ma.F. and L.M.) independently and in duplicate; disagreement was resolved by the senior author (M.D.). All the included studies were analyzed, and data related to topics of interest were extracted and summarized (Tables 1 and 2).

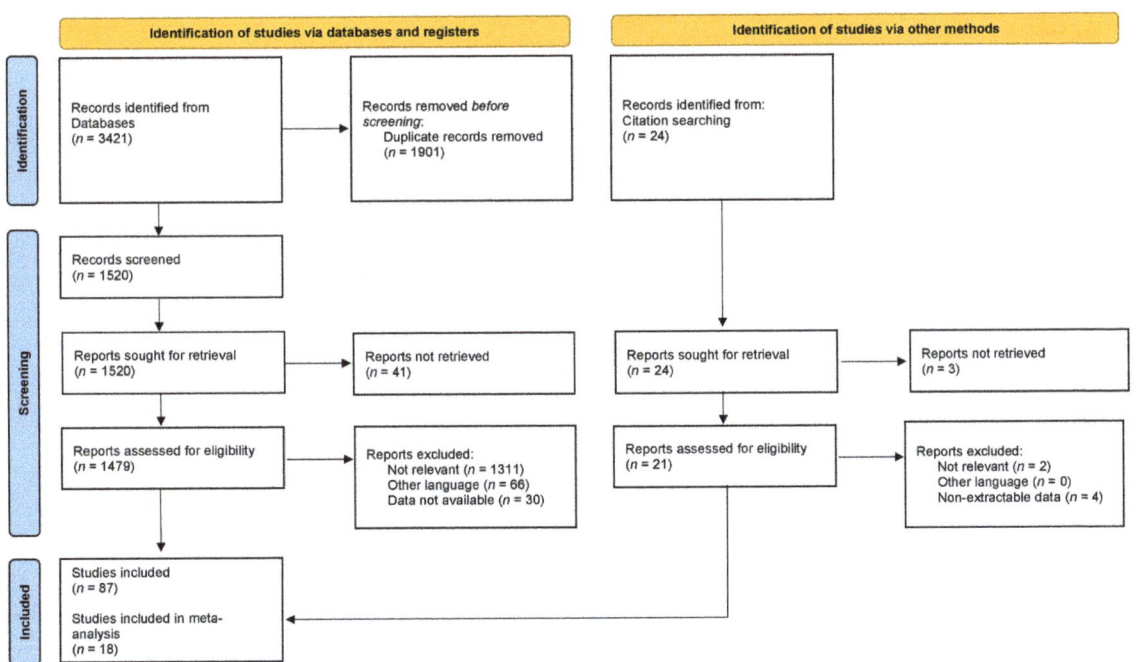

Figure 1. PRISMA 2020 flow diagram and the selection of studies.

Table 1. Data from series reporting on static spacers.

Article	Level of Evidence	Study Type	Patient N° (Spacer N°)	Mean Age (Year)	Mean Follow-Up (Months)	Mean Time of PJI Onset after Implant (Months)	Most Frequent Pathogens	Spacer Exchange: Repeated First Stage	Mean Time between First Stage and Second Stage (Months)	No Reimplantation (n°)	PJI Recurrence (n°)	Mean Time to Recurrence (Months)	Mean Duration of Antibiotic Therapy (Weeks)	Active Knee Flexion at Last Follow-Up (Degrees)	Functional Outcomes at Last Follow-Up: Score Type and Values	Peri-Operative Non-Infection Related-Complications (n°)
Akhtar et al., 2019 [21]	3	RCCS	17	81.3	46	N/A	N/A	2	9	N/A	1	N/A	N/A	N/A	N/A	6
Barrack et al., 2000 [22]	3	PCCS	28	68.5	36 (range 24–60)	N/A	N/A	0	0.9–1.4	2	2 (artrodesi)	N/A	N/A (range 4–7)	89	KSS: 115	N/A
Brunnekreef et al., 2013 [23]	3	RCCS	9	61	12	62.4	N/A	0	3.6 (range 1–10)	0	0	/	6	73.8	N/A	N/A
Chen et al., 2016 [24]	3	RCCS	8	73.9 (range 63–82)	40.8	N/A	N/A	0	5.1 (range 1.6–13.8)	0	2	17.5	6	74.3 (range 50–90)	KSS: 71.4 (range 60–81)	2
Chiang et al., 2011 [25]	3	PCCS	22	72 (range 67–80)	N/A	N/A	N/A	1	3.1 (range 2–4)	1	2	N/A	11.7	85 (range 70–100)	HSS: 82 (range 81–88)	7
Choi et al., 2012 [26]	3	RCCS	14	N/A	N/A	N/A	N/A	0	6	4	7	N/A	6	97 (range 75–130)	N/A	11
Emerson et al., 2002 [27]	3	RCCS	26	65.7	90 (range 33.6–152.4)	N/A	N/A	0	N/A (range 6–12)	0	8	N/A	6	93.7	N/A	N/A
Faschingbauer et al., 2016 [28]	4	RCS	133	70.1 ± 9.9	N/A	N/A	N/A	0	2.8	32	16	N/A	6	N/A	N/A	20
Fehring et al., 2000 [29]	3	RCCS	25	N/A	36 (range 24–72)	N/A	N/A	0	N/A	0	3	N/A	6	98 ± 17 (range 50–120)	HSS: 83 ± 17 (range 37–98)	2
Freeman et al., 2007 [30]	3	RCCS	28	71.2	86.6 (range 24–196.3)	N/A	N/A	0	N/A	0	3	N/A	6	N/A	KSS: 45 (range 35–80)	N/A
Ghanem et al., 2016 [31]	3	RCCS	5	N/A	N/A	N/A	N/A	N/A	N/A	0	3	N/A	range 4–6	N/A	N/A	N/A
Haleem et al., 2004 [32]	4	RCS	96	69 (range 37–89)	86.4 (range 30.0–158.4)	26.2 (range 0.5–177)	26.0% MSSA; 14.6% MRSA	N/A	1.4 (range 0.2–80.4)	0	9	12 (range 1.2–117.6)	5.3 (range 1–24)	90 (range 30–120)	KSS: 89 (range 35–97)	6
Hipfl et al., 2019 [33]	4	RCS	97	70 (range 30–88)	41 (range 27–56)	N/A	42% CoNS; 22% P. acnes	9	2.1 (range 1.4–5.5)	0	15	10 (range 1–26)	9 (range 6–24)	N/A	N/A	10
Hsu et al., 2007 [34]	3	RCCS	7	N/A	101 (range 63–120)	N/A	N/A	0	2.7 (range 1.8–3.5)	0	1	21	9.7 (range 6–12)	78 (range 60–100)	KSS: 81.4	N/A
Hsu et al., 2008 [35]	4	RCS	32	66 (range 50–78)	68.3 (range 8–197)	N/A	15.6% S. epidermidis; 12.5% MSSA	0	7.4 (range 2.3–29.7)	4	4	N/A (range: 2.5–7)	range 6–8	88 ± 19 (range 30–120)	KSS: 82 ± 14 (range 33–99)	22
Husted et al., 2002 [36]	4	RCS	17	72.2 (range 60–78)	25.7 (range 5–62)	17.2 (range 1–133)	41.2% S. aureus; 41.2% S. epidermidis	0	N/A	2	2	N/A	5.4	99.3 (range 70–130)	N/A	N/A
Ippolito et al., 2021 [37]	4	RCS	21	52.4 ± 20.6	123.6 ± 76.8 (range 20.4–291.6)	57.4 (range 3–246)	24% CoNS; 19% S. aureus	0	N/A	1	7	N/A	12	100 ± 17	N/A	18

Table 1. Cont.

Article	Level of Evidence	Study Type	Patient N° (Spacer N°)	Mean Age (Year)	Mean Follow-Up (Months)	Mean Time of PJI Onset after Implant (Months)	Most Frequent Pathogens	Spacer Exchange: Repeated First Stage	Mean Time between First Stage and Second Stage (Months)	No Reimplantation (n°)	PJI Recurrence (n°)	Mean Time to Recurrence (Months)	Mean Duration of Antibiotic Therapy (Weeks)	Active Knee Flexion at Last Follow-Up (Degrees)	Functional Outcomes at Last Follow-Up: Score Type and Values	Peri-Operative Non-Infection-Related-Complications (n°)
Johnson et al., 2012 [38]	3	RCCS	81	61 (range 58–64)	66 (range 12–121)	N/A	N/A	N/A	3.5 (range 2.7–4.3)	N/A	14	N/A	N/A	95 (range 30–130)	KSS: 84 (range 48–100)	0
Kong et al., 2021 [39]	3	RCCS	22	67.2 ± 10.1	43 (range 30–61)	N/A	N/A	1	3 (range 1.8–5.5)	0	1	N/A	N/A	80 (range 70–110)	KSS: 60 ± 6.3	0
Lichstein et al., 2016 [40]	4	RCS	109	67 (range 42–89)	44.4 (range 24.0–117.6)	N/A	51% Staphylococcus spp.; 19% Streptococcus spp.	0	N/A	N/A	7	N/A	11 (range 5–20)	100 (range 60–139)	KSS: 86 (range 65–98)	N/A
Lo Presti et al., 2021 [41]	4	RCS	12	64 (range 39–85)	34.3 (range 10–62)	N/A	25% MRSA; 16.7% E. faecalis	4	N/A	8	2	N/A	N/A (range 6–8)	N/A	N/A	0
Ma et al., 2020 [42]	3	RCCS	66	70.3 ± 11.0 (range 19–86)	75.3 ± 30.6 (range 24–133)	N/A	N/A	6	4	2	0	/	SHC: 0.7 STC: 14.7	N/A	N/A	5
Nahhas et al., 2020 [43]	1	RCT	24	64.9 ± 8.4	42 ± 14.4	N/A	N/A	2	2.4 ± 0.7 (range 2.1–2.6)	2	2	N/A	6	103 ± 12.7 (range 97.6–108.3)	KSS: 69.8 ± 14.1 (range 63.6–73.1)	13
Park et al., 2010 [44]	3	RCCS	20	66.5 (range 48–84)	36 (range 24–62)	N/A	30% MRSA; 20% MSSA	N/A	N/A	N/A	3	N/A	6	92 (range 65–140)	HSS: 80 (range 74–97)	N/A
Petis et al., 2019 [45]	4	RCS	240	N/A	N/A	N/A	N/A	0	N/A	0	0	/	N/A (range 6–8)	N/A	N/A	N/A
Preobrazhensky et al., 2019 [46]	3	RCCS	25	N/A	12	N/A	N/A	0	N/A	0	0	/	N/A	N/A	N/A	1
Rossi et al., 2021 [47]	3	RCS	13	N/A	18	N/A	N/A	0	N/A	0	0	/	N/A	100.8 ± 28	KSS: 76.9 ± 12	6
Schneider et al., 2022 [48]	3	RCCS	47	63 (range 9–36)	N/A	N/A	N/A	N/A	N/A	2	10	N/A	N/A	90.5	N/A	7
Silvestre et al., 2013 [49]	4	RCS	43 (45)	72 (63–81)	86 (range 60–132)	N/A	17.8% Staphylococcus spp.; 15.6% MRSA	N/A	4.4	2	2	N/A	6	92 (range 50–115)	KSS: 83 (range 43–95)	1
Skwara et al., 2016 [50]	3	RCCS	21	66.5 (range 48–84)	8.5	N/A	N/A	N/A	N/A	N/A	2	N/A	N/A	79 ± 26	N/A	N/A
Springer et al., 2004 [51]	4	RCS	34	N/A	N/A	N/A	61.7% CoNS; 17.6% S. aureus	N/A	N/A	1	3	N/A	6	N/A	N/A	9
Vasarhelyi et al., 2022 [52]	3	RCCS	76	69.4 ± 10.0	228 ± 75.6	51.4 (range 3–120)	N/A	4	3	N/A	10	N/A	6	82.1 ± 25.4	KSS: 72 ± 23.3	N/A
Vielgut et al., 2021 [53]	4	RCS	77	64.9 (range 31.3–82.4)	24.5 (range 6–107)	23.6 (range 6–336)	N/A	17	3.2 (range 1.8–7.3)	2	14	19.5 (range 0–63.9)	N/A (range 6–8)	N/A	N/A	N/A
Zamora et al., 2020 [54]	3	RCCS	14	N/A	N/A	N/A	N/A	1	N/A	2	2	N/A	N/A	N/A	N/A	N/A

Abbreviations: RCT, randomized controlled trial; PCCS, prospective comparative cohort study; PCS, prospective case series; RCS, retrospective case series; RCCS, retrospective comparative cohort study; CoNS, coagulase-negative staphylococci; MSSA/MRSA, methicillin-sensible/resistant *Staphylococcus aureus*; SHC, short-course antibiotic therapy; STD, standard-course antibiotic therapy; PJI, periprosthetic joint infection; FU, follow-up; KSS, Knee Society Score; HSS, Hospital for Special Surgery Knee-Rating Scale; N/A: data not available.

Table 2. Data from series reporting on articulated spacers.

Article	Level of Evidence	Study Type	Spacer Details	Patient N° (Spacer N°)	Mean Age (Year)	Mean Follow-Up (Months)	Mean Time to PJI Onset after Implant (Months)	Most Frequent Pathogens	Spacer Exchange: Repeated First Stage	Mean Time between First Stage and Second Stage (Months)	No Reimplantation (n°)	PJI Recurrence (n°)	Mean Time to Recurrence (Months)	Mean Duration of Antibiotic Therapy (Weeks)	Active Knee Flexion at Last Follow-Up (Degrees)	Functional Outcomes at Last Follow-Up: Score Type and Values	Peri-Operative Non-Infection-Related Complications (N°)
Ahmad et al., 2013 [55]	3	PCCS	C/C	75	67.5 (range 57–85)	51.6 (range 24–84)	N/A	27.9% S. aureus; 25.6% CoNS; 11.6%	0	N/A (range 0.7–5)	1	7	42	N/A (range 4–12)	115 (range 90–125)	KSS: 89.5 (range 74–95)	N/A
Akhtar et al., 2019 [21]	3	RCCS	C/C Pedestal C/C	13 14	69 73.4	32.9 52.5	N/A	N/A	2 1	9.6 7.7	N/A	2 1	N/A	N/A	N/A	N/A	10 2
Babis et al., 2008 [56]	4	PCS	C/C	24	71 (range 58–84)	72 (range 24–120)	N/A	58.3% S. aureus; 42.9% S. epidermidis	0	1.4	0	0	/	6	100	N/A	1
Boelch et al., 2021 [57]	4	RCS	C/C	60	67.8 (range 46–85)	35.6 (range 1–135)	53.5 (range 2–239)	N/A	8	N/A	4	12	N/A	6	N/A	N/A	N/A
Brunnekreef et al., 2013 [23]	3	RCCS	M/P	26	58	12	56.4	N/A	0	4.4	0	0	N/A	6	96.4	N/A	N/A
Buyuk et al., 2017 [58]	4	PCS	C/C	25	70 ± 9.7 (range 52–88)	39.8 ± 12.5 (range 22–73)	N/A	36% MRSE; 12% MSSE	2	3.8 ± 1.4 (range 2–6)	0	1	N/A	9.3 ± 3.4	N/A	KSS: 77 (range 32–96)	3
Carulli et al., 2013 [59]	4	PCS	M/P	9	66.5 (range 59–71)	55.2 (range 48–84)	15.5 (range 5–32)	67% S. aureus; 33% S. epidermidis	0	1.9 (range 1.6–2.3)	0	0	/	4.2 (range 3–7)	110 (range 105–125)	KSS: 86.4 (range 74–97)	0
Castelli et al., 2014 [60]	4	PCS	C/C	50	68 (range 54–80)	84 (range 24–156)	N/A	46% CoNS; 11% MSSA	0	3.7 (range 0.9–13.8)	0	4	12.8	6	94	KSS: 75.38	0
Chen et al., 2016 [24]	3	RCCS	M/P (autoclaved)	10	68.9 (range 20–88)	32 (range 24–46)	N/A	N/A	0	4.4 (range 2–9.7)	0	2	13 (range 11–15)	6	94.5 (range 70–125)	KSS: 74.7 (range 62–88)	3
Chiang et al., 2011 [25]	3	PCCS	C/C	23	71 (range 65–78)	N/A	N/A	N/A	0	3.4 (range 2.5–5)	0	1		11.2	113 (range 95–125)	HSS: 90 (range 86–94)	0
DeBoer et al., 2020 [15]	3	RCCS	C/C	77	63 (range 42–83)	N/A (range: 12–120)	N/A	N/A	0	4.4 (range 1.8–18.9)	2	14	N/A	6	N/A	N/A	N/A
Durbhakula et al., 2004 [61]	4	RCS	C/C	24	72 (range 44–94)	33 (range 28–51)	N/A	37.5% S. epidermidis; 25% S. aureus	0	2.8 (range 2.3–4.4)	2	3	/	6	104 (range 89–122)	HSS: 82 (range 63–96)	2
Evans 2004 [62]	4	RCS	C/C	31	64	>24	N/A	29% MRSA; 25.8% MSSA	0	2.4	2	3	21.3	6	111 (range 0–130)	N/A	1
Fehring et al., 2000 [29]	3	RCCS	C/C	30	N/A	27 (range 24–36)	N/A	N/A	0	N/A	1	1	N/A	6	105 ± 12 (range 90–126)	HSS: 84 ± 13 (range 45–95)	2

Table 2. Cont.

Article	Level of Evidence	Study Type	Spacer Details	Patient N° (Spacer N°)	Mean Age (Year)	Mean Follow-Up (Months)	Mean Time to PJI Onset after Implant (Months)	Most Frequent Pathogens	Spacer Exchange Repeated First Stage	Mean Time between First Stage and Second Stage (Months)	No Reimplantation (n°)	PJI Recurrence (n°)	Mean Time to Recurrence (Months)	Mean Duration of Antibiotic Therapy (Weeks)	Active Knee Flexion at Last Follow-Up (Degrees)	Functional Outcomes at Last Follow-Up: Score Type and Values	Peri-Operative Non-Infection-Related-Complications (N°)
Fei et al., 2022 [63]	3	RCCS	C/C	23	67.6 ± 9.4 (range 52–81)	46.6 ± 25.4 (range 14.4–91.3)	N/A	30.4% S. epidermidis; 17.4% S. aureus	0	3.6 ± 2 (range 2.2–10.9)	4	0	/	6	77.4 ± 9.2 (range 60–90)	KSS: 84.1 ± 5.6 (range 73–93)	0
			M/P (autoclaved)	24	67.8 ± 9.5 (range 37–80)	50.5 ± 28.8 (range 19.1–134.5)	N/A	33.3% S. epidermidis; 12.5% S. aureus	1	6.4 ± 4.6 (range 2.2–20.1)	4	0	/	6	85 ± 11.1 (range 60–100)	KSS: 83.4 ± 10 (range 52–93)	1
Freeman et al., 2007 [30]	3	RCCS	C/C	48	64.9	62.2 (range 25.7–119.6)	N/A	N/A	0	N/A	0	4	N/A	6	N/A	KSS: 70 (range 39.5–90)	N/A
Garg et al., 2011 [64]	4	RCS	C/C	36	62 (range 50-76)	62.4	10 (range 7–16)	N/A	0	18 (range 6–42)	7	0	/	N/A (range 10–12)	75.6	N/A	2
Ghanem et al., 2016 [31]	3	RCCS	C/C	30	N/A	N/A	N/A	N/A	N/A	N/A	2	8	N/A	N/A (range 4–6)	N/A	N/A	N/A
Ghanem et al., 2018 [65]	4	RCS	C/C	16	72.0 ± 8.3	22.5 ± 16.6	N/A	37.5% S. aureus; 31.2% S. epidermidis	0	6.2 ± 5.2	0	4	N/A	N/A (range 4–6)	103.3 ± 17.1	N/A	0
Gooding et al., 2011 [66]	4	RCS	M/P	115	68 (range 35–86)	108 (range 60–144)	N/A	32.2% S. epidermidis; 31.3% S. aureus	2	3.9 (range 1.2–28.3)	2	14	N/A	> 5	93.2 (range 30–140)	N/A	50
Ha 2006 [67]	4	RCS	C/C	12	65.7 (range 54–73)	N/A (range: 24–42)	N/A	25% MRSA; 16.7% MSSA	0	2.1 (range 0.9–3.7)	0	0	/	N/A	102 (range 75–140)	KSS: 87	8
Haddad et al., 2000 [68]	4	RCS	M/P	45	69 (range 26–83)	48 (range 20–112)	N/A	40% S. epidermidis; 20% S. aureus	N/A	3.6 (range 0.8–22.3)	1	4	N/A	N/A	94.5 (range 20–135)	HSS: 71.5 (range 32–96)	12
Hammerich et al., 2021 [69]	4	RCS	Reverse C/C (convex tibia + concave femur)	110	67.2 (range 43–89)	N/A	41.0 ± 3.4 (range 1–240)	N/A	3	1.8	0	0	/	N/A	N/A	N/A	0
Hart et al. 2006 [70]	4	RCS	C/C	48	68.2 (range 37.2–81.3)	48.5 (range 26–85)	39.6 (range 5–72)	62.5% CoNS; 10.4% S. aureus	0	4.3 (range 1.4–15)	2	6	N/A	2	92 (range 30–120)	N/A	N/A
Hoshino et al., 2021 [71]	4	PCS	C/C	7	77	54 ± 28 (range 11–90)	28 ± 16 (range 10–53)	N/A	0	6 ± 3 (range 3–12)	0	0	/	3	99 ± 22	KSS: 84 ± 10	0
Hsu et al. 2007 [34]	3	RCCS	C/C	21	N/A	58 (range 27–96)	N/A	N/A	0	3.2 (range 1.4–5.5)	0	2	17.3	8.4 (range 6–12)	95 (range 80–120)	KSS: 88.9	N/A
Incavo et al., 2009 [72]	4	RCS	C/C	11	61.1 (range 32–83)	N/A	37 (range 4–108)	45.5% S. aureus	0	N/A (range 1.4–5.5)	0	0	/	N/A (range 4–6)	N/A	N/A	2

Table 2. Cont.

Article	Level of Evidence	Study Type	Spacer Details	Patient N° (Spacer N°)	Mean Age (Year)	Mean Follow-Up (Months)	Mean Time to PJI Onset after Implant (Months)	Most Frequent Pathogens	Spacer Exchange: Repeated First Stage	Mean Time between First Stage and Second Stage (Months)	No Reimplantation (n°)	PJI Recurrence (n°)	Mean Time to Recurrence (Months)	Mean Duration of Antibiotic Therapy (Weeks)	Active Knee Flexion at Last Follow-Up (Degrees)	Functional Outcomes at Last Follow-Up: Score Type and Values	Peri-Operative Non-Infection-Related Complications (N°)
Jia et al., 2012 [73]	4	RCS	C/C	21	64.4	32.2 (range 17–54)	12.9 (range 8–26)	42.9% S. epidermidis; 19% S. aureus	1	2.7 (range 1.4–7.4)	0	0	/	4.9 (range 2–8)	94.3	KSS: 82.1	16
Johnson et al., 2012 [38]	3	RCCS	C/C or M/C	34	62 (range 59–65)	27 (range 12–72)	N/A	N/A	N/A	3.1 (range 2.4–3.7)	N/A	6	N/A	N/A	99 (range 60–120)	KSS: 83 (range 48–99)	4
Jung et al., 2022 [74]	3	RCCS	C/C	12	74.5 (range 63–85)	N/A	N/A	25% MSSA; 16.7% E. coli	0	1.9 (range 1.4–2.9)	0	0	/	N/A	N/A	N/A	0
			Spiked C/C	15	73.5 (range 60–81)			26.7% MSSA; 20% E. coli	1		0	0	/				1
Kalore et al., 2012 [75]	3	RCCS	M/P (autoclaved)	15	67.3	73 (range 37–105)	38.5	37.7% MSSA; 17% MRSA	1	4.9	2	2	N/A	> 6	95.7	N/A	1
			M/P (new)	16	63.6	19 (range 12–32)	31.9		1	2.7	1	1			98.3		0
			C/C	22	61.1	32 (range 14–56)	41.9		0	5.8	0	2			93.8		0
Kong et al., 2021 [39]	3	RCCS	C/C	20	65.5 ± 11.4	18 (range 8–28)	N/A	N/A	1	2.9 (range 2.1–5.1)	0	1	N/A	N/A	94 (range 80–115)	KSS: 75 ± 11.5	4
Kohl et al., 2011 [76]	4	PCS	C/C	16	73.1 (range 54–89)	> 24	N/A	43.8% CoNS; 12.5% S. aureus	0	3.5 (range 3–5)	0	0	/	N/A	114 (range 90–125)	KSS: 89.5 (range 78–95)	N/A
Lin et al., 2021 [77]	3	RCCS	C/C	CR: 66	64.4 (range 57–84)	58.3 (range 31–82)	N/A	31.9% Staphylococcus spp.; 21.3% Streptococcus spp.	5	3.5 (range 2.5–6.4)	4	8	N/A	> 4	N/A	N/A	37
			C/C	PS: 75	67.9 (range 58–87)	56.7 (range 35–81)			10	3.4 (range 2.3–6.0)	3	8					
Lu et al., 2018 [78]	4	RCS	C/P	11	69.9 (range 59–80)	24 (range 12–48)	N/A	63.6% S. aureus; 27.2% S. epidermidis	0	N/A	0	0	/	6	93.2 (range 80–105)	KSS: 84.9 (range 80–92)	0
MacAvoy et al., 2005 [79]	4	RCS	C/C	13	58 (range 36–71)	28 (range 15–44)	N/A	38.5% S. epidermidis; 30.8% S. aureus	0	N/A	2	4	/	6	98 (range 45–135)	N/A	5
Macheras et al., 2011 [80]	4	RCS	C/C	34	64 (range 45–73)	145.2 (range 120–168)	N/A	41.1% S. aureus; 20.6% S. epidermidis	0	N/A	1	3	N/A	6	105 (range 95–120)	KSS: 76 ± 18 (range 58–94)	1

Table 2. Cont.

Article	Level of Evidence	Study Type	Spacer Details	Patient N° (Spacer N°)	Mean Age (Year)	Mean Follow-Up (Months)	Mean Time to PJI Onset after Implant (Months)	Most Frequent Pathogens	Spacer Exchange: Repeated First Stage	Mean Time between First Stage and Second Stage (Months)	No Reimplantation (n°)	PJI Recurrence (n°)	Mean Time to Recurrence (Months)	Mean Duration of Antibiotic Therapy (Weeks)	Active Knee Flexion at Last Follow-Up (Degrees)	Functional Outcomes at Last Follow-Up: Score Type and Values	Peri-Operative Non-Infection-Related Complications (N°)
Marothi et al., 2016 [81]	4	RCS	C/C	28	70 (range 56–79)	4	N/A	N/A	0	N/A (range 1.4–1.8)	0	0	/	6	N/A	N/A	2
Mutimer et al., 2009 [82]	4	RCS	C/C	12	71	10	N/A	N/A	0	3.3 (range 2.4–9.0)	0	0	/	6	N/A	N/A	0
Nahhas et al., 2020 [43]	1	RCT	C/C	25	65.7 ± 8.9	42 ± 16.8	N/A	N/A	1	2.5 ± 1.2 (range 2.0–3.0)	1	1	N/A	6	114.0 ± 10.5 (range 109.7–118.3)	KSS: 79.4 ± 17.1 (range 72.4–86.3)	8
Nodzo et al., 2017 [16]	3	RCCS	Preformed C/C	58	65.3 ± 8.6	74.9 ± 35.1	N/A	N/A	N/A	2.5 (range 1.8–3.3)	N/A	10	N/A	6	N/A	N/A	N/A
			Molded C/C	43	66 ± 11.0	43.7 ± 16.7				2.3 (range 1.8–3.2)		5					
			M/P (autoclaved)	39	67.8 ± 10.2	52.4 ± 21.9				2.7 (range 2.2–3.5)		8					
Ocguder et al., 2010 [83]	4	RCS	C/C	17	63 (range 54–75)	20 (range 13–38)	7.7 (range 3–12)	29.4% Staphylococcus spp.; 23.5% S. epidermidis	0	4.2	1	2	12	6.8 (range 6–10)	85	KSS: 86 (range 40–97)	6
Ortola et al., 2017 [84]	4	RCS	C/C	112	56.2 ± 16.9	32.9 ± 12	36.8 ± 63.6	25.9%, S. aureus; 22.3% S. epidermidis	7	2.1 ± 0.4	15	3	N/A	N/A	N/A	N/A	N/A
Park et al., 2010 [44]	3	RCCS	C/C	16	60.2 (range 47–72)	29 (range 25–45)	N/A	25% MSSA; 25% C. Albicans	N/A	N/A	N/A	1	N/A	6	108 (range 85–140)	HSS: 87 (range 76–95)	N/A
Pascale et al., 2007 [85]	4	RCS	C/C	14	68 (range 60–76)	N/A	27.6 (range 12–36)	71.4% S. epidermidis	0	2.3	0	0	N/A	9 (range 6–9)	120 (range 97–130)	N/A	0
Pitto et al., 2005 [86]	4	RCS	C/C	21	67 (range 58–89)	24 (range 12–43)	N/A	57.1% Streptococcus spp.; 14.2% S. aureus	1	3	2	1	/	6	94	KSS: 81 (range 30–92)	0
Preobrazhensky et al., 2019 [46]	3	RCCS	M/P (autoclaved)	67	N/A	12	N/A	N/A	1	N/A	0	1	N/A	N/A (range 6–8)	N/A	N/A	N/A
Radoicic et al., 2016 [87]	4	RCS	C/C	18	66.6	N/A	N/A	Multi-bacterial	3	N/A	5	2	N/A	N/A	N/A	N/A	N/A
Roof et al., 2021 [88]	3	RCCS	C/C or M/P (new)	72	63.4 ± 11.7	24	N/A	N/A	6	N/A	5	8	N/A	N/A	93.7 ± 28	N/A	1
Rossi et al., 2021 [47]	3	RCCS	C/C or M/P (autoclaved)	27	N/A	18	N/A	N/A	1	N/A	0	1	N/A	N/A	114.8 ± 28	KSS: 80.8 ± 10	1

Table 2. Cont.

Article	Level of Evidence	Study Type	Spacer Details	Patient N° (Spacer N°)	Mean Age (Year)	Mean Follow-Up (Months)	Mean Time to PJI Onset after Implant (Months)	Most Frequent Pathogens	Spacer Exchange: Repeated First Stage	Mean Time between First Stage and Second Stage (Months)	No Reimplantation (n°)	PJI Recurrence (n°)	Mean Time to Recurrence (Months)	Mean Duration of Antibiotic Therapy (Weeks)	Active Knee Flexion at Last Follow-Up (Degrees)	Functional Outcomes at Last Follow-Up: Score Type and Values	Peri-Operative Non-Infection-Related Complications (N°)
Sakellariou et al., 2015 [89]	4	PCS	C/C	46	65.3 (range 32-84)	36 (range 8-60)	33.6 (range 4-84)	39.1% S. aureus; 26.1% Streptococcus spp.	0	N/A	0	6	N/A	N/A	N/A	N/A	3
Schneider et al., 2022 [48]	3	RCCS	M/P (new)	30	65.6 (range 11.4)	N/A	N/A	N/A	N/A	N/A	2	6	N/A	N/A	99.3	N/A	5
			C/C	19	64.6 (range 11.7)	N/A	N/A	N/A	N/A	N/A	2	6	N/A	N/A	77.2	N/A	5
Seo et al., 2020 [90]	4	RCS	C/C	14	70.2 ± 6.3	44.9 ± 6.5	N/A	21.4% Streptococcus spp.; 21.4% S. aureus	0	N/A	0	0	/	N/A	92.9	N/A	0
Shaikh et al., 2014 [91]	4	RCS	C/C	13	65	48	N/A (range 0.5-18)	15.4% MRSA; 15.4% C. Albicans	1	5.6 (range 2-29)	0	0	/	> 2	115 (range 75-150)	KSS: 83	0
Shen et al., 2010 [92]	4	RCS	C/C	17	67 (range 52-76)	31 (range 18-47)	N/A	23.5% Streptococcus spp.; 23.5% S. aureus	N/A	7.8	7	1	N/A	> 6	95.4 (range 90-105)	HSS: 83.6	10
Siebel et al., 2002 [93]	4	RCS	C/C	10	66.1	18.1	N/A	20% S. epidermidis; 10% S. aureus	0	1.9 (range 1.4-2.8)	0	0	/	N/A	86.5	HSS 63.8	0
Skwara et al., 2016 [50]	3	RCCS	C/C	16	N/A	8.5	N/A	N/A	N/A	N/A	N/A	1	N/A	N/A	102 ± 8.4	N/A	0
Struelens et al., 2013 [94]	4	RCS	C/C	154 (155)	66 ± 11	N/A	N/A	N/A	N/A	1.8 ± 0.79	N/A	N/A	N/A	N/A	N/A	N/A	82
Su et al., 2009 [95]	4	RCS	C/C	15	72 (range 65-79)	47.5 (range 37-61)	N/A	60% MRSA; 10% CoNS	0	3	2	1	N/A	N/A	110 (range 95-120)	HSS: 90.5 (range 82-92)	1
Thabe et al., 2007 [96]	4	RCS	C/C	20	72.3 (range 48-83)	73.2	N/A	N/A	0	0.9	0	0	/	N/A	106	N/A	0
Tian et al., 2018 [97]	4	RCS	C/C	25	64.9 (range 56-83)	64.2 (range 52-89)	N/A	20% MRSE; 16% MSSE	0	2.6 (range 1.4-7.3)	0	0	/	N/A	94 (range 90-98)	KSS: 83 (range 80-88)	8
Tigani et al., 2013 [98]	4	PCS	C/C	37 (38)	68 (range 36-86)	65 (range 24-139)	N/A	31.6% MSSE; 15.8% MRSE	5	2.4 (range 1.6-6.9)	2	9	N/A	6	101 (range 80-115)	N/A	1
Tsai et al., 2019 [99]	4	RCS	C/C	32	73.3 (range 58-93)	36.9 (range 30.1-45)	N/A	21.9% MSSA; 15.6% Enterococcus spp.	3	8.8 (range 4-12.5)	1	4	N/A	> 4	102 (range 80-122)	HSS ± 84.2 (range 78-90)	2

Table 2. Cont.

Article	Level of Evidence	Study Type	Spacer Details	Patient N° (Spacer N°)	Mean Age (Year)	Mean Follow-Up (Months)	Mean Time to PJI Onset after Implant (Months)	Most Frequent Pathogens	Spacer Exchange: Repeated First Stage	Mean Time between First Stage and Second Stage (Months)	No Reimplantation (n°)	PJI Recurrence (n°)	Mean Time to Recurrence (Months)	Mean Duration of Antibiotic Therapy (Weeks)	Active Knee Flexion at Last Follow-Up (Degrees)	Functional Outcomes at Last Follow-Up: Score Type and Values	Peri-Operative Non-Infection-Related-Complications (N°)
Van Thiel et al., 2011 [100]	4	RCS	C/C	60	66 (range 42–91)	35 (range 24–51)	N/A	20% MRSA; 20% MSSA	1	2.7	1	7	16.3 (range 2–30)	N/A	101.3 ± 18	KSS: 78.6 ± 17.8	1
Vasarhelyi et al., 2022 [52]	3	RCCS	C/C	104	68.6 ± 10.6	120 ± 49.2	43.8 (range 3–168)	N/A	7	3	N/A	17	N/A	6	110.6 ± 13.5	KSS: 86.8 ± 13.6	4
Vasso et al., 2016 [101]	4	RCS	C/C	46	69 (range 58–84)	144 (range 72–192)	N/A	37% MSSA; 28.3% CoNS	2	2.5 (range 2.3–3.1)	N/A	0	/	8	115 (range 100–128)	N/A	0
Vecchini et al., 2017 [102]	4	PCS	C/C	19 (20)	65.4 (range 30–82)	74.1 (range 10–112)	N/A	60% MSSA; 20% MRSA	0	9.1 (range 3–27)	1	0	/	3.6 (range 2–5)	N/A	N/A	4
Villanueva-Martinez et al., 2008 [103]	4	RCS	C/C	30	71 (range 64–82)	36 (range 24–60)	18 (range 1–144)	40% CoNS; 30% MSSA	1	3.5	1	N/A	N/A	N/A	107 (range 90–120)	N/A	6
Wan et al., 2012 [104]	4	RCS	C/C	33	70 ± 11	44 (range 24–62)	41 (range 1–192)	24.2% MSSA; 24.2% CoNS	8	3.2 (range 1.84–7.31)	2	3	N/A	6	N/A	N/A	N/A
Yi et al., 2015 [105]	4	RCS	C/C	17	63.7 (range 43–74)	45.6 (range 24–96)	N/A	23.5% S. epidermidis; 11.8% MSSA	1	3.9 (range 2.3–6.2)	1	1	N/A	4	105.9 (range 90–125)	HSS: 83.9 (range 77–91)	N/A
Zamora et al., 2020 [54]	3	RCCS	M/P (new)	3	N/A	N/A	N/A	N/A	1	N/A	N/A	0	/	N/A	N/A	N/A	N/A

Abbreviations: RCT, randomized controlled trial; PCCS, prospective comparative cohort study; PCS, prospective case series; RCS, retrospective case series; RCCS, retrospective comparative cohort study; C/C, cement on cement; C/P, cement on polyethylene; M/C, metal on cement; M/P, metal on polyethylene; CoNS, coagulase-negative staphylococci; MSSA/MRSA, methicillin-sensible/resistant Staphylococcus aureus; MSSE/MRSE, methicillin-sensible/resistant Streptococcus epidermidis; PJI, periprosthetic joint infection; CR, cruciate-retaining total knee arthroplasty; PS, posterior-stabilized total knee arthroplasty; FU, follow-up; KSS, Knee Society Score; HSS, Hospital for Special Surgery Knee-Rating Scale; N/A: data not available.

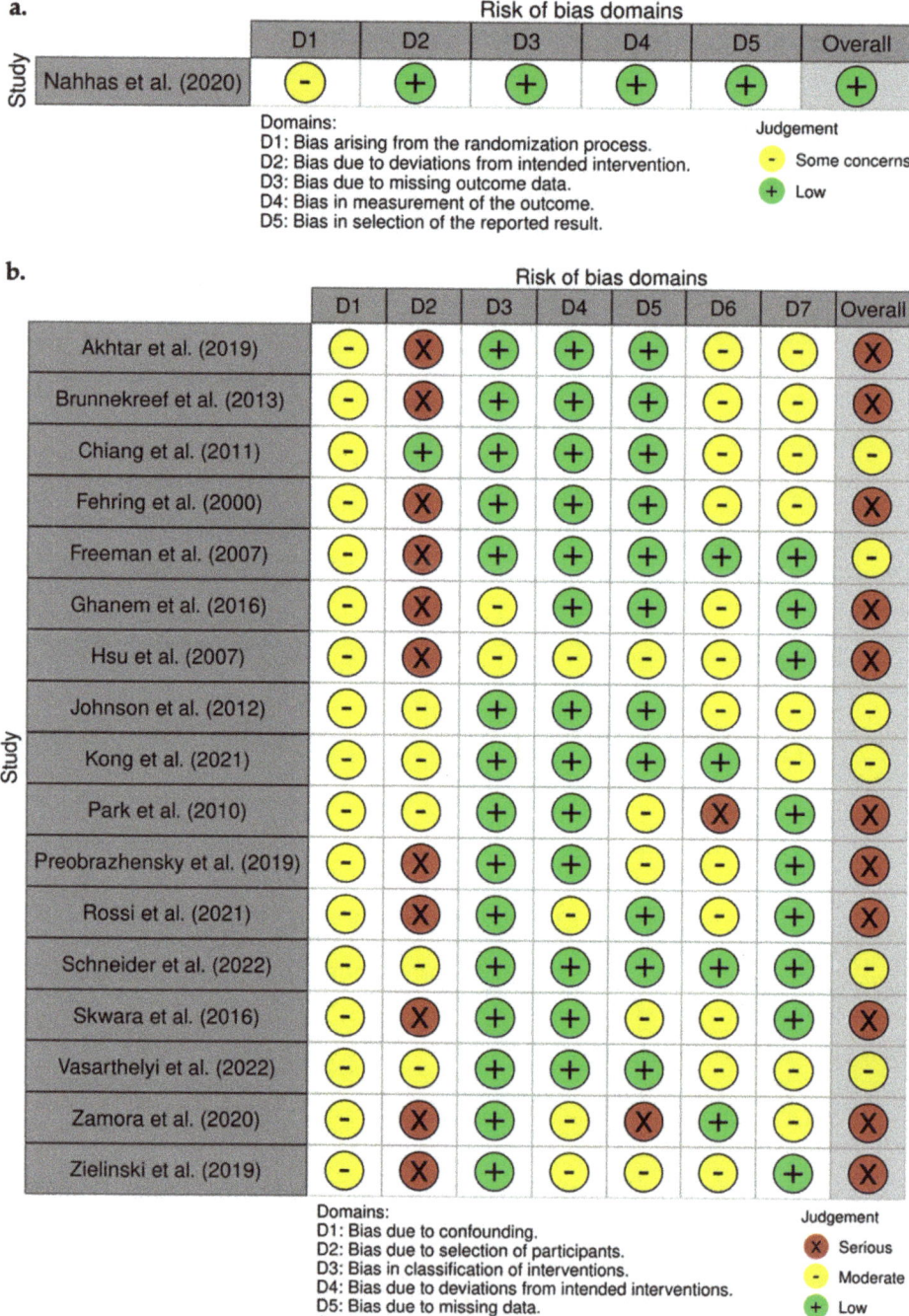

Figure 2. Cont.

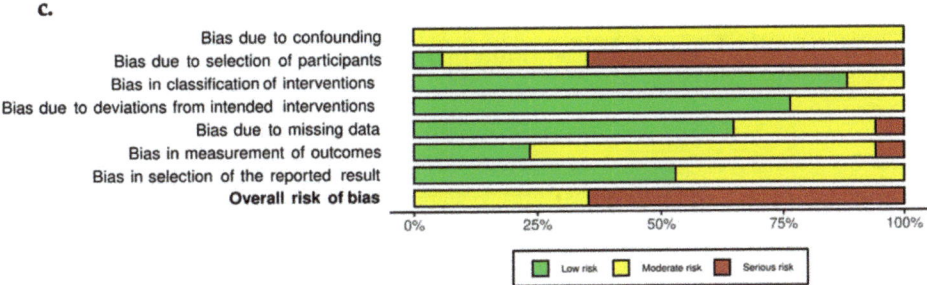

Figure 2. Quality assessment of the included studies in meta-analysis according to RoB2 [43] (a) and ROBINS-I [21,23,25,29–31,34,38,39,44,46–48,50,52,54,106] (b) tools: "traffic light" plots of the domain-level judgments for each individual result (**a**,**b**); weighted bar plots of the distribution of risk-of-bias judgments within each bias domain (**c**).

In detail, data extracted included study type, mean age, mean follow-up, number and details of spacers, mean time to infection onset, bacterial populations, number of spacers used, and repeated first stages, mean time between first stage and second stage, mean duration of antibiotic therapy, number of PJI recurrences, number of cases in which no reimplantation was performed, mean active knee flexion at last follow-up, functional outcome at last follow-up, and peri-operative non-infection-related local complications. Functional outcomes were reported according to the most reported scoring systems used in the studies analyzed in this review: Knee Society Score (KSS) and Hospital for Special Surgery Knee-Rating Scale (HSS). Local peri-operative complications not related to infection were reported, including extensor lag, spacer subluxation/fracture, extensor mechanism rupture, nerve palsy, periprosthetic fracture, dislocation, instability, arthrofibrosis, hematoma, and delayed wound healing. Success of the treatment was defined as the achievement of infection control at last follow-up (the absence of clinical and/or radiological and/or laboratory signs of infection, as mentioned in the individual papers). Failure of the treatment was defined as the persistence of infection, re-infection, or no reimplantation; the repetition of the first stage of the two-stage protocol due to persistence of infection was not considered a failure when it eventually resulted in successful control of the infection at last follow-up after the end of the treatment.

Studies with reported quantitative data were used for statistical analysis (Tables 3 and 4). Weighted means and standard deviations were calculated to summarize the values reported in the individual studies and to compare them. Chi-square statistics (Pearson Chi-square, Yates Chi-Square, Fisher exact test, Fisher–Freeman–Halton test) were used to assess associations and homogeneity among categorical variables. For quantitative variables, the Shapiro–Wilk test was used to verify normal distribution. The Levene test was used to assess the equality of variances. As a parametric test, the two-tailed unpaired Student T-test was used in case of equality of the variances; otherwise, the Welch T-test was used. The Mann–Whitney U-test was used as a non-parametric test in case of non-normal distribution of the variables. Spearman's rho was used to identify monotonic correlations between variables. Only comparative studies were included in the meta-analysis (Figures 3 and 4). Quantification of the extent of statistical heterogeneity across studies included in the meta-analysis employed the inconsistency statistic ($I^2 > 75\%$ was considered as high heterogeneity). Potential sources of heterogeneity by study level and clinically relevant characteristics were explored using stratified analysis and meta-regression. Publication bias was assessed using Egger's regression symmetry test. p-value < 0.05 was considered to be significant. All statistical analyses were performed with IBM SPSS v26.0 for MacOS (SPSS Inc., Chicago, Illinois) and ProMeta 3 (Internovi, Cesena, Italy) software.

Table 3. Summarized data from the included studies of this review.

	Static	Spacers with Data Available (n)	Articulated	Spacers with Data Available (n)	p-Value
Study series (n)	34		71		
• RCT	1		1		
• PCCS	2	-	2	-	0.111
• RCCS	19		23		
• PCS	0		9		
• RCS	12		36		
Spacers (n)	1511	-	2739	-	-
Mean age (years)	67 ± 5.6	1147	66.4 ± 3.5	2545	0.532
Mean follow-up (months)	68 ± 52.3	1002	53.5 ± 32.9	2163	0.117
Most frequent bacterial population	S. aureus CoNS S. epidermidis	347	S. aureus S. epidermidis CoNS	1303	-
Mean time to PJI (months)	34.8 ± 14.3	296	36.8 ± 11.9	737	0.735
Mean time between first and second stage (months)	3.1 ± 1.1	854	3.6 ± 2.3	2071	0.480
Mean duration of antibiotic therapy (weeks)	7.2 ± 1.9	870	6.1 ± 1	1170	0.007
Repeated first stage/spacer exchange (n)	47 (5.4%)	922	89 (4%)	2237	0.159
No reimplantation (n)	67 (7.1%)	947	94 (4.3%)	2198	0.001 *
PJI recurrence (n)	157 (12.4%)	1271	230 (9%)	2554	0.001 *
Mean time to PJI recurrence (months)	13.7 ± 3.9	285	23.2 ± 12.1	737	0.125
Mean active knee flexion at last FU	91.6 ± 7	763	100.3 ± 9.9	1549	<0.001 *
Mean KSS score at last FU	81.1 ± 13.1	569	81.9 ± 5.5	732	0.792
Mean HSS score at last FU	81.8 ± 0.7	67	81.7 ± 7	229	0.981
Peri-operative non-infection-related local complications (nn)	146 (16.7%)	872	318 (16.5%)	1932	0.852
Non-infection-related complications requiring revision surgery (n)	24 (2.9%)	820	58 (3.1%)	1876	0.819

* Statistically significant. Abbreviations: RCT, randomized controlled trial; PCCS, prospective comparative cohort study; RCCS, retrospective comparative cohort study; PCS, prospective case series; RCS, retrospective case series; CoNS, coagulase-negative staphylococci; PJI, periprosthetic joint infection; FU, follow-up; KSS, Knee Society Score; HSS, Hospital for Special Surgery Knee-Rating Scale.

Table 4. Correlations between time to second stage and outcomes.

	Static		Articulated		Total		Spacers with Data Available (n)
	Rho	p-Value	Rho	p-Value	Rho	p-Value	
PJI recurrence (n)	0.040	0.876	0.274	0.040 *	0.202	0.082	2786
Mean time to PJI recurrence	0.5	0.391	−0.772	0.072	0.092	0.789	474
Mean active knee flexion at last FU	−0.080	0.595	−0.361	0.019 *	−0.257	0.050 *	1656
Mean KSS score at last FU	−0.267	0.455	−0.073	0.759	−0.147	0.438	956

* Statistically significant. Abbreviations: PJI, periprosthetic joint infection; KSS, Knee Society Score; FU, follow-up.

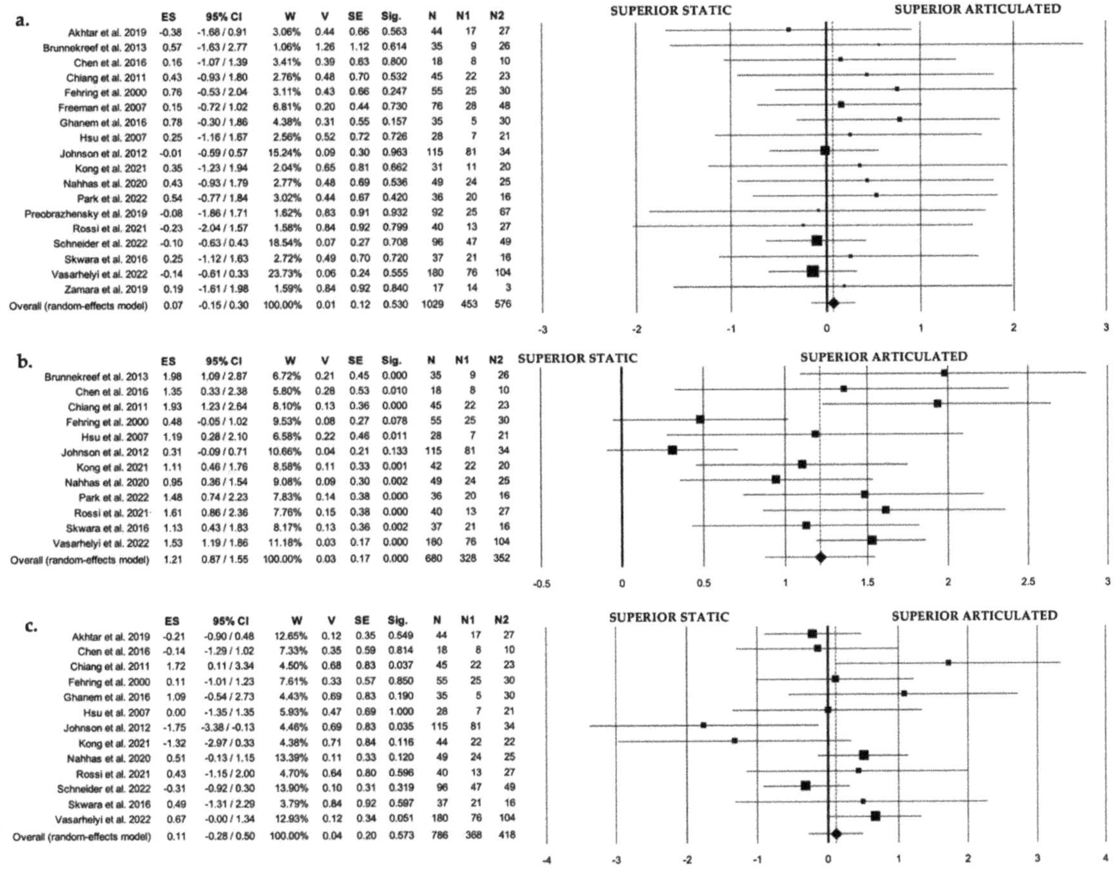

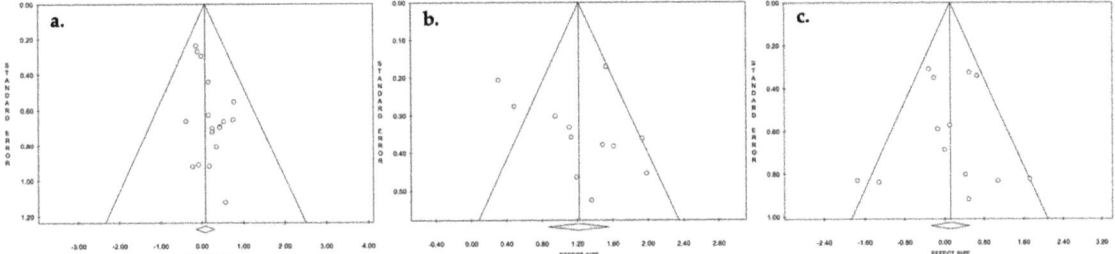

Figure 3. Forest plot of overall meta-analysis evaluating comparative studies (static spacers vs. articulated spacers) with data about PJI recurrences [21,23–25,29–31,34,38,39,43,44,46–48,50,52,54] (**a**), active knee flexion at last follow-up (**b**), and non-infection-related peri-operative local complications (**c**). Abbreviations: ES, effect size; 95% CI, 95% confidence interval; W, weight; V, variance; SE, standard error; N, sample size; N1, static spacer series sample size; N2, articulated spacer series sample size.

Figure 4. Funnel plot of effect sizes for publication bias of the comparative studies evaluating PJI recurrences (**a**), active knee flexion at last follow-up (**b**), and non-infection-related peri-operative local complications (**c**).

3. Results

A total of 3421 studies were found through the electronic search and 21 studies were added after the cross-referenced research on the bibliographies of the examined full-text articles. After a preliminary analysis, a total of 87 studies reporting series of knee spacers used for two-stage treatment of PJI were included in this systematic review (1 randomized controlled trial, 3 prospective comparative cohort studies, 26 retrospective comparative cohort studies, 9 prospective case series, 48 retrospective case series [18–102] (Tables 1 and 2; Figure 1)). Among these, eighteen studies were included in the meta-analysis (Figures 3 and 4). Studies comparing static vs. articulated spacers were 1 RCT [43], 1 PCCS [22], and 16 RCCS [18,20,21,26–28,31,35,36,41,43–45,47,49,51]. In total, 34 series on static spacers [18–51] and 71 on articulated spacers [18,20,21,26–28,31,35,36,41,43–45,47,49,51–102] were found (Figure 3).

The overall quality of the studies included in the meta-analysis, assessed by the RoB2 and the ROBINS-I tools [16,17], was high in only one case [40], moderate in 6 cases [22,27,35,36,45,49], and low in 11 cases [18,20,21,26,28,31,41,43,44,47,51] (Figure 2a–c).

A total of 4250 knee spacers were included: 1511 static spacers and 2739 articulated spacers (Table 3). The two groups were highly homogeneous considering a number of variables (Table 3). Mean age was comparable between static and articulated series (67 ± 5.6 years and 66.4 ± 3.5, respectively; $p = 0.532$) (Table 3). No statistical difference was found between the two groups also concerning the mean follow-up (68 ± 52.3 months for static group and 53.5 ± 32.9 months for articulated group; $p = 0.117$) (Table 3). The most frequent bacterial populations found were *Staphylococcus aureus*, *Streptococcus epidermidis*, and other coagulase-negative staphylococci in both groups (Table 3). Mean time to PJI onset from primary arthroplasty surgery was also similar (34.8 ± 14.3 months for static group and 36.8 ± 11.9 months for articulated group; $p = 0.735$) (Table 3). No significant difference was found in the time between first and second stage (3.1 ± 1.1 months for static group and 3.6 ± 2.3 months for articulated group; $p = 0.480$), nor in the number of spacer exchanges with repeated first stage before reimplantation (5.4% vs. 4% for static and articulated series, respectively; $p = 0.159$) (Table 3). Instead, a mismatch was found between the two groups in the mean duration of post-operative antibiotic therapy after first-stage surgery, being longer for static spacers (7.2 ± 1.9 vs. 6.1 ± 1 weeks; $p = 0.007$) (Table 3).

With respect to the results in terms of infection control, a significantly higher rate of both no reimplantation and PJI recurrence was found when static spacers were used. In detail, a revision knee arthroplasty was not performed in 7.1% of the PJIs in the static spacer group and in 4.3% of the cases in the articulated group ($p = 0.001$), while PJI recurrence was found in 12.4% vs. 9% of the two-stage procedures ($p = 0.001$) (Table 3). The time elapsed between the first and second stage appeared to directly influence the PJI recurrence rate (with a trend towards more recurrences in the case of longer time with a spacer in situ), although a significant correlation was only found for articulated spacers ($p = 0.040$) (Table 4). The meta-analysis performed on comparative studies evaluating the PJI recurrence with static vs. articulated spacers confirmed a trend for better infection control using articulated spacers, although no significant difference was found between the groups ($p = 0.530$) (Figure 3a). No significative heterogeneity ($I^2 \approx 0\%$, $p = 0.992$) or relevant publication bias (Figure 4a) was found regarding the PJI recurrence rate. No significant difference was found concerning the mean time to PJI recurrence between static and articulated spacers (13.7 ± 3.9 months and 23.2 ± 12.1 months, respectively; $p = 0.125$) (Table 3). Furthermore, no correlations between the mean time to second stage after spacer placement and the mean time to PJI recurrence were found (Table 4).

With regard to the functional outcomes, mean active knee flexion at last follow-up was found to be significantly higher using articulated spacers ($91.6° \pm 7°$ for static spacers vs. $100.3° \pm 9.9°$ for articulated spacers; $p < 0.001$) (Table 3). The meta-analysis also confirmed this strong significant difference ($p < 0.001$) (Figure 3b). Moderate heterogeneity ($I^2 = 69.1\%$, $p = 0.059$) and no relevant publication bias (Figure 4b) were found regarding the active knee flexion. A significant negative correlation was found between the mean time to second stage after spacer placement and the mean final active knee flexion, which appeared to be particularly marked when using articulated spacers ($p = 0.019$) (Table 4). However, when clinical scores were considered (KSS and HSS), no significant difference was found between static and articulated groups (81.1 ± 13.1 vs. 81.9 ± 5.5 for KSS, $p = 0.792$; 81.8 ± 0.7 vs. 81.7 ± 7 for HSS, $p = 0.981$) (Table 3).

No difference was found regarding the incidence of peri-operative local complications not related to the PJI between static and articulated spacers (complication rate: 16.7% vs. 16.5%; $p = 0.852$) (Table 3). The revision rate for non-infection-related complications was found to be also similar between static and articulated spacers (2.9% vs. 3.1%; $p = 0.819$) (Table 3). The meta-analysis did not find significant differences between the groups either ($p = 0.573$) (Figure 3c). Low heterogeneity ($I^2 = 41.3\%$, $p = 0.099$) and no relevant publication bias (Figure 4c) were found regarding the complication rate.

4. Discussion

Both static and articulated antibiotic-laden spacers have benefits and drawbacks, and the choice is based on multiple factors, including the clinical assessment of the patient's general functional status, general health, soft tissue envelope of the knee, virulence of the organism, and extent of bone loss [107]. The existing literature on the subject largely consists of small series with evidence levels III and IV and a limited number of randomized prospective trials.

In this review, we found, in the pooled analysis, a significantly lower number of PJI recurrences when an articulated spacer was used. This trend was also found in the meta-analysis of the comparative studies alone, though without a statistically significant difference. No significant differences were found either in the number of non-infection-related complications or in the functional results from the evaluation of the HSS and KSS scores, as already reported by previous studies [11].

Conversely, a strong difference emerged in favor of articulated spacers, both in the general pooled data analysis and the meta-analysis of comparative studies, regarding active knee flexion capability at the last follow-up after prosthesis reimplantation.

The main benefit of articulated spacers is that they enable movement of the joint between surgeries. Articulated spacers also allow a more comfortable position of the knee during sitting, standing, and car travel. Maintaining motion facilitates the recovery of limb function during treatment of infection. Knee flexion preserves the length and elasticity of the extensor mechanism and helps to prevent scarring of the soft tissue around the joint and capsular stiffening [96,108,109]. As a result, the extent of surgical exposure required and the overall difficulty of the second-stage surgery can be decreased [26,34,109]. Moreover, the findings of an in vitro study showed that cyclical loading of the cement spacers enhanced the elution of vancomycin and tobramycin [110]. A broad assortment of articulated spacers that can be placed after the removal of an infected total knee arthroplasty is available—for example, (1) handmade cement-on-cement spacers without molds, (2) premolded or preformed antibiotic cement spacers (with or without stems), (3) surgical molds for intraoperative fabrication (with or without metal femoral runners), and (4) autoclaved or new metal femoral and polyethylene components (Table 1) [111]. Most of the articulated spacers included in this study were found to be cement-on-cement spacers. Consequently, no further investigation was performed to reveal whether there are differences in outcomes depending on the subtype of mobile spacer.

Common indications for use of a static spacer are (1) patients with severe uncontrolled infections; (2) ligamentous laxity, particularly in the case of collateral ligament compromise, as an articulated spacer would not allow for multiplanar knee stability; (3) extensor mechanism disruption or insufficiency, as active flexion and control of the knee would not be achieved; (4) compromised soft tissue coverage over the joint, since motion might apply additional tension; (5) severe bone loss after prosthesis explant, as they can be customized to fill the gap and eventually stabilized using intramedullary dowels [9,108,109,112–114]. Moreover, static spacers are usually cheaper [115,116].

However, several shortcomings of static spacers have been suggested. Several studies have reported poor limb mobility with static spacers after reimplantation compared to articulated spacers [108,117,118]. In addition, unanticipated bone loss as a result of spacer migration has been observed. Using static spacers may also complicate exposure during the second-stage procedure due to the shortening of the ligaments and quadriceps, as well as wound closure [29].

A factor that is difficult to standardize within the two-stage protocol is the time of spacer persistence, before reimplantation. Longer intervals between the two stages are known to correlate with worse infectious and functional outcomes [7,119,120]. Elution of the antibiotic from any spacer reaches its peak in the first 72 h from placement: after this time, the function of any is mainly mechanical [13,121]. Moreover, a longer time of spacer persistence may increase the incidence of mechanical complications such as spacer rupture or dislocation, which can eventually lead to an interim spacer exchange [122].

We observed that, in the case of articulated spacers, a spacer persistence of more than 3 weeks increased the number of PJI recurrences. Furthermore, it was found that spacer persistence progressively decreases the ability of articulated spacers to preserve active flexion.

It was not possible to perform a detailed analysis of any inconsistencies in terms of the surgical and infectious complexity of the cases in order to exclude any selection bias whereby the more complex cases were preferentially treated with a static spacer. For example, the study by Guild et al., analyzing data on the existence of bone loss of any type, found no statistical difference in the placement of static vs. articulating spacers for the indication of bone loss [11]. However, when they classified bone loss according to the Anderson Orthopaedic Research Institute (AORI) classification [123], they found that static spacers were placed significantly more frequently for femoral bone loss than articulated spacers [11]. These data, however, may be biased as only a small minority of the studies specifically addressed pre-existing bone loss. However, not only bone deficiency has to be considered when assessing complexity. It depends on many other factors (type of microorganism, quality of soft tissue, comorbidity, etc.), and even within individual studies, it was almost never possible to effectively differentiate cases by complexity. A possible patient selection bias among the included studies represents the major limitation of this study. A previous review by Pivec et al. attempted to divide patients with an articulated spacer into complex and non-complex cases and compared the results between these two subgroups and patients with a static spacer [124]. They reported a slightly higher PJI recurrence rate in the articulated spacer group with only complex patients compared to the static spacer group, but no statistical significance was shown [124]. In the present review, considering the wide variability of the criteria used in the individual studies and the paucity of studies in which the individual patients could be characterized, we decided not to perform such an analysis. However, this review only considered primary infections, so it is reasonable to assume that tremendously destructive conditions of the knee that are unsuitable for dynamic spacers are a minority and probably not crucial in the interpretation of the overall emerging findings, also considering the high number of spacers included in this review. Unfortunately, only high-quality studies, with accurate assessment to ensure the homogeneity of patient selection, can help to solve this issue. A review, although systematic, can only state that it is reasonable to believe that the use of articulated spacers should definitely be considered in all cases where there are no significant contraindications, as it offers excellent results with respect to infection control and functional outcomes, with complications comparable to those expected with the use of static spacers. Unfortunately, it is difficult to establish the limit beyond which the use of a static spacer can guarantee greater benefit.

Among the limitations of this article, in addition to those already mentioned, the average low quality of the studies (for the majority consisting of case series or retrospective comparative studies) must be considered. In addition, this is certainly not the first review on the topic and essentially confirms evidence that has already emerged. The main strength is the amount of data collected and the depth of the analysis. In fact, to the best of our knowledge, it is the first review to provide a large-scale quantitative analysis. These aspects make it a very comprehensive and up-to-date review on the subject and reinforce the conclusion that only high-quality studies can clarify the elements still under discussion.

5. Conclusions

In conclusion, this review confirms that articulated spacers do not appear to be inferior to static spacers in terms of infection control, complications, and functional results, while they are superior in terms of active flexion granted after reimplantation. Statis spacers, often mostly used in more severe cases, can offer similar infection control in this scenario. However, despite the high number of included spacers, considering the average low quality of the studies included and the impossibility of determining the presence and extent of a selection bias in the choice of the spacers, it is not possible to generalize the results that emerged. Nevertheless, in cases that meet all the appropriate conditions for the placement of articulated spacers, optimal results can be expected, and their use can be recommended.

Author Contributions: Conceptualization, M.F. (Michele Fiore) and A.S.; methodology, M.F. (Michele Fiore); software, M.F. (Matteo Filippini); investigation, M.F. (Matteo Filippini) and L.M.; data curation, C.R. and A.P.; writing—original draft preparation, M.F. (Michele Fiore), M.F. (Matteo Filippini), L.M., R.Z. and C.G.; writing—review and editing, M.F. (Michele Fiore) and A.S.; supervision, P.V. and M.D.P. All authors have read and agreed to the published version of the manuscript.

Funding: This research received no external funding.

Institutional Review Board Statement: Not applicable.

Informed Consent Statement: Not applicable.

Data Availability Statement: The data reported in this study are available in the literature.

Conflicts of Interest: The authors declare no conflict of interest.

References

1. Gehrke, T.; Alijanipour, P.; Parvizi, J. The management of an infected total knee arthroplasty. *Bone Jt. J.* **2015**, *97*, 20–29. [CrossRef]
2. Lamagni, T. Epidemiology and burden of prosthetic joint infections. *J. Antimicrob. Chemother.* **2014**, *69* (Suppl. 1), i5–i10. [CrossRef] [PubMed]
3. Sambri, A.; Fiore, M.; Tedeschi, S.; De Paolis, M. The Need for Multidisciplinarity in Modern Medicine: An Insight into Orthopaedic Infections. *Microorganisms* **2022**, *10*, 756. [CrossRef] [PubMed]
4. Calanna, F.; Chen, F.; Risitano, S.; Vorhies, J.S.; Franceschini, M.; Giori, N.J.; Indelli, P.F. Debridement, antibiotic pearls, and retention of the implant (DAPRI): A modified technique for implant retention in total knee arthroplasty PJI treatment. *J. Orthop. Surg.* **2019**, *27*, 2309499019874413. [CrossRef]
5. Parvizi, J.; Tan, T.L.; Goswami, K.; Higuera, C.; Della Valle, C.; Chen, A.F.; Shohat, N. The 2018 Definition of Periprosthetic Hip and Knee Infection: An Evidence-Based and Validated Criteria. *J. Arthroplast.* **2018**, *33*, 1309–1314.e2. [CrossRef]
6. Osmon, D.R.; Berbari, E.F.; Berendt, A.R.; Lew, D.; Zimmerli, W.; Steckelberg, J.M.; Rao, N.; Hanssen, A.; Wilson, W.R.; Infectious Diseases Society of, A. Diagnosis and management of prosthetic joint infection: Clinical practice guidelines by the Infectious Diseases Society of America. *Clin. Infect. Dis.* **2013**, *56*, e1–e25. [CrossRef] [PubMed]
7. Izakovicova, P.; Borens, O.; Trampuz, A. Periprosthetic joint infection: Current concepts and outlook. *EFORT Open Rev.* **2019**, *4*, 482–494. [CrossRef]
8. Masters, J.P.; Smith, N.A.; Foguet, P.; Reed, M.; Parsons, H.; Sprowson, A.P. A systematic review of the evidence for single stage and two stage revision of infected knee replacement. *BMC Musculoskelet. Disord.* **2013**, *14*, 222. [CrossRef]
9. Charette, R.S.; Melnic, C.M. Two-Stage Revision Arthroplasty for the Treatment of Prosthetic Joint Infection. *Curr. Rev. Musculoskelet. Med.* **2018**, *11*, 332–340. [CrossRef]
10. Sambri, A.; Bianchi, G.; Parry, M.; Frenos, F.; Campanacci, D.; Donati, D.; Jeys, L. Is Arthrodesis a Reliable Salvage Option following Two-Stage Revision for Suspected Infection in Proximal Tibial Replacements? A Multi-Institutional Study. *J. Knee Surg.* **2018**, *32*, 911–918. [CrossRef]
11. Guild, G.N., III; Wu, B.; Scuderi, G.R. Articulating vs. Static antibiotic impregnated spacers in revision total knee arthroplasty for sepsis. A systematic review. *J. Arthroplast.* **2014**, *29*, 558–563. [CrossRef] [PubMed]
12. Anagnostakos, K.; Fink, B. Antibiotic-loaded cement spacers—Lessons learned from the past 20 years. *Expert Rev. Med. Devices* **2018**, *15*, 231–245. [CrossRef] [PubMed]

13. Anagnostakos, K.; Meyer, C. Antibiotic Elution from Hip and Knee Acrylic Bone Cement Spacers: A Systematic Review. *BioMed Res. Int.* **2017**, *2017*, 4657874. [CrossRef] [PubMed]
14. Risitano, S.; Sabatini, L.; Atzori, F.; Massè, A.; Indelli, P.F. Static antibiotic spacers augmented by calcium sulphate impregnated beads in revision TKA: Surgical technique and review of literature. *J. Orthop.* **2018**, *15*, 313–318. [CrossRef] [PubMed]
15. DeBoer, D.K. Comparison of Traditional Molded, First-Generation Premolded, and Second-Generation Premolded Antibiotic-Loaded Polymethylmethacrylate Articulating Spacers for Treatment of Chronic Prosthetic Joint Infection of the Knee. *J. Arthroplast.* **2020**, *35*, S53–S56. [CrossRef] [PubMed]
16. Nodzo, S.R.; Boyle, K.K.; Spiro, S.; Nocon, A.A.; Miller, A.O.; Westrich, G.H. Success rates, characteristics, and costs of articulating antibiotic spacers for total knee periprosthetic joint infection. *Knee* **2017**, *24*, 1175–1181. [CrossRef]
17. Romano, C.L.; Gala, L.; Logoluso, N.; Romano, D.; Drago, L. Two-stage revision of septic knee prosthesis with articulating knee spacers yields better infection eradication rate than one-stage or two-stage revision with static spacers. *Knee Surg. Sports Traumatol. Arthrosc.* **2012**, *20*, 2445–2453. [CrossRef]
18. Page, M.J.; McKenzie, J.E.; Bossuyt, P.M.; Boutron, I.; Hoffmann, T.C.; Mulrow, C.D.; Shamseer, L.; Tetzlaff, J.M.; Akl, E.A.; Brennan, S.E.; et al. The PRISMA 2020 statement: An updated guideline for reporting systematic reviews. *BMJ* **2021**, *372*, n71. [CrossRef]
19. Sterne, J.A.; Hernan, M.A.; Reeves, B.C.; Savovic, J.; Berkman, N.D.; Viswanathan, M.; Henry, D.; Altman, D.G.; Ansari, M.T.; Boutron, I.; et al. ROBINS-I: A tool for assessing risk of bias in non-randomised studies of interventions. *BMJ* **2016**, *355*, i4919. [CrossRef]
20. Sterne, J.A.C.; Savovic, J.; Page, M.J.; Elbers, R.G.; Blencowe, N.S.; Boutron, I.; Cates, C.J.; Cheng, H.Y.; Corbett, M.S.; Eldridge, S.M.; et al. RoB 2: A revised tool for assessing risk of bias in randomised trials. *BMJ* **2019**, *366*, l4898. [CrossRef]
21. Akhtar, A.; Mitchell, C.; Assis, C.; Iranpour, F.; Kropelnicki, A.; Strachan, R. Cement Pedestal Spacer Technique for Infected Two-stage Revision Knee Arthroplasty: Description and Comparison of Complications. *Indian J. Orthop.* **2019**, *53*, 695–699. [CrossRef] [PubMed]
22. Barrack, R.L.; Engh, G.; Rorabeck, C.; Sawhney, J.; Woolfrey, M. Patient satisfaction and outcome after septic versus aseptic revision total knee arthroplasty. *J. Arthroplast.* **2000**, *15*, 990–993. [CrossRef] [PubMed]
23. Brunnekreef, J.; Hannink, G.; Malefijt Mde, W. Recovery of knee mobility after a static or mobile spacer in total knee infection. *Acta Orthop. Belg.* **2013**, *79*, 83–89. [PubMed]
24. Chen, Y.P.; Wu, C.C.; Ho, W.P. Autoclaved metal-on-cement spacer versus static spacer in two-stage revision in periprosthetic knee infection. *Indian J. Orthop.* **2016**, *50*, 146–153. [CrossRef]
25. Chiang, E.R.; Su, Y.P.; Chen, T.H.; Chiu, F.Y.; Chen, W.M. Comparison of articulating and static spacers regarding infection with resistant organisms in total knee arthroplasty. *Acta Orthop.* **2011**, *82*, 460–464. [CrossRef]
26. Choi, H.R.; Malchau, H.; Bedair, H. Are prosthetic spacers safe to use in 2-stage treatment for infected total knee arthroplasty? *J. Arthroplast.* **2012**, *27*, 1474–1479.e1471. [CrossRef]
27. Emerson, R.H., Jr.; Muncie, M.; Tarbox, T.R.; Higgins, L.L. Comparison of a static with a mobile spacer in total knee infection. *Clin. Orthop. Relat. Res.* **2002**, *404*, 132–138. [CrossRef]
28. Faschingbauer, M.; Bieger, R.; Reichel, H.; Weiner, C.; Kappe, T. Complications associated with 133 static, antibiotic-laden spacers after TKA. *Knee Surg. Sports Traumatol. Arthrosc.* **2016**, *24*, 3096–3099. [CrossRef]
29. Fehring, T.K.; Odum, S.; Calton, T.F.; Mason, J.B. Articulating versus static spacers in revision total knee arthroplasty for sepsis. The Ranawat Award. *Clin. Orthop. Relat. Res.* **2000**, *380*, 9–16. [CrossRef]
30. Freeman, M.G.; Fehring, T.K.; Odum, S.M.; Fehring, K.; Griffin, W.L.; Mason, J.B. Functional advantage of articulating versus static spacers in 2-stage revision for total knee arthroplasty infection. *J. Arthroplast.* **2007**, *22*, 1116–1121. [CrossRef]
31. Ghanem, M.; Zajonz, D.; Bollmann, J.; Geissler, V.; Prietzel, T.; Moche, M.; Roth, A.; Heyde, C.E.; Josten, C. Outcome of total knee replacement following explantation and cemented spacer therapy. *GMS Interdiscip. Plast. Reconstr. Surg. DGPW* **2016**, *5*, Doc12. [CrossRef] [PubMed]
32. Haleem, A.A.; Berry, D.J.; Hanssen, A.D. Mid-term to long-term followup of two-stage reimplantation for infected total knee arthroplasty. *Clin. Orthop. Relat. Res.* **2004**, *428*, 35–39. [CrossRef]
33. Hipfl, C.; Winkler, T.; Janz, V.; Perka, C.; Müller, M. Management of Chronically Infected Total Knee Arthroplasty with Severe Bone Loss Using Static Spacers with Intramedullary Rods. *J. Arthroplast.* **2019**, *34*, 1462–1469. [CrossRef] [PubMed]
34. Hsu, Y.C.; Cheng, H.C.; Ng, T.P.; Chiu, K.Y. Antibiotic-loaded cement articulating spacer for 2-stage reimplantation in infected total knee arthroplasty: A simple and economic method. *J. Arthroplast.* **2007**, *22*, 1060–1066. [CrossRef] [PubMed]
35. Hsu, C.-S.C.-C.; Wang, J.-W.; Lin, P.-C. Two-stage revision of infected total knee arthroplasty using an antibiotic-impregnated static cement-spacer. *Chang. Gung Med. J.* **2008**, *31*, 583–591.
36. Husted, H.; Toftgaard Jensen, T. Clinical outcome after treatment of infected primary total knee arthroplasty. *Acta Orthop. Belg.* **2002**, *68*, 500–507.
37. Ippolito, J.A.; Thomson, J.E.; Rivero, S.M.; Beebe, K.S.; Patterson, F.R.; Benevenia, J. Management of Large Segmental Bone Defects at the Knee with Intramedullary Stabilized Antibiotic Spacers During Two-Stage Treatment of Endoprosthetic Joint Infection. *J. Arthroplast.* **2021**, *36*, 2165–2170. [CrossRef]
38. Johnson, A.J.; Sayeed, S.A.; Naziri, Q.; Khanuja, H.S.; Mont, M.A. Minimizing dynamic knee spacer complications in infected revision arthroplasty. *Clin. Orthop. Relat. Res.* **2012**, *470*, 220–227. [CrossRef]

39. Kong, L.; Mei, J.; Ge, W.; Jin, X.; Chen, X.; Zhang, X.; Zhu, C. Application of 3D Printing-Assisted Articulating Spacer in Two-Stage Revision Surgery for Periprosthetic Infection after Total Knee Arthroplasty: A Retrospective Observational Study. *BioMed Res. Int.* **2021**, *2021*, 3948638. [CrossRef]
40. Lichstein, P.; Su, S.; Hedlund, H.; Suh, G.; Maloney, W.J.; Goodman, S.B.; Huddleston, J.I., III. Treatment of Periprosthetic Knee Infection with a Two-stage Protocol Using Static Spacers. *Clin. Orthop. Relat. Res.* **2016**, *474*, 120–125. [CrossRef]
41. Lo Presti, M.; Costa, G.G.; Vasco, C.; Agrò, G.; Poggi, A.; Neri, M.P.; Zaffagnini, S. Küntscher nails with static cement spacer: A simple technique in periprosthetic knee infections with massive bone loss and instability. *Knee* **2021**, *29*, 580–588. [CrossRef] [PubMed]
42. Ma, H.H.; Chou, T.A.; Tsai, S.W.; Chen, C.F.; Wu, P.K.; Chen, C.M.; Chen, W.M. Is short-course systemic antibiotic therapy using an antibiotic-loaded cement spacer safe after resection for infected total knee arthroplasty? A comparative study. *J. Formos. Med. Assoc.* **2020**, *119*, 1070–1079. [CrossRef] [PubMed]
43. Nahhas, C.R.; Chalmers, P.N.; Parvizi, J.; Sporer, S.M.; Berend, K.R.; Moric, M.; Chen, A.F.; Austin, M.S.; Deirmengian, G.K.; Morris, M.J.; et al. A Randomized Trial of Static and Articulating Spacers for the Treatment of Infection Following Total Knee Arthroplasty. *J. Bone Jt. Surg. Am.* **2020**, *102*, 778–787. [CrossRef] [PubMed]
44. Park, S.J.; Song, E.K.; Seon, J.K.; Yoon, T.R.; Park, G.H. Comparison of static and mobile antibiotic-impregnated cement spacers for the treatment of infected total knee arthroplasty. *Int. Orthop.* **2010**, *34*, 1181–1186. [CrossRef] [PubMed]
45. Petis, S.M.; Perry, K.I.; Mabry, T.M.; Hanssen, A.D.; Berry, D.J.; Abdel, M.P. Two-Stage Exchange Protocol for Periprosthetic Joint Infection Following Total Knee Arthroplasty in 245 Knees without Prior Treatment for Infection. *J. Bone Jt. Surg. Am.* **2019**, *101*, 239–249. [CrossRef] [PubMed]
46. Preobrazhensky, P.M.; Bozhkova, S.A.; Kazemirsky, A.V.; Tikhilov, R.M.; Kulaba, T.A.; Kornilov, N.N. Functional outcome of two-stage reimplantation in patients with periprosthetic joint infection after primary total knee arthroplasty. *Int. Orthop.* **2019**, *43*, 2503–2509. [CrossRef]
47. Rossi, S.M.P.; Medetti, M.; Perticarini, L.; Ghiara, M.; Benazzo, F. Customized intraoperatively molded articulating cement spacers for two-stage revisions TKA with major bone defects. *Eur. J. Orthop. Surg. Traumatol.* **2021**, *31*, 1121–1128. [CrossRef]
48. Schneider, A.M.; Holzmeister, A.M.; Frazzett, A.J.; Adams, W.; Hopkinson, W.J.; Brown, N.M. New Primary Total Knee Arthroplasty Components Versus Other Contemporary Types of Spacers for the Treatment of Chronic Periprosthetic Knee Infection with a Two-Stage Protocol. *Orthopedics* **2022**, *45*, 109–115. [CrossRef]
49. Silvestre, A.; Almeida, F.; Renovell, P.; Morante, E.; López, R. Revision of infected total knee arthroplasty: Two-stage reimplantation using an antibiotic-impregnated static spacer. *Clin. Orthop. Surg.* **2013**, *5*, 180–187. [CrossRef] [PubMed]
50. Skwara, A.; Tibesku, C.; Paletta, R.J.; Sommer, C.; Krödel, A.; Lahner, M.; Daniilidis, K. Articulating spacers compared to fixed spacers for the treatment of infected knee arthroplasty: A follow-up of 37 cases. *Technol. Health Care* **2016**, *24*, 571–577. [CrossRef]
51. Springer, B.D.; Lee, G.C.; Osmon, D.; Haidukewych, G.J.; Hanssen, A.D.; Jacofsky, D.J. Systemic safety of high-dose antibiotic-loaded cement spacers after resection of an infected total knee arthroplasty. *Clin. Orthop. Relat. Res.* **2004**, *427*, 47–51. [CrossRef]
52. Vasarhelyi, E.; Sidhu, S.P.; Somerville, L.; Lanting, B.; Naudie, D.; Howard, J. Static vs. Articulating Spacers for Two-Stage Revision Total Knee Arthroplasty: Minimum Five-Year Review. *Arthroplast. Today* **2022**, *13*, 171–175. [CrossRef] [PubMed]
53. Vielgut, I.; Schwantzer, G.; Leithner, A.; Sadoghi, P.; Berzins, U.; Glehr, M. Successful Two-Stage Exchange Arthroplasty for Periprosthetic Infection Following Total Knee Arthroplasty: The Impact of Timing on Eradication of Infection. *Int. J. Med. Sci.* **2021**, *18*, 1000–1006. [CrossRef]
54. Zamora, T.; Garbuz, D.S.; Greidanus, N.V.; Masri, B.A. An articulated spacer made of new primary implants in two-stage exchange for infected total knee arthroplasty may provide durable results. *Bone Jt. J.* **2020**, *102*, 852–860. [CrossRef] [PubMed]
55. Ahmad, S.S.; Huber, K.; Evangelopoulos, D.S.; Kleer, B.; Kohlhof, H.; Schär, M.; Eggli, S.; Kohl, S. The cement prosthesis-like spacer: An intermediate halt on the road to healing. *Sci. World J.* **2013**, *2013*, 763434. [CrossRef]
56. Babis, G.C.; Zahos, K.A.; Tsailas, P.; Karaliotas, G.I.; Kanellakopoulou, K.; Soucacos, P.N. Treatment of stage III-A-1 and III-B-1 periprosthetic knee infection with two-stage exchange arthroplasty and articulating spacer. *J. Surg. Orthop. Adv.* **2008**, *17*, 173–178.
57. Boelch, S.P.; Jakuscheit, A.; Luedemann, M.; Heilig, P.; Kamawal, Y.; Arnholdt, J.; Rudert, M. Do not exchange the spacer during staged TKA exchange! *J. Orthop.* **2021**, *23*, 41–45. [CrossRef]
58. Buyuk, A.F.; Sofu, H.; Camurcu, I.Y.; Ucpunar, H.; Kaygusuz, M.A.; Sahin, V. Can Teicoplanin Be an Effective Choice for Antibiotic-Impregnated Cement Spacer in Two-Stage Revision Total Knee Arthroplasty? *J. Knee Surg.* **2017**, *30*, 283–288. [CrossRef] [PubMed]
59. Carulli, C.; Villano, M.; Civinini, R.; Matassi, F.; Nistri, L.; Innocenti, M. A novel technique to preserve range of motion in two-stage revision of infected total knee arthroplasty. *Int. Orthop.* **2013**, *37*, 1069–1074. [CrossRef]
60. Castelli, C.C.; Gotti, V.; Ferrari, R. Two-stage treatment of infected total knee arthroplasty: Two to thirteen year experience using an articulating preformed spacer. *Int. Orthop.* **2014**, *38*, 405–412. [CrossRef]
61. Durbhakula, S.M.; Czajka, J.; Fuchs, M.D.; Uhl, R.L. Antibiotic-loaded articulating cement spacer in the 2-stage exchange of infected total knee arthroplasty. *J. Arthroplast.* **2004**, *19*, 768–774. [CrossRef] [PubMed]
62. Evans, R.P. Successful treatment of total hip and knee infection with articulating antibiotic components: A modified treatment method. *Clin. Orthop. Relat Res.* **2004**, *427*, 37–46. [CrossRef] [PubMed]
63. Fei, Z.; Zhang, Z.; Wang, Y.; Zhang, H.; Xiang, S. Comparing the Efficacy of Articulating Spacers in Two-Stage Revision for Periprosthetic Joint Infection Following Total Knee Arthroplasty: All-Cement Spacers vs. Sterilized Replanted Metal-Polyethylene Spacers. *Int. J. Gen. Med.* **2022**, *15*, 3293–3301. [CrossRef] [PubMed]

64. Garg, P.; Ranjan, R.; Bandyopadhyay, U.; Chouksey, S.; Mitra, S.; Gupta, S.K. Antibiotic-impregnated articulating cement spacer for infected total knee arthroplasty. *Indian J. Orthop.* **2011**, *45*, 535–540. [CrossRef] [PubMed]
65. Ghanem, M.; Pempe, C.; Zajonz, D.; Roth, A.; Heyde, C.E.; Josten, C. Mid-term results of two-stage revision of total knee arthroplasty using a mobile (dynamic) cement spacer in the treatment of periprosthetic infections. *GMS Interdiscip. Plast. Reconstr. Surg. DGPW* **2018**, *7*, Doc02. [CrossRef] [PubMed]
66. Gooding, C.R.; Masri, B.A.; Duncan, C.P.; Greidanus, N.V.; Garbuz, D.S. Durable infection control and function with the PROSTALAC spacer in two-stage revision for infected knee arthroplasty. *Clin. Orthop. Relat. Res.* **2011**, *469*, 985–993. [CrossRef] [PubMed]
67. Ha, C.W. A technique for intraoperative construction of antibiotic spacers. *Clin. Orthop. Relat. Res.* **2006**, *445*, 204–209. [CrossRef]
68. Haddad, F.S.; Masri, B.A.; Campbell, D.; McGraw, R.W.; Beauchamp, C.P.; Duncan, C.P. The PROSTALAC functional spacer in two-stage revision for infected knee replacements. Prosthesis of antibiotic-loaded acrylic cement. *J. Bone Jt. Surg. Br.* **2000**, *82*, 807–812. [CrossRef]
69. Hammerich, K.; Pollack, J.; Hasse, A.F.; El Saman, A.; Huber, R.; Rupp, M.; Alt, V.; Kinne, R.W.; Mika, J. The Inverse Spacer-A Novel, Safe, and Cost-Effective Approach in Routine Procedures for Revision Knee Arthroplasty. *J. Clin. Med.* **2021**, *10*, 971. [CrossRef]
70. Hart, W.J.; Jones, R.S. Two-stage revision of infected total knee replacements using articulating cement spacers and short-term antibiotic therapy. *J. Bone Jt. Surg. Br.* **2006**, *88*, 1011–1015. [CrossRef]
71. Hoshino, T.; Watanabe, T.; Nakagawa, Y.; Katagiri, H.; Ozeki, N.; Ohara, T.; Shioda, M.; Kono, Y.; Sekiya, I.; Koga, H. Clinical outcomes of two-stage revision total knee arthroplasty in infected cases with antibiotic-loaded cement spacers produced using a handmade silicone mold. *Knee Surg. Relat. Res.* **2021**, *33*, 27. [CrossRef] [PubMed]
72. Incavo, S.J.; Russell, R.D.; Mathis, K.B.; Adams, H. Initial results of managing severe bone loss in infected total joint arthroplasty using customized articulating spacers. *J. Arthroplast.* **2009**, *24*, 607–613. [CrossRef]
73. Jia, Y.T.; Zhang, Y.; Ding, C.; Zhang, N.; Zhang, D.L.; Sun, Z.H.; Tian, M.Q.; Liu, J. Antibiotic-loaded articulating cement spacers in two-stage revision for infected total knee arthroplasty: Individual antibiotic treatment and early results of 21 cases. *Chin. J. Traumatol.* **2012**, *15*, 212–221.
74. Jung, K.H.; Lee, C.C.; Kim, T.H.; Han, J.W.; Park, K.B. Does spiked tibial cement spacer reduce spacer-related problems in two-stage revision total knee arthroplasty for infection? *Int. Orthop.* **2022**, *46*, 2009–2017. [CrossRef] [PubMed]
75. Kalore, N.V.; Maheshwari, A.; Sharma, A.; Cheng, E.; Gioe, T.J. Is there a preferred articulating spacer technique for infected knee arthroplasty? A preliminary study. *Clin. Orthop. Relat. Res.* **2012**, *470*, 228–235. [CrossRef]
76. Kohl, S.; Evangelopoulos, D.S.; Kohlhof, H.; Krueger, A.; Hartel, M.; Roeder, C.; Eggli, S. An intraoperatively moulded PMMA prostheses like spacer for two-stage revision of infected total knee arthroplasty. *Knee* **2011**, *18*, 464–469. [CrossRef]
77. Lin, T.L.; Tsai, C.H.; Fong, Y.C.; Shie, M.Y.; Chen, H.Y.; Chen, Y.W. Cruciate-Retaining vs Posterior-Stabilized Antibiotic Cement Articulating Spacers for Two-Stage Revision of Prosthetic Knee Infection: A Retrospective Cohort Study. *J. Arthroplast.* **2021**, *36*, 3750–3759. [CrossRef] [PubMed]
78. Lu, J.; Han, J.; Zhang, C.; Yao, Z.; Yang, Y. Polyethylene on Cement Spacers: An Economic Approach to an Effective Infection Eradication in a Two-Stage Knee Revision Articulating Spacers. *J. Knee Surg.* **2018**, *31*, 986–991. [CrossRef]
79. MacAvoy, M.C.; Ries, M.D. The ball and socket articulating spacer for infected total knee arthroplasty. *J. Arthroplast.* **2005**, *20*, 757–762. [CrossRef]
80. Macheras, G.A.; Kateros, K.; Galanakos, S.P.; Koutsostathis, S.D.; Kontou, E.; Papadakis, S.A. The long-term results of a two-stage protocol for revision of an infected total knee replacement. *J. Bone Jt. Surg. Br.* **2011**, *93*, 1487–1492. [CrossRef]
81. Marothi, D.P.; Sharma, V.; Sheth, A.N.; Shah, V.I.; Bharath, L.; Pachore, J.A. Management of Infected Total Knee Arthroplasty by a New Innovative Customized Articulating Knee Spacer: An Early Experience. *J. Orthop. Case Rep.* **2016**, *6*, 20–22. [CrossRef] [PubMed]
82. Mutimer, J.; Gillespie, G.; Lovering, A.M.; Porteous, A.J. Measurements of in vivo intra-articular gentamicin levels from antibiotic loaded articulating spacers in revision total knee replacement. *Knee* **2009**, *16*, 39–41. [CrossRef] [PubMed]
83. Ocguder, A.; Firat, A.; Tecimel, O.; Solak, S.; Bozkurt, M. Two-stage total infected knee arthroplasty treatment with articulating cement spacer. *Arch. Orthop. Trauma. Surg.* **2010**, *130*, 719–725. [CrossRef]
84. Ortola, D.J.; Fenga, D.; Marcellino, S.; Rosi, M.; Centofanti, F.; Rosa, M.A. Peri-Prosthetic Knee Infection Management: Spacers Loaded with Two or Three Antibiotic Agents. *Surg. Infect.* **2017**, *18*, 619–624. [CrossRef] [PubMed]
85. Pascale, V.; Pascale, W. Custom-made articulating spacer in two-stage revision total knee arthroplasty. An early follow-up of 14 cases of at least 1 year after surgery. *HSS J.* **2007**, *3*, 159–163. [CrossRef] [PubMed]
86. Pitto, R.P.; Castelli, C.C.; Ferrari, R.; Munro, J. Pre-formed articulating knee spacer in two-stage revision for the infected total knee arthroplasty. *Int. Orthop.* **2005**, *29*, 305–308. [CrossRef]
87. Radoicic, D.; Milanovic, M.; Marinkovic, J.; Radoicic, D. Ertapenem Articulating Spacer for the Treatment of Polymicrobial Total Knee Arthroplasty Infection. *Can. J. Infect. Dis. Med. Microbiol.* **2016**, *2016*, 5753489. [CrossRef]
88. Roof, M.A.; Baylor, J.L.; Bernstein, J.A.; Antonelli, B.J.; Kugelman, D.N.; Egol, A.J.; Melnic, C.M.; Chen, A.F.; Long, W.J.; Aggarwal, V.K.; et al. Comparing the Efficacy of Articulating Spacer Constructs for Knee Periprosthetic Joint Infection Eradication: All-Cement vs Real-Component Spacers. *J. Arthroplast.* **2021**, *36*, S320–S327. [CrossRef]

89. Sakellariou, V.I.; Savvidou, O.; Markopoulos, C.; Drakou, A.; Mavrogenis, A.F.; Papagelopoulos, P.J. Combination of Calcium Hydroxyapatite Antibiotic Carrier with Cement Spacers in Peri-Prosthetic Knee Infections. *Surg. Infect.* **2015**, *16*, 748–754. [CrossRef]
90. Seo, S.S.; Kim, C.W.; Lee, C.R.; Park, D.H.; Kwon, Y.U.; Jung, D.; Kim, D.S. Clinical outcomes of two-stage total knee arthroplasty using articulating cement spacer in patients with infected arthritic knee: A comparison with arthroscopic surgery. *Knee* **2020**, *27*, 444–450. [CrossRef]
91. Shaikh, A.A.; Ha, C.W.; Park, Y.G.; Park, Y.B. Two-stage approach to primary TKA in infected arthritic knees using intraoperatively molded articulating cement spacers. *Clin. Orthop. Relat. Res.* **2014**, *472*, 2201–2207. [CrossRef]
92. Shen, H.; Zhang, X.; Jiang, Y.; Wang, Q.; Chen, Y.; Wang, Q.; Shao, J. Intraoperatively-made cement-on-cement antibiotic-loaded articulating spacer for infected total knee arthroplasty. *Knee* **2010**, *17*, 407–411. [CrossRef]
93. Siebel, T.; Kelm, J.; Porsch, M.; Regitz, T.; Neumann, W.H. Two-stage exchange of infected knee arthroplasty with an prosthesis-like interim cement spacer. *Acta Orthop. Belg.* **2002**, *68*, 150–156.
94. Struelens, B.; Claes, S.; Bellemans, J. Spacer-related problems in two-stage revision knee arthroplasty. *Acta Orthop. Belg.* **2013**, *79*, 422–426.
95. Su, Y.P.; Lee, O.K.; Chen, W.M.; Chen, T.H. A facile technique to make articulating spacers for infected total knee arthroplasty. *J. Chin. Med. Assoc.* **2009**, *72*, 138–145. [CrossRef]
96. Thabe, H.; Schill, S. Two-stage reimplantation with an application spacer and combined with delivery of antibiotics in the management of prosthetic joint infection. *Oper. Orthop. Traumatol.* **2007**, *19*, 78–100. [CrossRef] [PubMed]
97. Tian, M.Q.; Yang, X.T.; Tian, X.B.; Sun, Y.B.; Duan, Y.H.; Sun, L. Short-term Follow-up of Antibiotic-loaded Articulating Cement Spacers in Two-stage Revision of Infected Total Knee Arthroplasty: A Case Series. *Orthop. Surg.* **2018**, *10*, 128–133. [CrossRef] [PubMed]
98. Tigani, D.; Trisolino, G.; Fosco, M.; Ben Ayad, R.; Costigliola, P. Two-stage reimplantation for periprosthetic knee infection: Influence of host health status and infecting microorganism. *Knee* **2013**, *20*, 9–18. [CrossRef] [PubMed]
99. Tsai, C.H.; Hsu, H.C.; Chen, H.Y.; Fong, Y.C.; Ho, M.W.; Chou, C.H.; Chen, Y.W.; Shie, M.Y.; Lin, T.L. A preliminary study of the novel antibiotic-loaded cement computer-aided design-articulating spacer for the treatment of periprosthetic knee infection. *J. Orthop. Surg. Res.* **2019**, *14*, 136. [CrossRef]
100. Van Thiel, G.S.; Berend, K.R.; Klein, G.R.; Gordon, A.C.; Lombardi, A.V.; Della Valle, C.J. Intraoperative molds to create an articulating spacer for the infected knee arthroplasty. *Clin. Orthop. Relat. Res.* **2011**, *469*, 994–1001. [CrossRef] [PubMed]
101. Vasso, M.; Del Regno, C.; Corona, K.; D'Apolito, R.; Schiavone Panni, A. Articulated spacer provides long-term knee improvement after two-stage reimplantation. *Knee Surg. Sports Traumatol. Arthrosc.* **2016**, *24*, 3100–3105. [CrossRef]
102. Vecchini, E.; Micheloni, G.M.; Perusi, F.; Scaglia, M.; Maluta, T.; Lavini, F.; Bondi, M.; Dall'Oca, C.; Magnan, B. Antibiotic-Loaded Spacer for Two-Stage Revision of Infected Total Knee Arthroplasty. *J. Knee Surg.* **2017**, *30*, 231–237. [CrossRef]
103. Villanueva-Martinez, M.; Rios-Luna, A.; Pereiro, J.; Fahandez-Saddi, H.; Villamor, A. Hand-made articulating spacers in two-stage revision for infected total knee arthroplasty: Good outcome in 30 patients. *Acta Orthop.* **2008**, *79*, 674–682. [CrossRef]
104. Wan, Z.; Karim, A.; Momaya, A.; Incavo, S.J.; Mathis, K.B. Preformed articulating knee spacers in 2-stage total knee revision arthroplasty: Minimum 2-year follow-up. *J. Arthroplast.* **2012**, *27*, 1469–1473. [CrossRef] [PubMed]
105. Yi, C.; Yiqin, Z.; Qi, Z.; Hui, Z.; Zheru, D.; Peiling, F.; Yuli, W.; Haishan, W. Two-Stage Primary Total Knee Arthroplasty with Well-Designed Antibiotic-Laden Cement Spacer Block for Infected Osteoarthritic Knees: The First Case Series from China. *Surg. Infect.* **2015**, *16*, 755–761. [CrossRef] [PubMed]
106. Zielinski, M.R.; Ziemba-Davis, M.; Warth, L.C.; Keyes, B.J.; Meneghini, R.M. Do Antibiotic Intramedullary Dowels Assist in Eradicating Infection in Two-Stage Resection for Septic Total Knee Arthroplasty? *J. Arthroplasty* **2019**, *34*, 2461–2465. [CrossRef] [PubMed]
107. Bowman, E.C.; Malkani, A.L. Point/Counterpoint: Static vs Articulating Spacers-Static Spacers for Resection Arthroplasty of the Knee. *J. Arthroplast.* **2020**, *35*, S35–S39. [CrossRef] [PubMed]
108. Mazzucchelli, L.; Rosso, F.; Marmotti, A.; Bonasia, D.E.; Bruzzone, M.; Rossi, R. The use of spacers (static and mobile) in infection knee arthroplasty. *Curr. Rev. Musculoskelet. Med.* **2015**, *8*, 373–382. [CrossRef]
109. Lu, J.; Han, J.; Zhang, C.; Yang, Y.; Yao, Z. Infection after total knee arthroplasty and its gold standard surgical treatment: Spacers used in two-stage revision arthroplasty. *Intractable Rare Dis. Res.* **2017**, *6*, 256–261. [CrossRef]
110. Rogers, B.A.; Middleton, F.R.; Shearwood-Porter, N.; Kinch, S.; Roques, A.; Bradley, N.W.; Browne, M. Does cyclical loading affect the elution of antibiotics from articulating cement knee spacers? *J. Bone Jt. Surg. Br.* **2011**, *93*, 914–920. [CrossRef]
111. Lachiewicz, P.F.; Wellman, S.S.; Peterson, J.R. Antibiotic Cement Spacers for Infected Total Knee Arthroplasties. *J. Am. Acad. Orthop. Surg.* **2020**, *28*, 180–188. [CrossRef] [PubMed]
112. Hasandoost, L.; Rodriguez, O.; Alhalawani, A.; Zalzal, P.; Schemitsch, E.H.; Waldman, S.D.; Papini, M.; Towler, M.R. The Role of Poly(Methyl Methacrylate) in Management of Bone Loss and Infection in Revision Total Knee Arthroplasty: A Review. *J. Funct. Biomater.* **2020**, *11*, 25. [CrossRef] [PubMed]
113. Kotwal, S.Y.; Farid, Y.R.; Patil, S.S.; Alden, K.J.; Finn, H.A. Intramedullary rod and cement static spacer construct in chronically infected total knee arthroplasty. *J. Arthroplast.* **2012**, *27*, 253–259. [CrossRef]
114. Voleti, P.B.; Baldwin, K.D.; Lee, G.C. Use of static or articulating spacers for infection following total knee arthroplasty: A systematic literature review. *J. Bone Jt. Surg. Am.* **2013**, *95*, 1594–1599. [CrossRef]

115. Antoci, V.; Phillips, M.J.; Antoci, V., Jr.; Krackow, K.A. Using an antibiotic-impregnated cement rod-spacer in the treatment of infected total knee arthroplasty. *Am. J. Orthop.* **2009**, *38*, 31–33. [PubMed]
116. Jiranek, W.A.; Hanssen, A.D.; Greenwald, A.S. Antibiotic-loaded bone cement for infection prophylaxis in total joint replacement. *J. Bone Jt. Surg. Am.* **2006**, *88*, 2487–2500. [CrossRef]
117. Kalore, N.V.; Gioe, T.J.; Singh, J.A. Diagnosis and management of infected total knee arthroplasty. *Open Orthop. J.* **2011**, *5*, 86–91. [CrossRef]
118. Jacobs, C.; Christensen, C.P.; Berend, M.E. Static and mobile antibiotic-impregnated cement spacers for the management of prosthetic joint infection. *J. Am. Acad. Orthop. Surg.* **2009**, *17*, 356–368. [CrossRef]
119. Golgelioglu, F.; Oguzkaya, S.; Misir, A.; Guney, A. The Effect of Time Spent with a Dynamic Spacer on Clinical and Functional Outcomes in Two-Stage Revision Knee Arthroplasty. *Indian J. Orthop.* **2020**, *54*, 824–830. [CrossRef]
120. Vielgut, I.; Sadoghi, P.; Wolf, M.; Holzer, L.; Leithner, A.; Schwantzer, G.; Poolman, R.; Frankl, B.; Glehr, M. Two-stage revision of prosthetic hip joint infections using antibiotic-loaded cement spacers: When is the best time to perform the second stage? *Int. Orthop.* **2015**, *39*, 1731–1736. [CrossRef]
121. Klinder, A.; Zaatreh, S.; Ellenrieder, M.; Redanz, S.; Podbielski, A.; Reichel, T.; Bösebeck, H.; Mittelmeier, W.; Bader, R. Antibiotics release from cement spacers used for two-stage treatment of implant-associated infections after total joint arthroplasty. *J. Biomed. Mater. Res. B Appl. Biomater.* **2019**, *107*, 1587–1597. [CrossRef] [PubMed]
122. Tan, T.L.; Goswami, K.; Kheir, M.M.; Xu, C.; Wang, Q.; Parvizi, J. Surgical Treatment of Chronic Periprosthetic Joint Infection: Fate of Spacer Exchanges. *J. Arthroplast.* **2019**, *34*, 2085–2090. [CrossRef] [PubMed]
123. Daines, B.K.; Dennis, D.A. Management of bone defects in revision total knee arthroplasty. *J. Bone Jt. Surg. Am.* **2012**, *94*, 1131–1139. [CrossRef] [PubMed]
124. Pivec, R.; Naziri, Q.; Issa, K.; Banerjee, S.; Mont, M.A. Systematic review comparing static and articulating spacers used for revision of infected total knee arthroplasty. *J. Arthroplast.* **2014**, *29*, 553–557. [CrossRef]

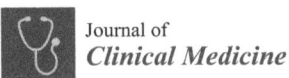

Editorial

Osteochondral Lesions of Ankle and Knee. Will Future Treatments Really Be Represented by Custom-Made Metal Implants?

Massimiliano Mosca, Alberto Grassi and Silvio Caravelli *

II Clinic of Orthopaedics and Traumatology, IRCCS Istituto Ortopedico Rizzoli, 40136 Bologna, Italy; massimiliano.mosca@ior.it (M.M.); alberto.grassi@ior.it (A.G.)
* Correspondence: doct.car@gmail.com

1. Introduction

Knee and ankle osteochondral lesions are structural defects of the cartilaginous surface and underlying subchondral bone which still represent a daily challenge for the orthopedic surgeon. Although etiology on a traumatic basis accounts for most cases, other causes are contemplated, including joint malalignments, instability, genetic predisposition, endocrine factors or avascular necrosis [1–3]. Optimal treatment is still the subject of debate.

Bone marrow stimulation procedures, osteochondral grafting and the osteochondral autograft transfer system (OATS) [4] are usually the first therapeutic step in young and active patients. However, these procedures are typically associated with donor site morbidity (pain, scar tissue and sensibility issues), incongruent grafts or graft resorption. Ferreira et al. [5] reported a complication rate of up to 41% after OATS surgery. Elderly patients with low functional requirements often benefit from a conventional joint replacement.

2. Discussion

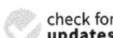

However, there is a pool of patients who fall into the so-called "gap of treatment"—active patients suffering from osteochondral lesions in the context of an otherwise healthy joint. These subjects have often passed the age for biological treatment but are not yet eligible for early knee or ankle joint prosthesis or come to our observation after a failed biological intervention [6]. In the last two decades, the interest in this type of patient has increased, leading to the development and production of small metal prosthetic devices of "focal joint replacement" or "focal resurfacing", with the aim of filling only the symptomatic cartilaginous lesion of the talar dome or femoral condyles. After the initial enthusiasm for good clinical and functional results, described in the literature in different studies [2,7–9], the complication rate reduced the expectations of these implants. The technical difficulties of the implant, the malpositioning and the particular and peculiar joint geometries of the ankle and knee can strongly influence the surgical result. Despite the design being developed to adapt to the joint surfaces, minimal changes in the implant positioning could create problems during walking and not be tolerated in biomechanically complex and congruent joints [2]. In addition, high rates of re-intervention have been described, whether or not related to the implant itself. In particular, repositioning or removal of the prosthesis, subchondral periprosthetic radiolucency, joint space narrowing and cyst formations around the implant screw have been reported [2,10].

In this panorama, new custom-made talar and condylar devices (Episealer®) have recently been designed and developed to address these technical issues. These CT-based patient-specific mini-metal prostheses are produced following the patient's joint anatomy, location and volumetric characteristics of the osteochondral lesion. They aim to represent the next step in advanced resurfacing techniques, improving clinical outcomes and avoiding the specific disadvantages of standard metal resurfacing. Despite being newly

Citation: Mosca, M.; Grassi, A.; Caravelli, S. Osteochondral Lesions of Ankle and Knee. Will Future Treatments Really Be Represented by Custom-Made Metal Implants? *J. Clin. Med.* 2022, 11, 3817. https://doi.org/10.3390/jcm11133817

Received: 24 June 2022
Accepted: 30 June 2022
Published: 1 July 2022

Publisher's Note: MDPI stays neutral with regard to jurisdictional claims in published maps and institutional affiliations.

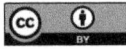

Copyright: © 2022 by the authors. Licensee MDPI, Basel, Switzerland. This article is an open access article distributed under the terms and conditions of the Creative Commons Attribution (CC BY) license (https://creativecommons.org/licenses/by/4.0/).

designed implants, good short-term results have already been published, reporting a failure rate of 2.5% [11,12]. A study by Moewis P et al. [6] evaluated these new implants at a 12-month follow-up, showing that after the condylar implantation, the knee kinematics were physiological with a medial pivot, lateral femoral rollback and coupled axial pattern, and external rotation during flexion.

This short editorial aims to ask questions and propose new long-term research approaches about the possibilities of custom-made metal implants, which are already revolutionizing the concept of total prosthetics, to improve clinical and radiological outcomes in patients suffering from primary or secondary osteochondral lesions following the failure of previous biological treatments. Moreover, we will focus on the duration and possible different complications, with respect to the biomechanics of large joints, pitfalls and technical tricks, and the cost/benefit ratio for the patient and the health protection entities.

Author Contributions: Conceptualization and Supervision: M.M. Review and editing: A.G. Writing and Draf preparation, Conceptualization: S.C. Review and editing: A.G. Writing and Draf preparation, Conceptualization: S.C. All authors have read and agreed to the published version of the manuscript.

Funding: This research received no external funding.

Conflicts of Interest: The authors declare no conflict of interest.

References

1. Bae, D.K.; Yoon, K.H.; Song, S.J. Cartilage healing after micro-fracture in osteoarthritic knees. *Arthroscopy* **2006**, *22*, 367–374. [CrossRef] [PubMed]
2. Maiorano, E.; Bianchi, A.; Hosseinzadeh, M.K.; Malerba, F.; Martinelli, N.; Sansone, V. HemiCAP implantation after failed previous surgery for osteochondral lesions of the talus. *Foot Ankle Surg.* **2021**, *27*, 77–81. [CrossRef] [PubMed]
3. Bollars, P.; Bosquet, M.; Vandekerckhove, B.; Hardeman, F.; Bellemans, J. Prosthetic inlay resurfacing for the treatment of focal, full thickness cartilage defects of the femoral condyle: A bridge between biologics and conventional arthroplasty. *Knee Surg. Sports Traumatol. Arthrosc.* **2012**, *20*, 1753–1759. [CrossRef] [PubMed]
4. Zanon, G.; Di Vico, G.; Marullo, M. Osteochondritis dissecans of the talus. *Joints* **2014**, *2*, 115–123. [CrossRef] [PubMed]
5. Ferreira, C.; Vuurberg, G.; Oliveira, J.M.; Espregueira-Mendes, J.; Pereira, H.; Reis, R.L.; Ripoll, P.L. Good clinical outcome after osteochondral autologous transplantation surgery for osteochondral lesions of the talus but at the cost of a high rate of complications: A systematic review. *J. ISAKOS* **2016**, *1*, 184–191. [CrossRef]
6. Moewis, P.; Kaiser, R.; Trepczynski, A.; von Tycowicz, C.; Krahl, L.; Ilg, A.; Holz, J.; Duda, G.N. Patient-specific resurfacing implant knee surgery in subjects with early osteoarthritis results in medial pivot and lateral femoral rollback during flexion: A retrospective pilot study. *Knee Surg. Sports Traumatol. Arthrosc.* **2021**, *3*, 1–12. [CrossRef] [PubMed]
7. Uribe, J.W.; Botto-van Bemden, A. Partial humeral head resurfacing for osteonecrosis. *J. Shoulder Elb. Surg.* **2009**, *18*, 711–716. [CrossRef] [PubMed]
8. Van Bergen, C.J.; Zengerink, M.; Blankevoort, L.; van Sterkenburg, M.N.; van Oldenrijk, J.; van Dijk, C.N. Novel metallic implantation technique for osteochondral defects of the medial talar dome. A cadaver study. *Acta. Orthop.* **2010**, *81*, 495–502. [CrossRef] [PubMed]
9. O'Loughlin, P.F.; Heyworth, B.E.; Kennedy, J.G. Current concepts in the diagnosis and treatment of osteochondral lesions of the ankle. *Am. J. Sports Med.* **2010**, *38*, 392–404. [CrossRef] [PubMed]
10. Vuurberg, G.; Reilingh, M.L.; van Bergen, C.J.A.; van Eekeren, I.C.M.; Gerards, R.M.; van Dijk, C.N. Metal Resurfacing Inlay Implant for Osteochondral Talar Defects After Failed Previous Surgery: A Midterm Prospective Follow-up Study. *Am. J. Sports Med.* **2018**, *46*, 1685–1692. [CrossRef] [PubMed]
11. Holz, J.; Spalding, T.; Boutefnouchet, T.; Means, P.; Eriksson, K.; Brittberg, M.; Konradsen, L.; Kösters, C.; Verdonk, P.; Högström, M.; et al. Patient-specific metal implants for focal chondral and osteochondral lesions in the knee; excellent clinical results at 2 years. *Knee Surg. Sports Traumatol. Arthrosc.* **2021**, *29*, 2899–2910. [CrossRef] [PubMed]
12. Martinez-Carranza, N.; Rockborn, P.; Roberts, D.; Högström, M.; Stålman, A. Successful Treatment of Femoral Chondral Lesions with a Novel Customized Metal Implant at Midterm Follow-Up. *Cartilage* **2021**, *13* (Suppl. 1), 1726S–1733S. [CrossRef] [PubMed]

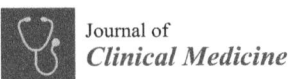

Systematic Review

Conservative vs. Surgical Management for Femoro-Acetabular Impingement: A Systematic Review of Clinical Evidence

Giuseppe Anzillotti [1,2], Alberto Iacomella [1,2,*], Matteo Grancagnolo [1,2], Enrico Maria Bertolino [1,2], Maurilio Marcacci [1,2], Cristiano Sconza [1,2], Elizaveta Kon [1,2] and Berardo Di Matteo [1,2]

1 Department of Biomedical Sciences, Humanitas University, 20072 Pieve Emanuele, MI, Italy
2 IRCCS Humanitas Research Hospital, 20089 Rozzano, MI, Italy
* Correspondence: albertoiacomella96@gmail.com

Abstract: Femoro-acetabular impingement (FAI) syndrome is one of the most studied conditions in sports medicine. Surgical or conservative approaches can be proposed for treating FAI, although the best standard of care is not established yet. Our aim is to provide a comprehensive review of the best treatment for FAI syndrome evaluating differences in outcomes between surgical and non-operative management. A literature search was carried out on the PubMed, EMBASE, Scopus, and PEDro databases, using the following keywords: "femoroacetabular impingement", "FAI", in association with "surgery", "arthroscopy", "surgical" and "conservative", "physiotherapy", "physical therapy", "rehabilitation", "exercise". Only Level I RCTs were included. Four articles were selected for this systematic review. Our analysis showed different therapeutic protocols, follow-up periods, and outcomes; however, three out of the four studies included favored surgery. Our study demonstrates beneficial effects for both arthroscopic treatment and a proper regimen of physical therapy, nevertheless a surgical approach seemed to offer superior short-term results when compared to conservative care only. Further trials with larger sample sizes and longer follow-ups are needed to assess the definitive approach to the FAI condition.

Keywords: femoro-acetabular impingement; hip; arthroscopy; cam; pincer; physical therapy

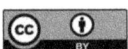

Citation: Anzillotti, G.; Iacomella, A.; Grancagnolo, M.; Bertolino, E.M.; Marcacci, M.; Sconza, C.; Kon, E.; Di Matteo, B. Conservative vs. Surgical Management for Femoro-Acetabular Impingement: A Systematic Review of Clinical Evidence. *J. Clin. Med.* 2022, 11, 5852. https://doi.org/10.3390/jcm11195852

Academic Editors: Massimiliano Mosca, Alberto Grassi, Silvio Caravelli and Moshe Salai

Received: 14 August 2022
Accepted: 29 September 2022
Published: 2 October 2022

Publisher's Note: MDPI stays neutral with regard to jurisdictional claims in published maps and institutional affiliations.

Copyright: © 2022 by the authors. Licensee MDPI, Basel, Switzerland. This article is an open access article distributed under the terms and conditions of the Creative Commons Attribution (CC BY) license (https://creativecommons.org/licenses/by/4.0/).

1. Introduction

Femoro-acetabular impingement (FAI) syndrome is defined as the triad of symptoms, clinical signs and imaging findings in which structural morphology results in conflict between the femoral head and the acetabulum [1]. First described during the 1990s [2–4], the incidence of FAI morphology, which could induce the syndrome, is estimated to be up to 37% and 67% in asymptomatic patients for cam and pincer, respectively [5]. Although FAI syndrome is one of the most studied conditions in sports medicine, its etiology still remains unknown [6].

Abnormal sphericity of the femoral head (cam or pistol grip), excessive protrusion of acetabular edge (pincer), or both, may lead to mechanical conflict leading to the syndrome [7].

Cam-type (Figure 1a) morphology results in impingement due to an abnormal-shaped femoral head that rotates into the acetabulum, especially during forceful flexion. Repetitive end-of-motion movements result in shearing and disruption of the acetabular cartilage from the labrum.

Pincer-type (Figure 1b) morphology is based on an abnormal acetabular component that overextends and can be localized (acetabular retroversion) or involve the whole acetabulum (coxa profunda or protrusio acetabuli). The pincer type is also characterized by labral degeneration caused by repeated impingement.

Subjective symptoms, and clinical and radiologic findings are the fundamental pillars to diagnose FAI syndrome. Clinical examination reveals pain in the hip region represented by the "C sign", decreased range of motion, and positivity to provocative tests (FADDIR and FABER) [8]. Radiologic findings are focused on X-ray measurements of the α angle (Figure 1c) for cam-type [1] (the angle between a line passing from the center of the femoral head to the center of the femoral neck and a second line passing from the center of the femoral head to a point where the distance from the bone to the center of the head is greater than the radius of the cartilage covered femoral head) [9] and detection of retroversion or over-coverage for pincer type [1,10].

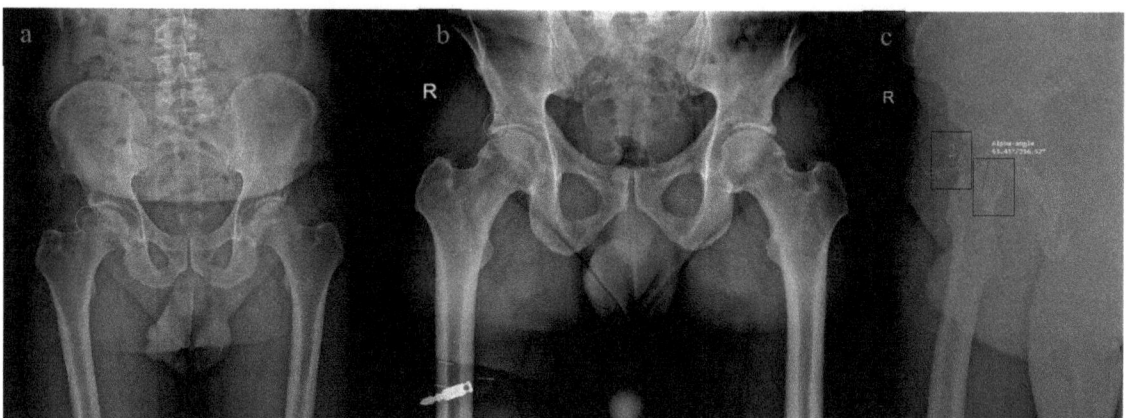

Figure 1. (**a**). FAI Cam type (**b**). FAI Pincer type (**c**). α angle in a lateral view: line 1 passing from the center of the femoral head to the center of the femoral neck and line 2 passing from the center of the femoral head to a point where the distance from the bone to the center of the head is greater than the radius of the cartilage covered femoral head.

Either surgical or conservative approaches can be proposed for treating FAI morphologies [11].

Conservative treatment mainly consists of supervised physical therapy, primarily tailored to the individual patient's needs and desired level of function. Commonly before starting the physical therapy, a detailed clinical examination is performed to assess the patient's impairments and adjust the exercise regimen that will be administered. Pain, function, and range of motion are established during the clinical examination [12,13]. During this initial evaluation, the physician has to train the patient on the condition and its management, including pain relief advice. Milestones of the therapy include joint mobilization, therapeutic exercises, soft tissue mobility, stretching, and motor control exercises. Avoiding impingement positions is also suggested. The frequency and number of exercise sessions vary among different rehabilitative centers. The exercises are usually first performed under the guidance of an experienced physiotherapist and can then be continued either in rehabilitative centers or at home [14,15]. Surgical treatment is also tailored to the patient's type of impingement and is performed arthroscopically [16,17].

Arthroscopic treatments adopted are acetabuloplasty, femoroplasty, labral repair or debridement, and treatment of articular cartilage and ligament teres lesions, depending on the type of impingement present and damage to the adjacent structures. To date, the standard of care for the treatment of FAI has not been encoded and appears urgent to better define the most congruous approach to this disease [18].

The aim of the present systematic review is to provide a comprehensive analysis of the treatment of FAI syndrome, focusing exclusively on all the published Level I evidence studies available to elucidate the difference in outcomes between surgical and non-operative management.

2. Materials and Methods

The present systematic review was performed according to "PRISMA guidelines" [Preferred Reporting Items for Systematic Reviews and Meta-analyses]. A literature search was carried out on the PubMed, EMBASE, Scopus, and PEDro databases, on June 30th, 2022, by two independent investigators, using the following keywords that were combined to achieve maximum search strategy sensitivity: "femoroacetabular impingement", "FAI", in association with: "surgery", "arthroscopy", "surgical" and "conservative", "physiotherapy", "physical therapy", "rehabilitation", "exercise". Manual research throughout the reference lists of all retrieved articles was further conducted. A PRISMA flowchart of the selection and screening method is provided in Figure 2.

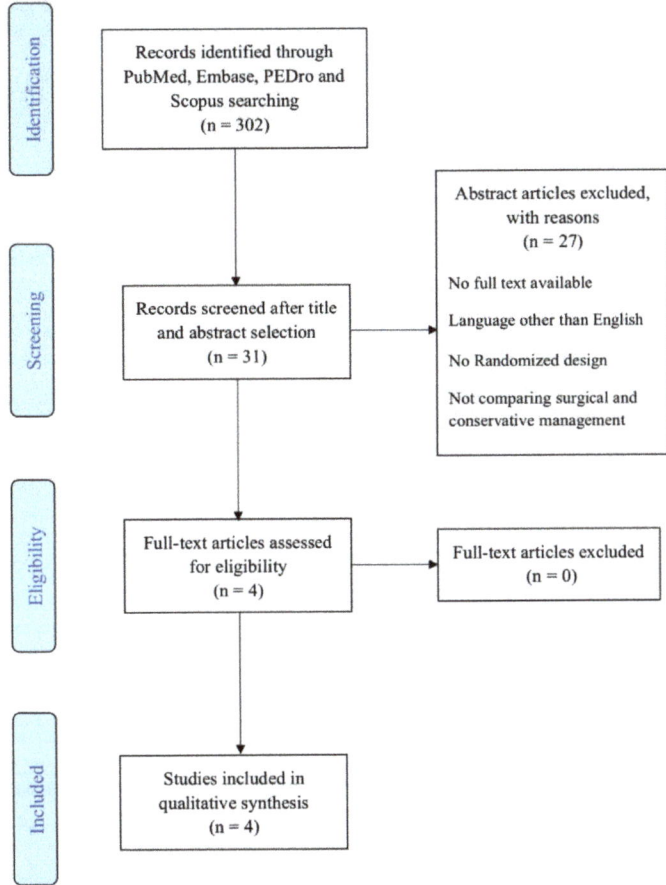

Figure 2. PRISMA Flowchart summarizing the selection process.

First, all the retrieved articles were screened by title and abstract, using the following inclusion criteria for article selection: (1) clinical reports with randomized design (level I) comparing conservative management to surgery; (2) written in the English language; (3) published from 2000 to 2022; (4) dealing with the treatment of patients affected by FAI syndrome. "Treatment" meant both surgery and conservative management, including exercise therapy, physical therapy (e.g., laser therapy, ultrasounds, shockwave therapy) and injective treatment as well. Exclusion criteria were: (1) case series or comparative non-randomized trials; (2) written in languages other than English; (3) not dealing with the treatment of FAI syndrome. We further excluded all duplicate articles, articles from nonpeer reviewed journals or articles lacking access to the full text. Conference presentations, narrative reviews, editorials, and expert opinions were also excluded. Two investigators extracted relevant data independently. The following data were extracted from each study: demographics, study design and level of evidence, follow-up times, treatment groups, evaluation scores adopted, and overall clinical findings. Discrepancies between the two reviewers were resolved by discussion and consensus, and the results were reviewed by the senior investigators. The final list of the selected studies is presented in Table 1.

Table 1. Synopsis of the main features of the RCTs included in the systematic review.

Study	Study Design	Treatment Groups	Outcome Measures	Follow-Up	Rehabilitation Program	Main Results	Comments on Results
Griffin et al. [11]	RCT	171 surgical and 177 PT	iHOT-33 EuroQol EQ-5D-5L SF-12	12mo	6 to 10 sessions over 12 to 24 weeks with physiotherapist personalized hip therapy with an assessment of pain, function, and range of hip motion; patient education; an exercise program that has the key features of individualization, progression, and supervision; help with pain relief, which could include one X-ray or ultrasound-guided intra-articular steroid injection	At 12 mo follow-up, there was a mean adjusted difference of 6·8 points in the iHOT-33 score between groups, in favor of hip arthroscopy. This is a statistically significant difference that also exceeded the minimum clinically important difference for iHOT-33.	Hip arthroscopy is more clinically effective than best conservative care
Mansell et al. [12]	RCT	38 surgical and 40 PT	HOS iHOT-33 GRC	24mo	12 sessions over 6 weeks with joint mobilizations, mobilization with motion, therapeutic exercise, soft tissue mobility, stretching, motor control exercises and home exercise program.	There was no significant difference between the surgery and no surgery groups at any time point out to 2 years on the HOS ADL and sport subscales or the iHOT-33. There was a statistically significant improvement from baseline to 1 and 2 years on the HOS ADL subscale and the iHOT-33 in the surgery group only.	Despite improvements over time, no meaningful change was perceived by most patients. A high rate of crossover to the surgery group affected the power of the study and prevents us from making definitive conclusions.
Palmer et al. [15]	RCT	112 surgical and 110 PT	HOS ADL HOS sport NAHS HAGOS OHS iHOT-33 EQ-5D-3L PainDETECT HADS	8mo	Up to 8 physiotherapy sessions over 5 mo with physiotherapist personalized hip therapy, with emphasis on improving core stability and movement control.	The mean HOS ADL in the arthroscopic surgery group was 10.0 points (95% confidence interval 6.4 to 13.6, $p = 0.001$) higher than in the physiotherapy program group at 8mo follow-up.	Patients with FAI syndrome experience a greater improvement in symptoms with arthroscopic hip surgery than with physiotherapy and activity modification at 8mo follow-up.
Hunter et al. [14]	RCT	49 surgical and 50 PT	dGEMRIC score HOAMS iHOT-33 HOOS SF-12 GIS Modified UCLA	12mo	6 PT sessions over 12 weeks. If needed 4 more PT sessions were added between 12 weeks and 6 months. 1. An individualized and progressive exercise program supervised by a physiotherapist. 2. Education about the condition and its Management. 3. Advice regarding pain relief which could include referral to the participants' General Practitioner or ultrasound-guided intra-articular steroid injection.	The primary outcome of hip cartilage metabolism dGEMRIC showed no statistically significant difference Between PHT and arthroscopic hip surgery at 12 months follow-up. the range of secondary outcomes demonstrated statistically and clinically important improvements with significance between group differences favoring surgery.	This trial adds new information that shows the patient reported benefits of surgery are not explained by nor linked to better hip cartilage metabolism at 12 months.

The quality of the randomized controlled trials (RCTs) included was assessed independently by two reviewers using the Cochrane Risk of Bias Assessment Tool. The risk of bias was assessed as a judgment (high, low, or unclear) for individual elements from seven domains, as detailed in Table 2.

Table 2. Cochrane Risk of Bias assessment for all the included studies. + Low risk of bias; − High risk of bias.

	Selection Bias Random Sequence Generation	Selection Bias Allocation Concealment	Reporting Bias Selective Reporting	Performance Bias Blinding (Participants and Personnel)	Detection Bias Blinding (Outcome Assessment)	Attrition Bias Incomplete Outcome Data	Other Bias
Griffin et al. [11]	+	+	+	−	+	+	+
Mansell et al. [12]	+	+	−	−	−	−	−
Palmer et al. [15]	+	+	+	−	+	+	+
Hunter et al. [14]	+	−	+	−	+	−	−

3. Results

In the present review, data from 749 patients were retrieved: 418 right side (55.8%) and 392 males (52.3%). Furthermore, 532 (71.0%) cases were classified as CAM impingement, 47 (6.3%) as Pincer FAI, 90 (12%) as mixed FAI and 80 cases (10.7%) were not specified. The mean follow-up was 14 months, and the weighted mean age was 34.7 years.

In the arthroscopy cluster 372 (49.7%) patients were analyzed: 213 right side (56.5%) and 190 males (51.1%). Moreover, 263 (70.7%) cases were classified as CAM impingement, 23 (6.2%) as Pincer FAI, 46 (12.4%) as mixed FAI and 40 (10.7%) cases were not specified. The weighted mean age was 34.7 years. The physiotherapy cluster accounts for 377 (50.3%) patients: 205 (54.4%) right side and 202 (53.6%) male gender; 269 (71.4%) cases were classified as CAM impingement, 24 (6.4%) as Pincer FAI, 44 (11.6%) as mixed FAI and 40 (10.6%) cases were not specified. The weighted mean age was 35.10 years.

From 749 patients enrolled in our review, only 620 (83.0%) completed the aimed follow-up: 55 (7.4%) were lost at follow-up in the arthroscopy cluster and 72 (9.6%) in the physiotherapy one. Furthermore, among all the studies included, 52 patients crossed over from conservative to surgical treatment, which represents 70% of non-surgical patients from the study conducted by Mansell et al. [12], 5% from Palmer et al. [15], 8% from Griffin et al. [11], and the 6% from Hunter et al. [14]

4. Reported Clinical Outcomes

4.1. International Hip Outcome Tool (iHOT-33)

The 33-item International Hip Outcome Tool (iHOT-33) is a questionnaire designed for self-administration which uses a visual analog scale format and can be provided to young active patients with pathologies affecting the hip.

Mansell et al. [12] reported a statistically significant improvement in iHOT-33 from baseline to 2 years in both groups, but the mean difference was not significant.

Similar results were reported by Griffin et al. [11] who documented an increase in the iHOT-33 score in both groups. Conversely to Mansell et al. [12], in the primary intention-to-treat analysis at 12 months, the iHOT-33 score was significantly higher in the hip arthroscopy group compared to the conservative group.

These results were consistent with the study by Palmer et al. [15] that confirmed a significantly higher iHOT-33 score in participants who received arthroscopic surgery compared to those who received the physiotherapy approach. Again, similar findings were found in the study by Hunter et al. [14] who showed a significant difference between the two groups at 12 months in favor of surgical treatment.

4.2. Hip Outcome Score of Daily Living (HOS-ADL) and Sports (HOS-Sports)

The Hip Outcome Score (HOS) activities of daily living (ADL) and sports subscales are self-reported outcomes with evidence of reliability and responsiveness for patients who are treated for arthroscopic hip surgery.

Mansell et al. [12] did not report any statistically significant difference between the surgery and physical therapy groups in HOS-ADL and HOS-sports at 6-month, 1-year and

2-year follow-ups. Conversely, Palmer et al. [15] found a significant difference of 10.0 points in HOS ADL in favor of the surgical group. Furthermore, 32% of patients treated in the physical therapy group and 51% of surgical patients reached the MCID (at least 9 points) in HOS-ADL, thus confirming the superior outcomes of the surgical group. Similarly, PASS (Patient acceptable symptomatic state, -defined as HOS-ADL $\geq$ 87 points-) was obtained in 19% of patients receiving physical therapy compared to 48% of patients receiving surgery.

4.3. EQ-5D 3L/5L and EQ-5D-5L-VAS

The EQ-5D 3L/5L and EQ-5D-5L-VAS are health surveys that can be used to compare improvement across different interventions by measuring changes in health-related quality of life over time.

Griffin et al. [11] found a statistically significant difference at 6 months in EQ-5D 3L/5L and EQ-5D 5L-VAS scores between the arthroscopy and conservative treatment group.

Hunter et al. [14] measured the baseline to 6-month and baseline to 12-month differences of these scores: comparing surgical and conservative groups, they reported significant improvement at 12 months relative to baseline in EQ-5D-5L, but not in EQ5D-VAS score, in favor of the surgical treatment. Finally, Palmer et al. [15] reported a statistically significant improvement at 6 months in the EQ-5D-3L index and EQ-5D-3L-VAS score in favor of arthroscopy.

4.4. Other Health-Related Scores

The global rating of change (GRC) is a score used to assess functional change over time in the clinical setting.

Mansell et al. [12] considered a GRC (Global Rating of Change) score to verify an eventual improvement of quality of life: 45.2% of patients in the arthroscopy group compared to 25.0% in the conservative treatment showed a GRC > 13, considered as the threshold for a satisfactory outcome. However, the relative risk of perceiving a statistically significant improvement was not different between the groups.

The Hip Disability and Osteoarthritis Outcome Score (HOOS) is a 40-item questionnaire used to assess patient-relevant outcomes in five separate subscales (pain, symptoms, activity of daily living, sport and recreation function and hip-related quality of life).

Hunter et al. [14] reported an improvement in the perceived quality of life in favor of the arthroscopy group compared to physiotherapy at 12 months by analyzing the Hip Disability and Osteoarthritis Outcome Score (HOOS) subscales: pain ($p = 0.001$), symptoms ($p = 0.007$), ADL ($p = 0.000$), sport ($p = 0.003$) and quality of life ($p = 0.004$). In all cases, better results were documented for the surgical group.

4.5. Delayed Gadolinium-Enhanced Magnetic Resonance Imaging (MRI) of Cartilage (dGEMRIC)

Hunter et al. [14] compared the dGEMRIC index between arthroscopy and physiotherapy groups at baseline and 12 months and showed no significant inter-group difference: although patients with symptomatic FAI experienced better outcomes after arthroscopic surgery, no imaging difference was detected to support these clinical findings.

5. Discussion

The present review highlighted the differences between surgical and conservative approaches in the treatment of femoro-acetabular impingement syndrome.

Formerly, Mok et al. [19], Dwyer et al. [20], and Gatz et al. [18] analyzed the three RCTs available until then. Our research added the latest RCT in literature (Hunter et al. [14]) and found the arthroscopic approach to be the preferred treatment for femoro-acetabular impingement syndrome in young and active patients. Our findings are comparable to results recently obtained in the work of Mahmoud et al. [21]

The subjective scores considered by the authors included iHOT-33, SF-12, EQ-5D-5L and HOS. iHot 33 is a clinical assessment tool for active patients which consists of symptoms, functional limitations, recreational activities, and sports and is, therefore, considered one of the main questionnaires to quantitatively evaluate patients' symptoms [22]. The iHOT 33 tool demonstrated significantly better results for arthroscopic treatment in three out of the four studies included. Despite these notable results in favor of arthroscopy, potential biases should not be underestimated: Mansell et al. [12] enrolled military patients, thus introducing a potential bias in the generalizability of results. The study conducted by Mansell et al. [12] suffered from a high rate of crossover to surgery, lowering the statistical power of the results coming from the non-operative group. Moreover, both arthroscopy and physical therapy are predisposed to a performance bias since the administration of treatments could induce a placebo effect. To date, no blinded study has been conducted for the treatment of FAI: indeed, ethical considerations usually prevent from receiving approval to perform sham procedures, such as merely diagnostic arthroscopy or even skin incisions, which would be necessary to blind the patients. In an attempt to overcome this flaw, one study is currently ongoing and aims to compare arthroscopic treatment to sham surgery [23].

Furthermore, the role played by post-operative rehabilitation should not be underestimated [24]. The strength of the index hip has been recently demonstrated to be inferior in flexion, extension and adduction, up to 16 weeks following the arthroscopic procedure, compared to the contralateral healthy hip [25]. Therefore, effective postoperative rehabilitation could benefit from enhancing recovery after hip arthroscopy, thus speeding up the full healing of the patient [26]. The beneficial role of the surgical procedure was evident in most of the scores analyzed and these findings are in line with other similar studies on the topic [18]. Nonetheless, even if Griffin et al. [11] and Hunter et al. [14] adopted the same physiotherapy regimen based on an International Consensus, the large heterogeneity of the rehabilitation protocols adopted and the little evidence supporting the various programs, remarkably complicate a definitive conclusion in favor of arthroscopy. Looking at our results, three out of four high-quality evidence studies suggested the superiority of the arthroscopic treatment compared to the best conservative care, yet the optimal non-surgical treatment still lacks consensus. In everyday clinical practice, conservative treatment is usually proposed as a first-line approach although different regimens are proposed. Exercises focused on core strengthening are usually administered, even if their efficacy was proven only in small cohorts with different follow-up periods [27–30]. The rationale behind physiotherapy lies in relieving pain due to impingement by allowing the strengthening of the muscles and impeding unfavorable movements. However, the exact timing of the commonly administered exercises is not known, and duration displays large variability among the studies (Mansell et al. 12 sessions [12], Palmer et al. 8 sessions [15], Griffin et al. 10 sessions [11], Hunter et al. 6 sessions [14]). The trials conducted by Griffin et al. [11] and Hunter et al. [14] allowed intra-articular corticosteroids injection for pain relief in the non-operative group, which may have garbled the outcomes.

Many authors suggested a possible association between FAI syndrome and idiopathic hip osteoarthritis [31–33]: although hip arthroscopy seemed to provide superior functional results and better pain control, there are insufficient data to support the preventive role of surgery [34]. In fact, there is limited evidence on the long-term outcomes of hip arthroscopy in terms of OA progression: surgery might be not able to delay joint degeneration and relapse of symptoms compared to conservative treatment. Any surgical procedure is indeed able to impair the joint environment, so long-term evaluation is needed to understand the real risk/benefit ratio of hip arthroscopy over time; however, larger long-term studies are usually burdensome and their prohibitive costs will most likely affect the future evidence available. Furthermore, when considering such surgical procedures, one should not neglect the possible surgery-related complications: although in the cohort of patients analyzed (total number = 395), just two had notable complications (one fracture and one septic arthritis), previous studies found an adverse event rate following hip arthroscopy in up to 5% of patients [35].

Based on these findings, the optimal treatment for FAI remains uncertain.

Although we included only randomized controlled trials, several methodological limitations must be acknowledged: first, the small number of papers selected prevents the assessment of a definitive conclusion on the best standard of care for the FAI syndrome. The number of patients studied is still too small and not representative of the real incidence of the disease in the general population, estimated to be up to 17% of patients with groin pain [26]. Furthermore, FAI includes a wide spectrum of anatomical morphologies, requiring a tailored surgical approach. In the present analysis, no stratification was made based on the different subtypes of FAI and different surgical procedures performed. Furthermore, when considering physical therapy, we need to consider the compliance of the patients, which is must higher in the context of clinical trials compared to the real-world setting, where physiotherapy regimens are often discontinued due to working or social habits of patients; therefore, in real life, the outcomes following conservative treatment might be inferior to those reported in the RCTs.

6. Conclusions

Femoro-acetabular impingement syndrome is a common cause of pain and groin dysfunction in young active adults. Both arthroscopic treatment and a proper regimen of physical therapy are effective for pain relief and restoring functional status. However, the surgical approach seems to offer superior short-term results when compared to conservative care only. Further evaluations are needed to clarify whether surgery might prevail even at middle to long-term follow-up.

Author Contributions: G.A. wrote the paper; A.I., M.G., E.M.B. contributed to writing and searching for the articles; M.M., C.S. and E.K. critically revised the manuscript, B.D.M. provided the work project, coordinated the writing, and revised the last version of the paper. All authors have read and agreed to the published version of the manuscript.

Funding: The authors received no financial support for the research, authorship, and/or publication of this article.

Conflicts of Interest: The authors declare no conflict of interest.

References

1. Griffin, D.R.; Dickenson, E.J.; O'Donnell, J.; Agricola, R.; Awan, T.; Beck, M.; Clohisy, J.C.; Dijkstra, H.P.; Falvey, E.; Gimpel, M.; et al. The Warwick Agreement on femoroacetabular impingement syndrome (FAI syndrome): An international consensus statement. *Br. J. Sports Med.* **2016**, *50*, 1169–1176. [CrossRef] [PubMed]
2. Ganz, R.; Bamert, P.; Hausner, P.; Isler, B.; Vrevc, F. Cervico-acetabular impingement after femoral neck fracture. *Unfallchirurg* **1991**, *94*, 172–175. [PubMed]
3. Myers, S.R.; Eijer, H.; Ganz, R. Anterior femoroacetabular impingement after periacetabular osteotomy. *Clin. Orthop. Relat. Res.* **1999**, *363*, 93–99. [CrossRef]
4. Ometti, M.; Schipani, D.; Conte, P.; Pironti, P.; Salini, V. The efficacy of intra-articular HYADD4-G injection in the treatment of femoroacetabular impingement: Results at one year follow up. *J. Drug Assess.* **2020**, *9*, 159–166. [CrossRef]
5. Frank, J.M.; Harris, J.D.; Erickson, B.J.; Slikker, W., III; Bush-Joseph, C.A.; Salata, M.J.; Nho, S.J. Prevalence of Femoroacetabular Impingement Imaging Findings in Asymptomatic Volunteers: A Systematic Review. *Arthroscopy* **2015**, *31*, 1199–1204. [CrossRef] [PubMed]
6. Zadpoor, A.A. Etiology of Femoroacetabular Impingement in Athletes: A Review of Recent Findings. *Sports Med.* **2015**, *45*, 1097–1106. [CrossRef] [PubMed]
7. Dimmick, S.; Stevens, K.J.; Brazier, D.; Anderson, S.E. Femoroacetabular impingement. *Radiol Clin. N. Am.* **2013**, *51*, 337–352. [CrossRef] [PubMed]
8. Dooley, P.J. Femoroacetabular impingement syndrome: Nonarthritic hip pain in young adults. *Can. Fam. Physician* **2008**, *54*, 42–47.
9. Laborie, L.B.; Lehmann, T.G.; Engesæter, I.Ø.; Sera, F.; Engesæter, L.B.; Rosendahl, K. The alpha angle in cam-type femoroacetabular impingement: New reference intervals based on 2038 healthy young adults. *Bone Joint J.* **2014**, *96*, 449–454. [CrossRef]
10. Fioruzzi, A.; Acerbi, A.; Jannelli, E.; Ivone, A.; Fontana, A. Interobserver and intraobserver reliability of a new radiological classification for femoroacetabular impingement syndrome. *Musculoskelet Surg.* **2020**, *104*, 279–284. [CrossRef]
11. Griffin, D.R.; Dickenson, E.J.; Wall, P.D.; Achana, F.; Donovan, J.L.; Griffin, J.; Hobson, R.; Hutchinson, C.E.; Jepson, M.; Parsons, N.R.; et al. Hip arthroscopy versus best conservative care for the treatment of femoroacetabular impingement syndrome (UK FASHIoN): A multicentre randomised controlled trial. *Lancet* **2018**, *391*, 2225–2235. [CrossRef]

12. Mansell, N.S.; Rhon, D.I.; Meyer, J.; Slevin, J.M.; Marchant, B.G. Arthroscopic Surgery or Physical Therapy for Patients with Femoroacetabular Impingement Syndrome: A Randomized Controlled Trial With 2-Year Follow-up. *Am. J. Sports Med.* **2018**, *46*, 1306–1314. [CrossRef] [PubMed]
13. Mansell, N.S.; Rhon, D.I.; Marchant, B.G.; Slevin, J.M.; Meyer, J.L. Two-year outcomes after arthroscopic surgery compared to physical therapy for femoracetabular impingement: A protocol for a randomized clinical trial. *BMC Musculoskelet. Disord.* **2016**, *17*, 60. [CrossRef] [PubMed]
14. Hunter, D.J.; Eyles, J.; Murphy, N.J.; Spiers, L.; Burns, A.; Davidson, E.; Dickenson, E.; Fary, C.; Foster, N.E.; Fripp, J.; et al. Multi-centre randomised controlled trial comparing arthroscopic hip surgery to physiotherapist-led care for femoroacetabular impingement (FAI) syndrome on hip cartilage metabolism: The Australian FASHIoN trial. *BMC Musculoskelet. Disord.* **2021**, *22*, 697. [CrossRef] [PubMed]
15. Palmer, A.J.; Gupta, V.A.; Fernquest, S.; Rombach, I.; Dutton, S.J.; Mansour, R.; Wood, S.; Khanduja, V.; Pollard, T.C.; McCaskie, A.W.; et al. Arthroscopic hip surgery compared with physiotherapy and activity modification for the treatment of symptomatic femoroacetabular impingement: Multicentre randomised controlled trial. *BMJ* **2019**, *364*, 185. [CrossRef]
16. Hartwell, M.J.; Morgan, A.M.; Nelson, P.A.; Fernandez, C.E.; Nicolay, R.W.; Sheth, U.; Tjong, V.K.; Terry, M.A. Isolated Acetabuloplasty for Femoroacetabular Impingement: Favorable Patient-Reported Outcomes and Sustained Survivorship at Minimum 5-Year Follow-Up. *Arthroscopy* **2021**, *37*, 3288–3294. [CrossRef]
17. Byrd, J.W.T.; Jones, K.S. Arthroscopic femoroplasty in the management of cam-type femoroacetabular impingement. *Clin. Orthop. Relat. Res.* **2009**, *467*, 739–746. [CrossRef]
18. Gatz, M.; Driessen, A.; Eschweiler, J.; Tingart, M.; Migliorini, F. Arthroscopic surgery versus physiotherapy for femoroacetabular impingement: A meta-analysis study. *Eur. J. Orthop. Surg. Traumatol.* **2020**, *30*, 1151–1162. [CrossRef]
19. Mok, T.N.; He, Q.Y.; Teng, Q.; Sin, T.H.; Wang, H.J.; Zha, Z.G.; Zheng, X.F.; Pan, J.H.; Hou, H.G.; Li, J.R. Arthroscopic Hip Surgery versus Conservative Therapy on Femoroacetabular Impingement Syndrome: A Meta-Analysis of RCTs. *Orthop Surg.* **2021**, *13*, 1755–1764. [CrossRef]
20. Dwyer, T.; Whelan, D.; Shah, P.S.; Ajrawat, P.; Hoit, G.; Chahal, J. Operative Versus Nonoperative Treatment of Femoroacetabular Impingement Syndrome: A Meta-analysis of Short-Term Outcomes. *Arthroscopy* **2022**, *36*, 263–273, Erratum in *Arthroscopy* **2021**, *37*, 784. [CrossRef]
21. Mahmoud, S.S.S.; Takla, A.; Meyer, D.; Griffin, D.; O'Donnell, J. Arthroscopic hip surgery offers better early patient-reported outcome measures than targeted physiotherapy programs for the treatment of femoroacetabular impingement syndrome: A systematic review and meta-analysis of randomized controlled trials. *J. Hip. Preserv. Surg.* **2022**, *9*, 107–118. [CrossRef] [PubMed]
22. Mohtadi, N.G.; Griffin, D.R.; Pedersen, M.E.; Chan, D.; Safran, M.R.; Parsons, N.; Sekiya, J.K.; Kelly, B.T.; Werle, J.R.; Leunig, M.; et al. The Development and validation of a self-administered quality-of-life outcome measure for young, active patients with symptomatic hip disease: The International Hip Outcome Tool (iHOT-33). *Arthroscopy* **2012**, *28*, 595–605. [CrossRef] [PubMed]
23. Risberg, M.A.; Ageberg, E.; Nilstad, A.; Lund, B.; Nordsletten, L.; Løken, S.; Ludvigsen, T.; Kierkegaard, S.; Carsen, S.; Kostogiannis, I.; et al. Arthroscopic Surgical Procedures Versus Sham Surgery for Patients with Femoroacetabular Impingement and/or Labral Tears: Study Protocol for a Randomized Controlled Trial (HIPARTI) and a Prospective Cohort Study (HARP). *J. Orthop. Sports Phys. Ther.* **2018**, *48*, 325–335. [CrossRef]
24. Bennell, K.L.; Spiers, L.; Takla, A.; O'Donnell, J.; Kasza, J.; Hunter, D.J.; Hinman, R.S. Efficacy of adding a physiotherapy rehabilitation programme to arthroscopic management of femoroacetabular impingement syndrome: A randomised controlled trial (FAIR). *BMJ* **2017**, *7*, e014658. [CrossRef] [PubMed]
25. Wierks, C.H.; Boersma, J.B.; Pate, M.J.; Davis, A.T. Hip Strength Before and After Arthroscopic Femoroacetabular Impingement Surgery. *Orthopedics* **2021**, *44*, 148–153. [CrossRef] [PubMed]
26. O'Connor, M.; Minkara, A.A.; Westermann, R.W.; Rosneck, J.; Lynch, T.S. Return to Play After Hip Arthroscopy: A Systematic Review and Meta-analysis. *Am. J. Sports Med.* **2018**, *46*, 2780–2788. [CrossRef]
27. Harris-Hayes, M.; Czuppon, S.; Van Dillen, L.R.; Steger-May, K.; Sahrmann, S.; Schootman, M.; Salsich, G.B.; Clohisy, J.C.; Mueller, M.J. Movement-Pattern Training to Improve Function in People With Chronic Hip Joint Pain: A Feasibility Randomized Clinical Trial. *J. Orthop. Sports Phys. Ther.* **2016**, *46*, 452–461. [CrossRef]
28. Kemp, J.L.; Coburn, S.L.; Jones, D.M.; Crossley, K.M. The Physiotherapy for Femoracetabular Impingement Rehabilitation STudy (physioFIRST): A Pilot Randomized Controlled Trial. *J. Orthop. Sports Phys. Ther.* **2018**, *48*, 307–315. [CrossRef]
29. Smeatham, A.; Powell, R.; Moore, S.; Chauhan, R.; Wilson, M. Does treatment by a specialist physiotherapist change pain and function in young adults with symptoms from femoroacetabular impingement? A pilot project for a randomised controlled trial. *Physiotherapy* **2017**, *103*, 201–207. [CrossRef]
30. Röling, M.A.; Mathijssen, N.M.C.; Bloem, R.M. Incidence of symptomatic femoroacetabular impingement in the general population: A prospective registration study. *J. Hip. Preserv. Surg.* **2016**, *3*, 203–207. [CrossRef]
31. Ganz, R.; Parvizi, J.; Beck, M.; Leunig, M.; Nötzli, H.; Siebenrock, K.A. Femoroacetabular impingement: A cause for osteoarthritis of the hip. *Clin. Orthop. Relat. Res.* **2003**, *417*, 112–120. [CrossRef] [PubMed]
32. Tannast, M.; Goricki, D.; Beck, M.; Murphy, S.B.; Siebenrock, K.A. Hip damage occurs at the zone of femoroacetabular impingement. *Clin. Orthop. Relat. Res.* **2008**, *466*, 273–280. [CrossRef] [PubMed]

33. Condello, V.; Zdanowicz, U.; Di Matteo, B.; Spalding, T.; Gelber, P.E.; Adravanti, P.; Heuberer, P.; Dimmen, S.; Sonnery-Cottet, B.; Hulet, C.; et al. Allograft tendons are a safe and effective option for revision ACL reconstruction: A clinical review. *Knee Surg. Sports Traumatol. Arthrosc.* **2019**, *27*, 1771–1781. [CrossRef] [PubMed]
34. Collins, J.A.; Ward, J.P.; Youm, T. Is prophylactic surgery for femoroacetabular impingement indicated? A systematic review. *Am. J. Sports Med.* **2014**, *42*, 3009–3015. [CrossRef] [PubMed]
35. Matsuda, D.K.; Carlisle, J.C.; Arthurs, S.C.; Wierks, C.H.; Philippon, M.J. Comparative systematic review of the open dislocation, mini-open, and arthroscopic surgeries for femoroacetabular impingement. *Arthroscopy* **2011**, *27*, 252–269. [CrossRef]

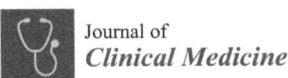

Article

Custom-Made 3D-Printed Implants for Anterior Column Reconstruction in the Upper Cervical Spine after Intralesional Extracapsular Excision—Report of 2 Cases and Literature Review

Marco Girolami [1], Cristiana Griffoni [1,*], Emanuela Asunis [1], Luigi Falzetti [1], Stefano Bandiera [1], Giovanni Barbanti Brodano [1], Riccardo Ghermandi [1], Valerio Pipola [1], Silvia Terzi [1], Eleonora Pesce [1], Donato Monopoli Forleo [2], Marco Cianchetti [3], Maria Rosaria Fiore [4], Livio Presutti [5,6], Milena Fini [7] and Alessandro Gasbarrini [1]

1   Department of Spine Surgery, IRCCS Istituto Ortopedico Rizzoli, 40136 Bologna, Italy
2   Instituto Tecnológico de Canarias (ITC), 35003 Las Palmas Gran Canaria, Spain
3   Proton Therapy Unit, Hospital of Trento, Azienda Provinciale per i Servizi Sanitari (APSS), 38122 Trento, Italy
4   Radiotherapy Unit, National Center of Oncological Hadrontherapy (CNAO), 27100 Pavia, Italy
5   Otolaryngology and Audiology Unit, IRCCS Azienda Ospedaliero-Universitaria Policlinico di Sant'Orsola, 40138 Bologna, Italy
6   Department of Experimental, Diagnostic and Specialty Medicine—DIMES, Alma Mater Studiorum University, 40126 Bologna, Italy
7   Scientific Direction, IRCCS Istituto Ortopedico Rizzoli, 40136 Bologna, Italy
*   Correspondence: cristiana.griffoni@ior.it; Tel.: +39-0516366130

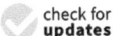

Abstract: The use of three-dimensional (3D)-printed custom-made implants is spreading in the orthopedics field for the reconstruction of bone losses or for joint replacement, thanks to their unparalleled versatility. In particular, this novel technology opens new perspectives to formulate custom-made fixation strategies for the upper cervical region, sacrum and pelvis, where reconstruction is challenging. We report and analyze the literature concerning upper cervical reconstruction with 3D-printed personalized implants after tumor surgery, and discuss two cases of patients where this technology was used to reconstruct the anterior column after extracapsular debulking of C2 recurrent chordoma at our institution.

Keywords: 3D-printing; anterior reconstruction; upper cervical region

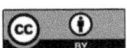

1. Introduction

In the past three decades, there have been tremendous technical and technological advances that have profoundly changed spine surgery, allowing what seemed to be impossible before. The spread of rigid segmental fixation paved the way for more complex reconstructions, thus, allowing more aggressive approaches in the treatment of primary bone tumors. Given the encouraging results achieved in terms of local control and overall survival, increasing interest has grown towards more refined reconstructions of the spine.

The advent of three-dimensional (3D) printing techniques, also known as additive manufacturing, with their unparalleled versatility, have offered a very attractive prospective in the reconstruction of substance losses, such as those produced by the resection of musculoskeletal neoplasms [1].

Three-dimensional printing refers to the process of fabricating a physical model through successive layering of powder-like materials (including Ti6Al4V, cobalt-chromium alloy, and stainless steel) based on a volumetric digital image generated by computer-aided design (CAD). It can fabricate an implant tailored to the specific anatomy of the individual patient in a controllable manner to enhance the primary immediate postoperative stability. It can also produce size-controllable micropore structures, which can lower the elastic modulus of the metals, decrease the stress at the solid parts of the implant, and promote integration between metal and bone at the contact surface.

We recently reported a prospective observational study on custom-made 3D-printed titanium reconstruction of vertebral bodies performed in 13 patients who underwent en bloc resection for primary spinal tumors [2]. The results from this series suggested that 3D printing can be effectively used to produce custom-made prosthesis for anterior column reconstruction.

In particular, the upper cervical region has a unique biomechanical function that makes reconstruction in this region challenging. Instrumentation-related complications, such as construct subsidence, migration, and pseudoarthrosis are common due to the lack of an optimal implant. Thus, the novel 3D technology is helpful for spine surgeons to perform safer and more adequately planned cervical surgeries.

We present here two cases of patients affected by C2 chordoma treated by means of extracapsular debulking and reconstruction of the spine with customized 3D-printed prosthesis.

A chordoma is a low-grade, slow-growing but locally invasive and locally aggressive tumor that belongs to the sarcoma family of tumors. Chordomas arise from remnants of the notochord and occur along the midline spinal axis between the clivus and the sacrum, anterior to the spinal cord. The location distribution of chordomas is 50% sacral, 35% skull base, and 15% occur in the vertebral bodies of the mobile spine (most commonly the C2 vertebrae followed by the lumbar then thoracic spine). Overall 5-year survival is approximately 50%, and treatment is en bloc surgical resection (if technically feasible) followed by high-dose conformal radiation therapy such as proton beam radiation [3].

2. Materials and Methods

In 2017 and 2018, two patients with C2 chordoma (Enneking stage IB), underwent extracapsular debulking at our institution, with upper cervical reconstruction using customized 3D-printed vertebral bodies. Demographic data of the two patients are reported in Table 1.

Table 1. Patients' demographics.

Patient	Age (Years), Sex	Diagnosis	Enneking	WBB	Previous Treatments	Approach	Margin	Local Control (Months)	Overall Survival (Months)	Oncological Status
1	65, M	Recurrent chordoma C2	IB	8-5/A-D	RT (70.4 Gy carbon-ion, $\Delta t = 4$ y) Extracapsular debulking and reconstruction w/ allograft and carbon-fiber buttress plate ($\Delta t = 2$ y)	A	Intralesional	18	20	DOC
2	75, M	Recurrent chordoma C2	IB	8-3/A-D	Extracapsular debulking ($\Delta t = 8$ m) RT (74 Gy proton-ion, $\Delta t = 2$ m)	A+P	Intralesional	12	32	DOD

RT, radiation therapy; DOD, died of the disease; DOC, died of complications.

Design of the Implant

Prior to surgery, the design of the prosthesis started from a preoperative thin-cut (1–1.5 mm) computed tomography (CT) that allowed evaluation of the patient-specific anatomy such as shape, width, and length of the endplates, to the extent of the planned resection. Based on these data, a CAD model of the spine was generated, and a virtual implant was designed.

The virtual model was visualized prior to production, to allow further refinements (i.e., fixation technique) until the production of the final version of the prosthesis. Finally, the approved model was fabricated by successive layering of melted Ti_6Al_4V powder (Arcam AB, Mölndal, Sweden). The design and the fabrication of the implant were performed at Instituto Tecnològico de Canarias, Las Palmas, Spain, in a time span that was kept within

2 weeks from initial consultation with the senior author (AG). The images showing this procedure are reported as Supplementary Materials.

3. Results

3.1. Case Report 1

The first case that we report, is of a 65-year-old man in whom a local recurrence of chordoma was detected at the site of an extracapsular debulking (and reconstruction with allograft stabilized with a carbon plate) at C2 that he underwent 2 years before. That first surgical treatment had been performed due to local progression after heavy-particles radiation therapy (70.4 Gy/16 ft. of carbon-ion) that the patient underwent 2 years before that surgery. MRI showed (Figure 1) recurrence of the tumor in the site of the previous surgery, surrounding the fibular graft and the plate (Figure 2), extending into the epidural space (Bilski grade 1C). Vertebral arteries (layer F) were not involved by the tumor as well as the posterior elements.

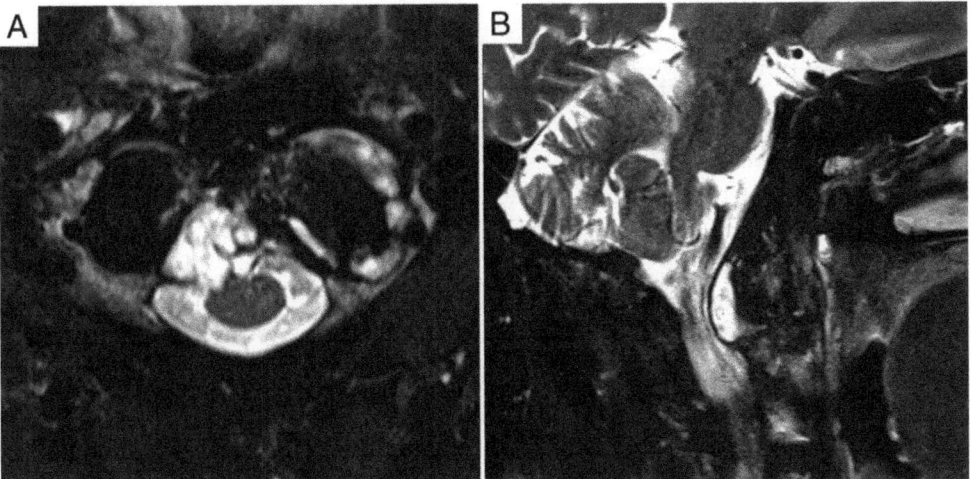

Figure 1. Case report 1: pre-operative MRI. (**A**) Axial view showing Bilski grade 1C epidural involvement. (**B**) Sagittal view showing extracompartimental extension.

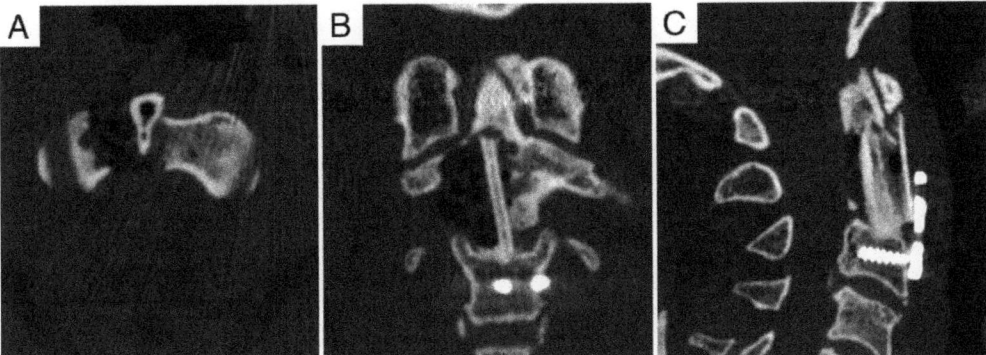

Figure 2. Case report 1: previous reconstruction of the anterior column with fibular graft and buttress plating. (**A**) Axial view. (**B**) Coronal view. (**C**) Sagittal view.

Despite these findings, the patient was complaining of only mild neck pain and was neurologically intact. Revision surgery consisted of hardware (and graft) removal and extracapsular tumor debulking through a single anterior submandibular extraoral-retropharyngeal pre-vascular approach [4]. A custom-made titanium 3D-printed prosthesis was used for reconstruction (Figure 3) (see Section 3.3 for details). Post-operative course was uneventful, and the patient was able to return to work (dentist) after 4 weeks. Pathological examination of the surgical specimen confirmed the diagnosis of CHO without evidence of de-differentiation.

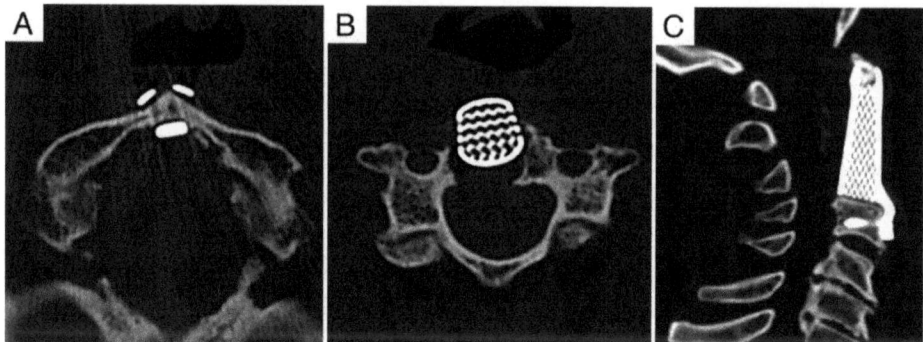

Figure 3. Case report 1: post-operative CT-scan. (**A**,**B**) Axial views, showing the prosthesis and its hooking to C1. (**C**) Sagittal view.

At 3, 6, 9 and 12 months follow-up, the implant showed good stability suggesting firm osteointegration (Figure 4). At 18 months follow up, a second recurrence of tumor was detected for which another revision surgery was performed for tumor debulking and spinal cord decompression through a double (anterior and posterior) approach (Figure 5). This allowed exploration of the implant–bone interface and direct visualization from which strong osteointegration could be confirmed. The patient experienced a severe neurological complication (ischemic brain injury) due to a major intraoperative vascular injury of carotid artery. The patient died after 2 months for the sequelae of the surgery.

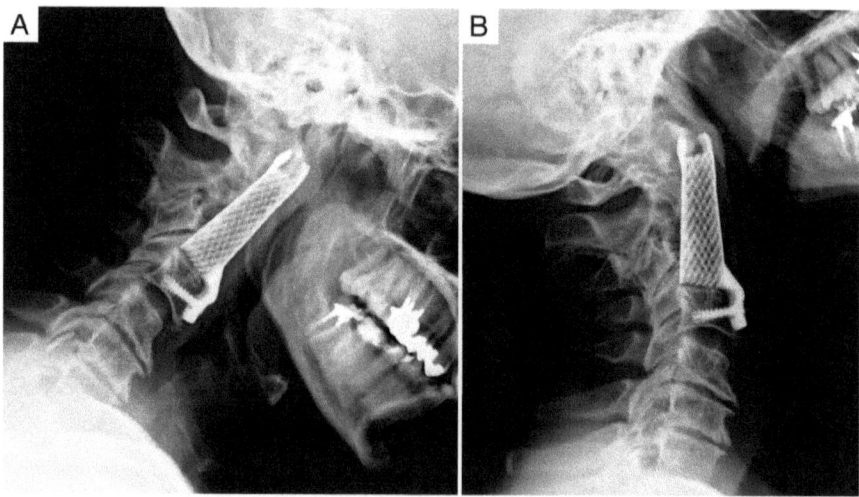

Figure 4. Case report 1: follow up at 9 months. (**A**,**B**) Dynamic X-rays showing no subsidence or displacement of the implant and stability of the spine.

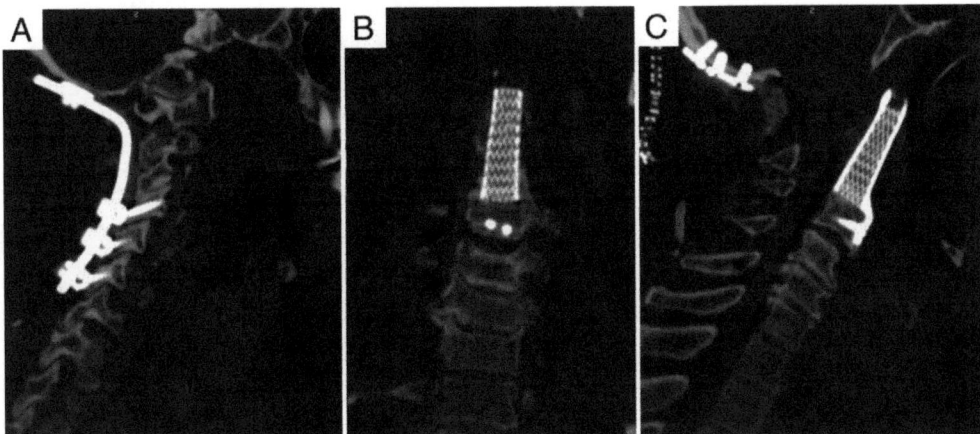

Figure 5. Case report 1: post-operative CT scan after revision. (**A**) Posterior instrumented C0-C6 fixation. (**B**,**C**) 3D-printed implant firmly osteo-integrated.

3.2. Case Report 2

The second case that we report, is of a 75-year-old man in whom a recurrent C2 chordoma progressed locally despite heavy-particles radiation therapy (74 Gy/37 ft. of proton-ion). The patient had already been submitted to extracapsular debulking (without reconstruction), after frozen-section diagnosis of chordoma, 6 months before the radiation therapy. The CT scan showed pathological fracture due to progression of disease (Figure 6).

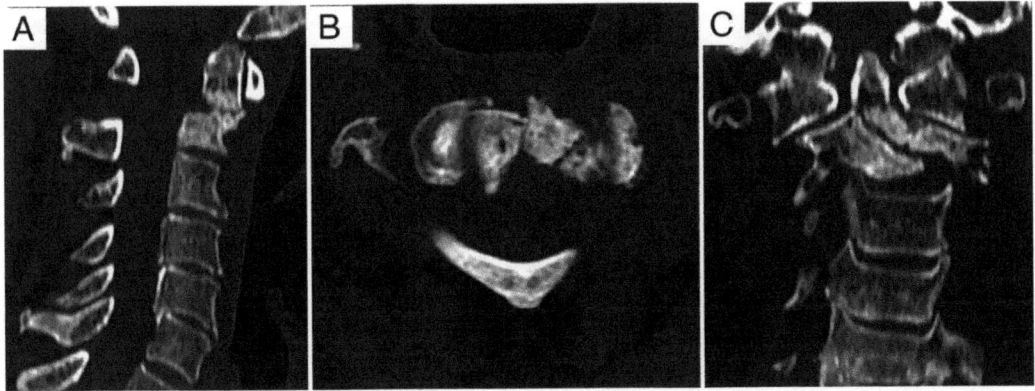

Figure 6. Case report 2: pre-operative CT. Pathological C2 fracture after surgery and radiation therapy for chordoma. (**A**) Sagittal view. (**B**) Axial view. (**C**) Coronal view.

MRI showed the lesion replacing the vertebral body and the *dens*, extending into the posterior elements via the pedicles and extracompartimentally both into the epidural space causing spinal cord compression (Bilski grade 2) and in the prevertebral (layer A) space. Vertebral arteries (layer F) were not involved by the tumor (Figure 7).

Despite these findings, physical examination showed only chronic sequelae (mild swallowing deficit, right facial nerve palsy and mild ataxia) of a previous right cerebellar infarction that the patient suffered from 20 years before.

Taking into account the involvement of both the anterior and posterior columns, revision surgery was planned to be performed through a double (anterior and posterior) approach. The first stage consisted of tumor debulking, ventral decompression of the spinal cord and anterior column reconstruction with a custom-made titanium 3D-printed prosthesis (see Section 3.3 for details) thorough an anterior submandibular extraoral-retropharyngeal pre-vascular approach [4]. The second stage consisted of posterior decompression, debulking of the posterior extension of the tumor and occiput to C4 instrumented fusion with occipital plate and lateral mass screws (Figure 8). Post-operative course was uneventful.

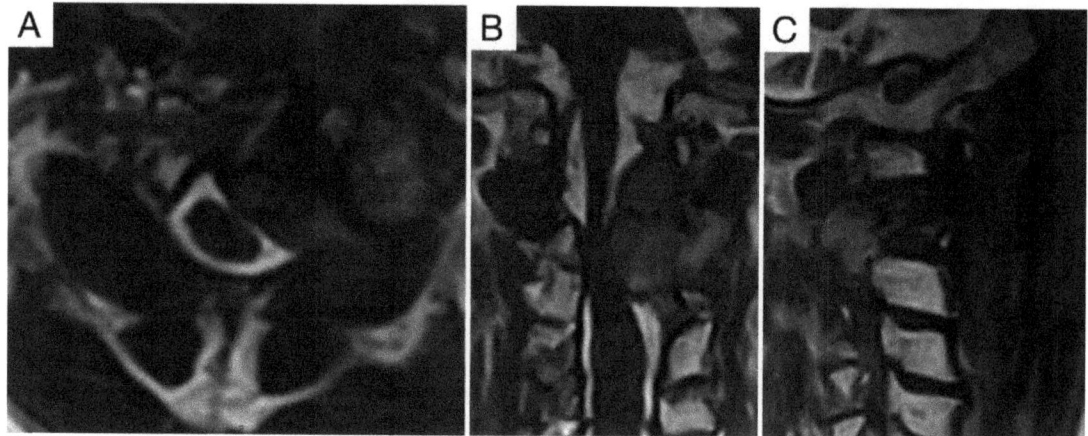

Figure 7. Case report 2: pre-operative MRI. (**A**) Axial view showing Bilski grade 2 epidural involvement (thus, causing spinal cord compression). (**B**) Coronal view. (**C**) Sagittal view.

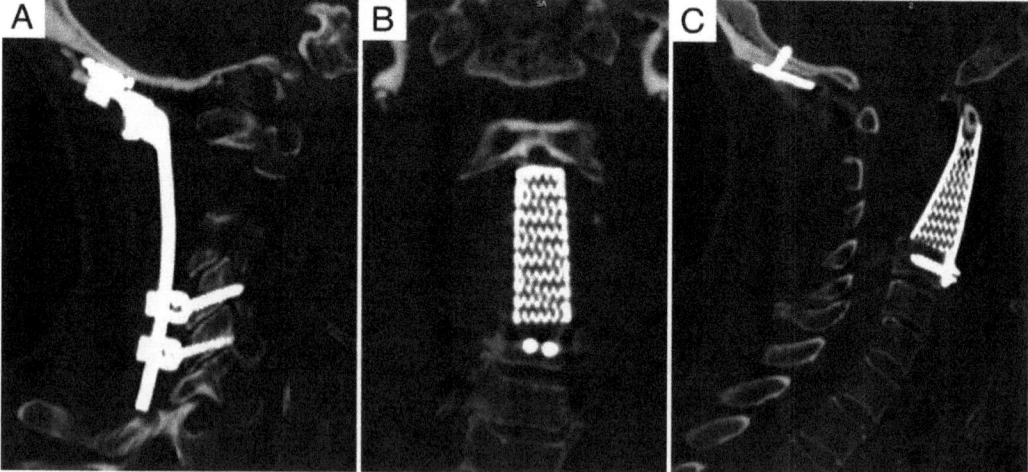

Figure 8. Case report 2: post-operative CT scan. (**A**) Posterior instrumented occipito–cervical fixation. (**B,C**) Anterior column reconstruction with 3D-printed custom made prothesis: distal fixation in C3 with integrated plate–screw system stabilized to the implant, proximal fixation obtained with a saddle that fitted the anterior arch of C1.

At 6 and 12 month follow-ups, CT-scan and X-ray showed good stability of the implant from which osteointegration can be assumed. The patient died 32 months after the surgery.

3.3. Reconstruction

In both cases, after thorough extracapsular tumour debulking, reconstruction was performed with a custom-made 3D-printed titanium implant.

The prosthesis was inserted accommodating the anterior arch of C1 into a saddle (proximally) and with progressively increasing length until slight distraction of the anterior column could be felt, indicative of a good fitting. Distally, the base of the implant was laid on the upper endplate of the adjacent vertebral body (C3) to which it was secured with two convergent screws through an integrated anterior plate.

To ensure proper fitting of the prosthesis, a series of three implants was produced for each case: one of the expected length (measured on the preoperative CT scan), one shorter by 2 mm, and one longer by 2 mm.

4. Discussion

In this study, we assessed the effectiveness and safety of spinal reconstruction using customized 3D-printed patient-specific implants in the upper cervical region in two patients affected by C2 chordoma. It might appear to be misleading to compare the present report of the treatment of chordoma, with others that include other primary bone tumors of spinal metastases. However, because of the complex regional anatomy of the high cervical spine (which includes important and functionally relevant structures such as vertebral arteries, esophagus, trachea, spinal cord and cervical spinal nerves) en-bloc resection with wide/marginal *tumor-free* margins (which would be the recommended treatment for malignant primary bone tumors, such as chordoma or chondrosarcoma) is technically unfeasible in most cases. Therefore, intralesional extracapsular (or gross total) excision remains the only reasonable option, thus, bridging the gap in the surgical treatment of such different entities. These limitations to fulfill oncologic appropriateness, along with the difficult exposure (that makes incomplete excisions more likely) explains why oncological outcomes (local control and overall survival) tend to be poorer for primary bone tumors arising in this region. Since oncologic outcomes of the treatment of chordoma goes beyond the scope of the present report, they are briefly summarized in Table 1.

Anterior column reconstruction at this level is as well limited by the same constraints, especially, achievement of a reliable and firm proximal fixation might be hard to obtain, thus, making additional posterior stabilization indispensable. Several techniques have been described such as fashioning of the proximal end of a bone graft (auto- or allogenic) into the shape of a clothespin, along with a proper length selection, as the most classical way to achieve primary stability [4]. In this way a saddle is created into which the anterior arch of C1 can be accommodated.

In case reconstruction is performed with a mesh cage, it can be opened and shaped as a "T" allowing an analogous saddle mechanism and, at the same time, creating a plate through which screws can be inserted (into the anterior arch or directed to the lateral masses) to provide more rigid fixation [5,6].

The same fixation strategy can be used when a plate is used with a neutralizing principle, but it can be limited if C1 has to be excised as well, since the thickness of the clivus is such that only very short screws can be inserted [7].

Alternatively, plates can be used with a buttress principle and fixated only distally to limit migration of the graft/mesh cage.

Anecdotal use of full thickness osteo-cutaneous flaps has been reported, particularly after radiotherapy [8].

Three-dimensional printing technology opened a crack to the development of custom-made fixation strategies, this being particularly intriguing in the upper cervical spine, as in the sacrum and pelvis.

In both the reported cases, a titanium prosthesis was taken into consideration for the reconstruction (allowing a tailored solution for proximal fixation), since further radiation was prevented by having already reached spinal cord tolerance.

A total of 26 cases of cervical spine reconstruction using personalized 3D-printed prosthesis after debulking (for both primary and metastatic tumors) were reported in 11 papers listed in the PubMed database (search: "cervical C2 tumor reconstruction") between 1 January 2016 and 30 August 2022 (Table 2). The most common proximal fixation strategy reported was by including trajectories for divergent screws in the lateral masses of C1 within the implant (four reports), or through integrated plates (one report), while only one reported the use of a "saddle". In those cases where C1 had been excised, completely or partially, because infiltrated by the tumor, primary stability was achieved using the occipital condyles as a proximal point of fixation (two reports) or, through an integrated plate, on the clivus (one report). For reconstructions below C2, the reported strategies for fixation became the same as those used distally: at least two screws into the vertebral body through the implants, or through integrated plates (one report each).

In addition to these macroscopic details, it must be considered that the progressive layering process allows production of a lattice structure of such regularity and with predetermined surface characteristics that the potential for bone ingrowth is high, leaving only a minimal percentage (up to <10%) of the actual volume of the implant being occupied by titanium.

All the authors described combined (anterior–posterior, or posterior–anterior) approaches, most frequently staging the procedures. Surgical planning is primarily to be taken depending to the local extension of the disease, but additional posterior approach might be not necessary for stability if a 3D-printed implant is used. Of the reported cases, one underwent excision and reconstruction through a single anterior approach and did not experience any mechanical consequence.

Mismatch between the size of the implant and that of the gap produced by the resection might be an unsolvable problem with 3D-printed implants. To overcome this potential problem we produced three differently sized implants of 2 mm height increase. Other authors [10,13,14,16,17] were reported to have produced more implants of different sizes ranging from 2 [14] to 32 [10]. This needs to be taken into consideration in an eventual cost-effectiveness analysis on the use of 3D-printed implants [20,21].

The role of 3D-printing is growing both in orthopedics and neurosurgery. Among the benefits of 3D-printing, it must be mentioned that it requires detailed planning preoperatively and commits surgeons to its meticulous respect. Furthermore, this same technology can be used to produce models that can be used for patient counselling, or training for follow up, or even experienced surgeons [22–24].

Table 2. Literature review.

Authors	Year	Article Type	n	Diagnosis	Age, Sex	Previous Treatments	Surgical Treatment	Approach	Adjuvant Treatments	Proximal Fixation	Distal Fixation	Follow-Up
Xu N et al. [9]	2016	Case report	1	C2 Ewing sarcoma	12, M	None	Single-level (C2) IL spondylectomy	P (C0-C6) + A (extraoral retropharyngeal) staged (2 weeks)	CHT + RT	Divergent TI-screws in C1 lateral masses	Titanium wiring in DVB (C3; TI-screws insertion not possible)	1 year
Li X et al. [10]	2017	Case report	1	C2-C3-C4 thyroid ca. metastasis	53, F	None	3-level (C2-C4) IL corpectomy + thyroidectomy and lateral lymph nodes dissection	A and P (C1-C6)	Radioiodine I[131]	Divergent TI-screws in C1 lateral masses	2 TI-screws in DVB (C5)	1 year
Mobbs RJ et al. [11]	2017	Case report	1	C1-C2 chordoma	63, M	CT-guided transoral biopsy	2-level (C1-C2) IL excision	P (C0-C3) and A (transoral)	RT	2 TiP-screws in the clivus	2 TI-screws in DVB (C3)	9 months
He S et al. [12]	2019	Case report	1	C2-C7 chondrosarcoma	27	Posterior open biopsy	6-level (C2-C7) IL en bloc resection	P (C0-T2) and A (retropharyngeal) staged (1 week)	Local cisplatinum intra-op.	Divergent TI-screws in C1 lateral masses	2 TiP-screws in DVB (T1)	14 months
He S et al. [13]	2019	Case series	7	C1-C3 (4 patients) C1-C2 (3 patients) - 5 chordoma - 1 Langerhans cell histiocytosis - 1 plasmocytoma	Average 47.6 ± 19.0 (range 12–72)	---	Multi-level IL spondylectomy (4 3-level, 3 2-level)	P and A (retropharyngeal) staged	---	TI-screws in occipital condyles	2 TiP-screws in DVB	Average 14.8 (range 7.3–24.2)
Parr WHC et al. [14]	2020	Case report	1	C3-C4-C5 chordoma	45, M	CT-guided biopsy	3-level IL spondylectomy	P (C2-C6) and A staged (3 days)	RT (proton-beam)	2 TI-screws in C2	2 TI-screws in DVB (C6)	17 months
Li Y et al. [15]	2020	Case report	1	C1 plasmocytoma	57, M	CT-guided transoral biopsy	IL tumor debulking	A (retropharyngeal) and P (C0-C3)	RT (57 Gy/27 fr.)	1 TI-screw in occipital condyle	1 TI- and 1 TiP-screw in DVB (C2)	(Not reported)

Table 2. Cont.

Authors	Year	Article Type	n	Diagnosis	Age, Sex	Previous Treatments	Surgical Treatment	Approach	Adjuvant Treatments	Proximal Fixation	Distal Fixation	Follow-Up
Wei F et al. [16]	2020	Case series	9	7 C2 2 C2-C3 - 4 giant cell tumor - 2 chordoma - 1 Ewing sarcoma - 1 paraganglioma - 1 hemangioendothelioma	Average 31.4 (range 12–59)	CT-guided biopsy	Single- and multi-level IL spondylectomy	P (4 cases to C0, 5 to C1) and A (retropharyngeal) staged (average 14.4 days)	RT, CHT (in 2 cases)	Divergent TI-screws in C1 lateral masses	2 TIP-screws in DVB (not possible in 2 cases)	Average 28.6 (range 12–42)
Yang X et al. [17]	2020	Case report	1	C3-C4-C5-C6-C7-T1 chordoma	40, F	2 tumor debulkings	6-level IL extracapsular excision	A (retropharyngeal) and P (C1-T3)	None	3 TIP-screws in vertebral body of C2	3 TIP-screws in DVB (T2)	9 months
Hunn SAM et al. [18]	2020	Case report	2	C2 thyroid ca. metastasis	56, F	None	Single-level (C2) IL corpectomy	A (retropharyngeal) and P (C1-C3)	RT and CHT	2 TIP-screws in C1 lateral masses	3 TIP-screws in DVB (C3)	14 months
				C2-C3 myeloma	63, M	None	2-level (C2-C3) IL corpectomy	and P (C1-C4)	(Not reported)		3 TIP-screws in DVB (C4)	4 months
Baldassarre BM et al. [19]	2021	Case report	1	C1-C2 chordoma	45	Biopsy	IL excision	P (C0-C4) and A (retropharyngeal) staged (1 day)	RT (proton beam)	Saddle for anterior arch of C1	2 TIP-screws in DVB (C3)	12 months

CHT, chemotherapy; RT, radiation therapy; IL, intralesional; TI, through-the-implant (0-profile); TIP, through integrated plate; DVB, distal vertebral body.

5. Conclusions

Location of spinal tumors in the upper cervical spine provides challenges both for tumor excision, since satisfactory exposure is difficult to achieve (often requiring multiple approaches), and reconstruction, especially for proximal fixation. Three dimensional printing allowed the reported authors to design patient-specific solutions, not only for shape and size of the implants, but also for the method to achieve proximal fixation. Despite this, in cases of tumor extension to posterior elements, anterior fixation alone is limited, and posterior stabilization is generally required.

Supplementary Materials: The following supporting information can be downloaded at: https://www.mdpi.com/article/10.3390/jcm11206058/s1, File S1: Brochure of the implant for cervical reconstruction.

Author Contributions: Conceptualization, M.G.; validation, L.F.; investigation, M.G., E.P.; resources, M.G., S.B., R.G., G.B.B., V.P., S.T., D.M.F., M.C., M.R.F.; writing—original draft preparation, C.G., E.A.; writing—review and editing, M.G., C.G., L.F.; visualization, C.G., E.A.; supervision, L.P., M.F., A.G.; funding acquisition, M.F. All authors have read and agreed to the published version of the manuscript.

Funding: This study was partly funded by National Funding Organizations (Ministero della Salute—IMH) under the framework of the EuroNanoMed III Project "Next generation antibacterial nanostructured osseointegrated customized vertebral replacement—NANOVERTEBRA" Joint Transnational call for proposals (JTC 2018).

Institutional Review Board Statement: Data were collected as part of an observational prospective study approved by the Ethics Committee of IRCCS Istituto Ortopedico Rizzoli in 2016. The study was conducted in accordance with the Declaration of Helsinki.

Informed Consent Statement: Informed consent was obtained from all subjects involved in the study.

Data Availability Statement: Data supporting reported results can be found in the electronic medical records of the Institute.

Acknowledgments: The authors acknowledge the invaluable contribution of Carlo Piovani for patients' image storage and data collection.

Conflicts of Interest: The authors declare no conflict of interest.

References

1. Girolami, M.; Sartori, M.; Bandiera, S.; Barbanti-Brodano, G.; Evangelisti, G.; Ghermandi, R.; Pipola, V.; Tedesco, G.; Terzi, S.; Asunis, E.; et al. 3D Vertebral Prosthesis. In *3D Printing in Bone Surgery*; Zoccali, C., Ruggeri, P., Benazzo, F., Eds.; Springer Nature: Basel, Switzerland, 2022; pp. 97–104.
2. Girolami, M.; Boriani, S.; Bandiera, S.; Barbanti-Bródano, G.; Ghermandi, R.; Terzi, S.; Tedesco, G.; Evangelisti, G.; Pipola, V.; Gasbarrini, A. Biomimetic 3D-printed custom-made prosthesis for anterior column reconstruction in the thoracolumbar spine: A tailored option following en bloc resection for spinal tumors: Preliminary results on a case-series of 13 patients. *Eur. Spine J.* **2018**, *27*, 3073–3083. [CrossRef]
3. Tenny, S.; Varacallo, M. Chordoma. In *WHO Classification of Tumours, Soft Tissue and Bone Tumours*, 5th ed.; Statpearls Publishing: Tampa, FL, USA, 2022. Available online: https://www.ncbi.nlm.nih.gov/books/NBK430846/ (accessed on 12 February 2022).
4. McAfee, P.C.; Bohlman, H.H.; Riley, L.H., Jr.; Robinson, R.A.; Southwick, W.O.; Nachlas, N.E. The anterior retropharyngeal approach to the upper part of the cervical spine. *J. Bone Jt. Surg. Am.* **1987**, *69*, 1371–1383.
5. Singh, P.K.; Agrawal, M.; Mishra, S.; Agrawal, D.; Sawarkar, D.; Jagdevan, A.; Verma, S.; Doddamani, R.; Meena, R.; Garg, K.; et al. Management of C2 Body Giant Cell Tumor by Innovatively Fashioned Iliac Crest Graft and Modified Cervical Mesh Cage Used as Plate. *World Neurosurg.* **2020**, *140*, 241–246. [CrossRef]
6. Yang, J.; Yang, X.H.; He, S.H.; Jiao, J.; Jia, Q.; Hu, J.B.; Xiao, J.R. A Novel Reconstruction Using a Combined Anterior and Posterior Approach After Axis Tumor Spondylectomy. *Clin. Spine Surg.* **2020**, *33*, E299–E306. [CrossRef]
7. Suchomel, P.; Buchvald, P.; Barsa, P.; Froehlich, R.; Choutka, O.; Krejzar, Z.; Sourkova, P.; Endrych, L.; Dzan, L. Single-stage total C-2 intralesional spondylectomy for chordoma with three-column reconstruction. Technical note. *J. Neurosurg. Spine* **2007**, *6*, 611–618. [CrossRef] [PubMed]
8. Kaltoft, B.; Kruse, A.; Jensen, L.T.; Elberg, J.J. Reconstruction of the cervical spine with two osteocutaneous fibular flap after radiotherapy and resection of osteoclastoma: A case report. *J. Plast. Reconstr. Aesthet. Surg.* **2012**, *65*, 1262–1264. [CrossRef]
9. Xu, N.; Wei, F.; Liu, X.; Jiang, L.; Cai, H.; Li, Z.; Yu, M.; Wu, F.; Liu, Z. Reconstruction of the Upper Cervical Spine Using a Personalized 3D-Printed Vertebral Body in an Adolescent with Ewing Sarcoma. *Spine* **2016**, *41*, E50–E54. [CrossRef]

10. Li, X.; Wang, Y.; Zhao, Y.; Liu, J.; Xiao, S.; Mao, K. Multilevel 3D Printing Implant for Reconstructing Cervical Spine with Metastatic Papillary Thyroid Carcinoma. *Spine* **2017**, *42*, E1326–E1330. [CrossRef]
11. Mobbs, R.J.; Thompson, R.; Sutterlin, I.I.I.C.E.; Phan, K. The utility of 3D printing for surgical planning and patient-specific implant design for complex spinal pathologies: Case report. *J. Neurosurg. Spine* **2017**, *26*, 513–518. [CrossRef]
12. He, S.; Yang, X.; Yang, J.; Ye, C.; Liu, W.; Wei, H.; Xiao, J. Customized "Whole-Cervical-Vertebral-Body" Reconstruction After Modified Subtotal Spondylectomy of C2-C7 Spinal Tumor Via Piezoelectric Surgery. *Oper. Neurosurg.* **2019**, *17*, 580–587. [CrossRef] [PubMed]
13. He, S.; Ye, C.; Zhong, N.; Yang, M.; Yang, X.; Xiao, J. Customized anterior craniocervical reconstruction via a modified high-cervical retropharyngeal approach following resection of a spinal tumor involving C1-2/C1-3. *J. Neurosurg. Spine* **2019**, *32*, 432–440. [CrossRef] [PubMed]
14. Parr, W.C.H.; Burnard, J.L.; Singh, T.; McEvoy, A.; Walsh, W.R.; Mobbs, R.J. C3-C5 Chordoma Resection and Reconstruction with a Three-Dimensional Printed Titanium Patient-Specific Implant. *World Neurosurg.* **2020**, *136*, 226–233. [CrossRef]
15. Li, Y.; Zheng, G.; Liu, T.; Liang, Y.; Huang, J.; Liu, X.; Huang, J.; Cheng, Z.; Lu, S.; Huang, L. Surgical Resection of Solitary Bone Plasmacytoma of Atlas and Reconstruction with 3-Dimensional-Printed Titanium Patient-Specific Implant. *World Neurosurg.* **2020**, *139*, 322–329. [CrossRef]
16. Wei, F.; Li, Z.; Liu, Z.; Liu, X.; Jiang, L.; Yu, M.; Xu, N.; Wu, F.; Dang, L.; Zhou, H.; et al. Upper cervical spine reconstruction using customized 3D-printed vertebral body in 9 patients with primary tumors involving C2. *Ann. Transl. Med.* **2020**, *8*, 332. [CrossRef]
17. Yang, X.; Wan, W.; Gong, H.; Xiao, J. Application of Individualized 3D-Printed Artificial Vertebral Body for Cervicothoracic Reconstruction in a Six-Level Recurrent Chordoma. *Turk. Neurosurg.* **2020**, *30*, 149–155. [CrossRef]
18. Hunn, S.A.M.; Koefman, A.J.; Hunn, A.W.M. AWM. 3D-printed Titanium Prosthetic Reconstruction of the C2 Vertebra: Techniques and Outcomes of Three Consecutive Cases. *Spine* **2020**, *45*, 667–672. [CrossRef]
19. Baldassarre, B.M.; Di Perna, G.; Portonero, I.; Penner, F.; Cofano, F.; Marco, R.; Marengo, N.; Garbossa, D.; Pecorari, G.; Zenga, F. Craniovertebral junction chordomas: Case series and strategies to overcome the surgical challenge. *J. Craniovertebr. Junction Spine* **2021**, *12*, 420–431.
20. Lannon, M.; Algird, A.; Alsunbul, W.; Wang, B.H. Cost-Effective Cranioplasty Utilizing 3D Printed Molds: A Canadian Single-Center Experience. *Can. J. Neurol. Sci.* **2022**, *49*, 196–202. [CrossRef]
21. Czyżewski, W.; Jachimczyk, J.; Hoffman, Z.; Szymoniuk, M.; Litak, J.; Maciejewski, M.; Kura, K.; Rola, R.; Torres, K. Low-Cost Cranioplasty-A Systematic Review of 3D Printing in Medicine. *Materials* **2022**, *15*, 4731. [CrossRef]
22. Park, C.K. 3D-Printed Disease Models for Neurosurgical Planning, Simulation, and Training. *J. Korean Neurosurg. Soc.* **2022**, *65*, 489–498. [CrossRef] [PubMed]
23. Błaszczyk, M.; Jabbar, R.; Szmyd, B.; Radek, M. 3D Printing of Rapid, Low-Cost and Patient-Specific Models of Brain Vasculature for Use in Preoperative Planning in Clipping of Intracranial Aneurysms. *J. Clin. Med.* **2021**, *10*, 1201. [CrossRef]
24. Garcia, J.; Yang, Z.; Mongrain, R.; Leask, R.L.; Lachapelle, K. 3D printing materials and their use in medical education: A review of current technology and trends for the future. *BMJ Simul. Technol. Enhanc. Learn.* **2018**, *4*, 27–40. [CrossRef] [PubMed]

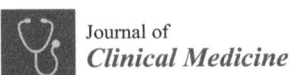

Systematic Review

Bilateral Knee Arthroplasty in Patients Affected by Windswept Deformity: A Systematic Review

Eugenio Cammisa [1], Iacopo Sassoli [2], Matteo La Verde [2], Stefano Fratini [2], Vito Gaetano Rinaldi [2], Giada Lullini [3], Vittorio Vaccari [2], Stefano Zaffagnini [2] and Giulio Maria Marcheggiani Mucciolo [2,*]

1. Orthopedic Unit, Imola Hospital, 40026 Imola, Italy
2. II Orthopaedic and Traumatology Clinic, IRCCS Istituto Ortopedico Rizzoli—DIBINEM, University of Bologna, Via di Barbiano, 1/10, 40100 Bologna, Italy
3. UOC Medicina Riabilitativa e Neuroriabilitazione, IRCCS Istituto delle Scienze Neurologiche di Bologna, 40139 Bologna, Italy
* Correspondence: giulio.marcheggiani2@unibo.it; Tel.: +39-051-6366509; Fax: +39-051-583789

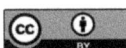

Citation: Cammisa, E.; Sassoli, I.; La Verde, M.; Fratini, S.; Rinaldi, V.G.; Lullini, G.; Vaccari, V.; Zaffagnini, S.; Marcheggiani Mucciolo, G.M. Bilateral Knee Arthroplasty in Patients Affected by Windswept Deformity: A Systematic Review. *J. Clin. Med.* **2022**, *11*, 6580. https://doi.org/10.3390/jcm11216580

Academic Editor: Robert Hube

Received: 14 July 2022
Accepted: 3 November 2022
Published: 6 November 2022

Publisher's Note: MDPI stays neutral with regard to jurisdictional claims in published maps and institutional affiliations.

Copyright: © 2022 by the authors. Licensee MDPI, Basel, Switzerland. This article is an open access article distributed under the terms and conditions of the Creative Commons Attribution (CC BY) license (https://creativecommons.org/licenses/by/4.0/).

Abstract: Background: "Windswept" deformity (WSD) consists of a non-frequent condition in which the patient presents a valgus deformity in one knee and a varus deformity in the other. We performed a review of the available literature to aggregate the accessible data on the outcomes of bilateral knee arthroplasty in patients with WSD and to discuss the surgical challenges that this condition might pose. Methods: A systematic review of the literature following the PRISMA guidelines was conducted. The relevant studies between 1979 and 2021 were identified. Four studies with a total of 68 patients were included for analysis. The mean follow-up for varus knees was 3.3 years, 3.1 years for valgus knees. The quality and rigor of the included studies was assessed using the Methodological index for non-randomized studies (MINORS). Results: All the studies reported improvement in knee function following knee replacement surgery, and a reduction in axial deviation of both knees, with similar results in valgus and varus knees in terms of patient satisfaction. The most relevant data were that unicompartmental knee arthroplasty (UKA) allowed for limited axial correction with slightly inferior functional results. Kinematic alignment (KA) allowed for similar results in both knees. Conclusion: The present review shows how satisfactory results can be achieved in both knees in patients with WSD and osteoarthrosis (OA). However, the operating surgeon should be aware of the importance of the implant choice in terms of functional outcomes. In the absence of extra-articular deformities, calipered KA total knee arthroplasty (TKA) can be performed on both knees with good axial correction and functional outcome. Level of evidence: II —Systematic review of cohort studies.

Keywords: knee arthroplasty; TKA; windswept; varus knee; valgus knee; kinematic alignment

1. Introduction

"Windswept" deformity (WSD) consists of a non-frequent condition in which the patient presents a valgus deformity in one knee and a varus deformity in the other. These concomitant deformities present some unique challenges when performing knee arthroplasty on these patients [1].

The patients with WSD knees have opposite deformities in the coronal plane, and each knee may present different insufficiencies of bone and soft tissue [2]. Windswept deformities (WSD) can be recognized on anterior-posterior (AP) radiography, where the alignment of the knees can be obtained with the use of the hip-knee-ankle angle (HKA) or the femorotibial angle (FTA), and an opposite axial deviation is present in the same patient [3].

The underlying cause of WSD can vary. It often correlates with skeletal dysplasia, physeal disturbances, metabolic bone disorders, rheumatic arthritis, and post-trauma, while it remains an unusual condition in patients with primary arthritis [4].

In WSD, medial compartment osteoarthritis (OA) on the side of varus deformity and lateral compartment OA on the side of the valgus deformity can be found. There is also a contracture of the soft tissues on the medial side of the knee, which often need to be released in varus knees to achieve satisfactory results. The same is true for the lateral ligaments and soft tissues in valgus knees [5,6]. Other crucial challenges are the different degrees of patellofemoral arthritis and the patellar tracking that should be optimized to gain superior outcomes: This is especially important in valgus knees, which can require an extensive lateral retinacular release. In bilateral OA in WSD, knee arthroplasty can be performed in one or two stages, and the choice depends on the clinical criteria of the patient and the will of the surgeon [7,8].

In literature, few studies analyzed windswept deformities and their outcomes after bilateral knee arthroplasty.

The purpose of our study is to perform a review of the available literature to aggregate the accessible data on the outcomes of bilateral knee arthroplasty in patients with WSD and to discuss the surgical challenges that this condition might pose to the surgeon.

2. Materials and Methods

2.1. Search Strategy

The literature search was operated on Medline, EMBASE and Cochrane CENTRAL on 20 September 2022 by two researchers. The string used for the search was: "(windswept OR (valgus AND varus)) AND (tka OR (('arthroplasty'/exp OR arthroplasty) AND ('knee'/exp OR knee)) OR (('total'/exp OR total) AND ('knee'/exp OR knee))) AND bilateral".

All relevant studies were identified in accordance with the Preferred Reporting Items for Systematic review and Meta-Analysis (PRISMA) guidelines (Figure S1). The authors also evaluated the references of the included articles, so it was possible to trace a further study that was added to our review as it met all the inclusion and exclusion criteria. The selected articles adhered to the systematic reviews' Population, Intervention, Comparison and Outcomes (PICO) criteria. The review was registered on the International prospective register of systematic reviews (PROSPERO) with the following registration number: CRD42022361781.

2.2. Eligibility Criteria

Our inclusion criteria for the study were as follows: (1) the studies about knee arthroplasty as a treatment modality in WSD, (2) the patients of each article with WSD must have been treated with arthroplasty in both knees, (3) the articles should report functional outcomes before and after knee arthroplasty.

Our exclusion criteria were: (1) articles not reporting on the functional outcomes, (2) articles not reporting on the preoperative and postoperative knee alignment, and (3) articles that included other treatments for WSD instead of knee arthroplasty. After the removal of duplicate articles, a full-text review of the selected studies was undertaken by two independent junior authors (IS and MLV).

2.3. Data Extraction

The data were extrapolated from the selected documents using a standardized data collection form. Information on the number of patients, their demographic data, the follow-up period, the type of implant, and if the arthroplasty was made in one stage or two stages were reported in a spreadsheet. In order to simplify data collection and facilitate readability, the preoperative and postoperative clinical and functional outcomes were compiled into two spreadsheets, one for the preoperative valgus knee and one for the preoperative varus knee. There were no inconsistencies in the results.

2.4. Quality Assessment and Risk of Bias

Two authors assessed the quality and rigor of the included studies using the Methodological Index for Non-randomized Studies (MINORS) [9]. The global ideal score is 16 for non-comparative studies. The items were scored 0 if not reported; 1 when reported but inadequate; and 2 when reported and adequate. Consensus was reached by the two reviewers (IS/MLV) when there was no difference in opinion on an item. If no consensus was reached, the independent opinion of a third reviewer was decisive (EC). The individual scores are reported in Table 1.

Table 1. Individual MINORS score.

	MINORS Criteria	Howell et al. [10]	Song et al. [11]	Meding et al. [12]	Tanaka et al. [13]
1	A clearly stated aim	2	2	2	2
2	Inclusion of consecutive patients	2	2	2	2
3	Prospective collection of data	2	1	2	2
4	Endpoints appropriate to the aim of the study	2	1	2	2
5	Unbiased assessment of the study endpoint	0	0	1	2
6	Follow-up period appropriate to the aim of the study	2	2	2	2
7	Loss to follow up less than 5%	2	1	1	2
8	Prospective calculation of the study size	2	2	2	2
9	An adequate control group				
10	Contemporary groups				
11	Baseline equivalence of groups				
12	Adequate statistical analyses				
	TOT	14	11	14	16

2.5. Statistical Analysis

The results were summarized using descriptive statistics for continuous variables, frequencies, and percentages for categorical variables. Microsoft Excel, 2016 version (Microsoft Corporation, Redmond, WA, USA) was used for data analysis.

3. Results

3.1. Search Results

Initially, the search identified 128 articles, 38 of which were duplicates. Of the remaining 91 articles, 65 were eliminated because they did not fit the study's inclusion criteria.

From the remaining 26 articles, two were not included because it was not possible to retrieve the complete text. At the same time, another 20 were eliminated after a full-text analysis for the following reasons: patients included in the study did not present WSD, the patients did not undergo bilateral knee arthroplasty, patients were not treated with arthroplasty, articles that presented only the abstracts, articles without any score measuring the clinical outcome.

All four studies met the inclusion criteria and reported clinical and functional outcome scores to evaluate the treatment results and preoperative and postoperative knee alignment.

Population data and additional relevant data are included in Table 2.

The results are summarized in Table 3 for the valgus knees and Table 4 for the varus knees.

Table 2. TKA: Total Knee Arthroplasty; CR: Cruciate Retaining; PS: Posterior Stabilized; MA: Mechanical Aligned; KA: Kinematic Aligned; DVT: Deep Vessel Thrombosis, dMCL: deep Medial Collateral Ligament, PC: Posterior Capsule, LPR: Lateral Patellar Retinalculum, ITB: Ileotibial Band.

	Year	Journal	N. Patients	Implant Used	Simultaneous Bilateral Procedures	Two Stage Procedures	MINORS	Surgery Associated Releases	Complications
Howell et al. [10]	2019	KSSTA	19	Varus; 17 TKA CR KA, 2 TKA PS KA Valgus: 15 TKA CR KA, 4 TKA PS KA	0	19	14/16		
Song et al. [11]	2008	Kor Knee Surg	14	PS TKA MA	3	11 (within 7 days)	11/16	Varus: 11 dMCL, 2 PC, 1 ITB Valgus: 14 dMCL, 5 PC, 4 ITB	Valgus: 1 patellar clunk syndrome
Meding et al. [12]	2000	Jour Arthrop	22	TKA CR	22	0	14/16	Varus: 19 dMCL, 9 PC, 6 LPR Valgus: 22 dMCL, 9PC, 3 ITB, 8 LPR	Varus: 1 patella revision, 1 TKA revision, 1 patella subluxation Valgus: 1 patella revision, 1 superficial wound infection
Tanaka et al. [13]	2020	The Knee	13	UKA	13	0			1 DVT

Table 3. Valgus knees.

Authors	Age at Surgery (y)	FU (y)		Knee Motion			PROMS			Valgus Alignment Pre-op	Valgus Alignment Post-op
				Pre-op	Post-op		Pre-op	Post-op			
Howell et al. [12]	68 ± 7	2.3 (range 1–4)	Flexion (°)	114 ± 6	NA	KSS	34 ± 15	NA		11 ± 5 *	1 ± 2.3 *
			Extension (°)	10 ± 8	NA	FJS	NA	90 [69–96] **			
						OKS	24 ± 8	47 [39–47] **			
Song et al. [11]	66 ± 6.3	2.1 ± 0.9	Flexion (°)	NA	NA	HSS	64.7 ± 5.8	86 ± 4.9		10.21 ± 5.8	6.8 ± 1.4
			Extension (°)	NA	NA						
Meding et al. [10]	72.5 ± 9.32	5.6 ± 3.8	Flexion (°)	111.41 ± 11.97	111.5 ± 18	KSS	45.81 ± 18.70	87.64 ± 6.47		15.95 ± 5.88	6.09 ± 1.93
			Extension (°)	−5.23 ± 9.82	0.95 ± 2.59	KSS	40.68 ± 16.21	72.95 ± 17.23			
Tanaka et al. [13]	73 ± 7.8	2.6 ± 1.4	Flexion (°)	137 ± 10.7	132.9 ± 9.4	OKS	25.3 ± 9.7	34.9 ± 5.8		8.3 ± 5.3	4.3 ± 3.4
			Extension (°)	−3.8 ± 4.8	−1.7 ± 3.3						

KSS: Knee Society Score; OKS: Oxford Knee Score; FJS: Forgotten Joint Score; HSS: Hospital for Special Surgery knee score; NA: Not Available. If not otherwise specified, varus alignment is measured on standing anteroposterior radiograph as a deviation of the FTA from 180°. * measured on HKA. ** median and interquartile range.

Table 4. Varus knees.

Authors	Age at Surgery (y)	FU (y)		Knee Motion			PROMS			Varus Alignment Pre-op	Varus Alignment Post-op
				Pre-op	Post-op		Pre-op	Post-op			
Howell et al. [12]	68 ± 7	2.3 (range 1–4)	Flexion (°)	112 ± 5	NA	KSS	30 ± 11	NA		3 ± 2 *	0 ± 2.1 *
			Extension (°)	10 ± 8	NA	FJS	NA	90 [73–100] **			
						OKS	22 ± 8	47 [41–47] **			
Song et al. [11]	66 ± 6.3	2.1 ± 0.9	Flexion (°)	NA	NA	HSS	61.5 ± 5.9	86.9 ± 5.24		7.8 ± 6.7	−5.4 ± 3.2
			Extension (°)	NA	NA						
Meding et al. [10]	72.5 ± 9.32	5.6 ± 3.8	Flexion (°)	109.77 ± 14.60	110.59 ± 9.91	KSS	37.59 ± 18.05	86.09 ± 9.07		5.90 ± 5.29	−5.91 ± 4.62
			Extension (°)	−5.23 ± 14.01	0.45 ± 2.13	KSS	40.23 ± 15.7	73.86 ± 17			
Tanaka et al. [13]	73 ± 7.8	2.6 ± 1.4	Flexion (°)	133.5 ± 17.7	130.00 ± 7.7	OKS	25.3 ± 9.7	34.9 ± 5.8		0.6 ± 5.1	−1 ± 4.2
			Extension (°)	−4.6 ± 4.8	−1.3 ± 2.3						

KSS: Knee Society Score; OKS: Oxford Knee Score; FJS: Forgotten Joint Score; HSS: Hospital for Special Surgery knee score; NA: Not Available. If not otherwise specified, varus alignment is measured on standing anteroposterior radiograph as a deviation of the FTA from 180°. * measured on HKA. ** median and interquartile range.

Each study included in the review was a retrospective case series of patients affected by windswept deformity of the knee and treated with joint replacement surgeries, for a total of 68 patients and 136 knees.

Three studies were considered at low risk of bias (MINORS higher than or equal to 14), one was considered at high risk of bias. The four studies included were all retrospective case series. The biggest one was Meding et al. [10] with 22 patients. The mean follow-up was at least two years for every study.

In three papers, total knee replacement was employed. Meding et al. [10] used cruciate-retaining (CR) implants, Song et al. [11] used a posterior stabilized (PS) design, while Howell et al. [12] used both designs with a prevalence of CR (79% of valgus knees, 89% of varus knees).

Tanaka et al. [13] only used unicompartmental knee implants for treating both types of deformity.

The follow-up time was greater than two years for all studies.

Only one author, Howell et al. [12], performed all the surgeries in a staged fashion. In 11 patients (58%), the valgus side was addressed first. All other authors reported either bilateral one-stage procedures or a combination of the two.

Howell et al. [12] performed the arthroplasties using a calipered kinematic alignment (KA), while the other authors used a mechanical alignment (MA).

Meding et al. [10] and Song et al. [11] described the necessity for ligament releases in some patients, summarized in Table 2.

Howell et al. [12] performed patellar resurfacing in all patients. Tanaka et al. [13] and Song et al. [11] do not mention any patellar treatment. Meding et al. [10] performed two patellar resurfacing procedures with metal backed component in the same patient, both required a revision.

3.2. Outcome Analysis

All authors reported increased clinical and functional scores after surgery; the individual scores are reported in Tables 3 and 4.

Meding et al. [10] and Tanaka et al. [13] evaluated the range of motion in terms of flexion and extension of the knee before surgery and at follow-up. Although there was no significant difference in the flexion range after surgery, hyperextension was reduced after the surgery in varus and valgus knees in both sides.

All the studies in the review reported alignment through the accurate calculation of the FTA or the HKA before and after surgery; each study describes angles of both the varus and valgus knee.

The most significant alignment changes in the varus knees were reported by Song et al. [11], which went from a mean varus alignment of 7.8 ± 6.7 degrees (measured with FTA) to a mean valgus alignment of 5.4 ± 3.2, for an overall mean change of 13.2 degrees.

Regarding the valgus knees, each study demonstrated a more significant correction than the paired varus knees; Howell et al. [12] reported a mean correction of more than 10 degrees to a mean after surgery of $1° \pm 2.3°$ (calculated with HKA angle).

Tanaka et al. [13] reported one case of deep-vessel thrombosis, which was fully treated with antithrombotic therapy. One case of radiolucency under the tibial component at follow-up was also reported and treated conservatively. Meding et al. [10] reported in the varus group one case of patella revision, one case of TKA revision, and one case of patella subluxation. In the valgus group, there was one case of patella revision and one superficial infection.

4. Discussion

The most important finding of this systematic review was that there was no significant difference in paired knees' outcomes.

As is known, initial valgus and varus deformity affects the difficulty of TKA. Both bone tissue deformities and soft tissue imbalances concur to determine the success of the knee alignment correction [10]. Recently, Baldini et al. also demonstrated that contralateral limb alignment could affect the operated side, especially in great preoperative deformities. That is supposedly due to the adduction moment in association with extensive releases [14].

There is growing interest in the KA technique as an alternative to mechanical alignment (MA) for small and big deformities. KA allows the preservation of the native knee kinematics in minor deformities without affecting the ligament balance. KA is a more difficult choice in more significant deformities due to compromised ligaments and the increased risk of mechanical failure if an insufficient constraint is chosen. However, it is certainly interesting that in 19 patients with both varus and valgus deformity, Howell et al. [12] found no differences in the OKS and FJS between the paired knees at a mean follow-up of 2.3 years, and better results than some reported for MA TKAs [15].

Two studies in this review analyzed MA TKA. All the paired knee results were similar. A slight greater improvement from baseline is shown for varus knees due to lower PROMs scores reported before surgery. This difference is, however, well within the confidence intervals.

It must be noted that KA can correct for intra-articular deformities, while any extra-articular deformity remains unaddressed. Because of that, the authors suggest a careful study of the deformity when choosing KA over MA.

Since the WSD is a bilateral deformity often requiring bilateral surgical intervention, all the considerations usually made for bilateral TKA apply. The comparison between simultaneous (one-stage) and staged (two-stage) TKA is difficult because surgical indications for a one-stage procedure are mostly given to younger and healthier patients [16]. This represents a selection bias, which limits most of the studies in literature. What is currently known is that one-stage TKA costs less and has better rehabilitation outcomes than two-stage. The single hospitalization and physical therapy cycles are cheaper because of the shorter length of stay, but due to the double surgical trauma, the patient would need twice as many blood transfusions [17]. Moreover, Richardson et al. found higher mechanical complications and infection rates in two-stage TKA [18]. This could be explained by an orthopedic, mechanical concept: knee osteoarthritis is often associated with axial deformities and limb shortening [19], so their simultaneous correction maintains lower limb equal length, preventing pelvis and spine asymmetry imbalance. Patients' selection could represent a limit because of different comorbidities between the two cohorts, as explained before. The indication must be given in function of each patient [20] and requires the approval of the colleague anesthesiologists. In both orthopedic and anesthesiologist complex cases, the choice should be two-stage, so it was in three of the WSD studies we included in this review.

Howell et al. [12] analyzed a cohort of 19 patients who underwent two-stage KA-TKAs, finding no differences in the OKS and FJS between paired knees with varus and valgus deformity at a mean follow-up of 2.3 years, and better results than MA-TKA [15].

Song et al. [11] studied a cohort composed of both simultaneous and staged TKAs for a total of 14 patients, eight of whom presented degenerative scoliosis associated with knee deformity. They found satisfactory clinical outcomes and overall patient satisfaction regarding pain relief and function, with no differences between kind of deformity and postoperative result.

Meding et al. [10] especially analyzed simultaneous bilateral TKAs (20 patients of 22), finding no differences between clinical outcomes in the varus and valgus groups postoperatively. Patients noted no side-to-side differences concerning pain or function at the final follow-up.

The cohort of Tanaka et al. [13] consisted of 13 patients subjected to bilateral one-staged unicompartmental knee arthroplasty. Two considerations must be made: the knees had smaller axial deformities compared to the other studies, and the postoperative OKS scores are significantly lower than what Howell et al. [12] reported. This is to be expected since UKA allows for smaller axial corrections.

Given these results, the authors suggest caution when choosing UKA in patients with WSD; even in carefully selected patients, the achieved results can be less than optimal.

Two studies reported on the ligament releases performed during surgery. It can be noted that valgus knees required more ligament releases to be correctly balanced. Deep medial collateral ligament releases for tight medial compartment, iliotibial band release, posterior capsule release and lateral patellar retinaculum release were all more frequent in valgus knee.

This review has several limitations. Firstly, the small amount of literature available on this rare condition makes the collectible data relatively unabundant. Only four studies for a total of 68 patients and 136 knees had met the inclusion criteria.

WSD is a rare condition not often found in clinical practice, and in the literature there is a lack of studies with larger sample sizes. Two studies did not fully report the pre- and postoperative data, posing a risk of bias. This furthermore highlights the importance of review studies to better compile and interpret all the available data from different sources.

The heterogeneity of treatment choices, such as implant design and prosthesis alignment, between the available studies hindered the possibility of a quantitative aggregate analysis. As a result, a meta-analysis was not performed. Nevertheless, the comprehensive comparative analysis of the results of the studies presented provides a good scope on the subject and a good starting point for further discussion. More studies on the subject are needed.

5. Conclusions

The present review shows how knee arthroplasty can achieve satisfactory results in both knees in patients with WSD and OA. However, the operating surgeon should be aware of the importance of the implant choice in terms of functional outcomes, given that UKA functional outcomes were inferior to TKA. In the absence of extra-articular deformities, calipered KA TKA can be performed on both knees with good axial correction and functional outcome.

Supplementary Materials: The following supporting information can be downloaded at: https://www.mdpi.com/article/10.3390/jcm11216580/s1 Figure S1: PRISMA Flowchart.

Author Contributions: E.C. and G.M.M.M. designed the research, developed the concept of the article. E.C. and M.L.V. acquired the data and revised it critically for important intellectual content. E.C., S.F. and I.S. analyzed the data. G.M.M.M., S.Z., G.L. and V.V. contributed to interpretation of data. E.C., M.L.V. and V.G.R. drafted the manuscript. All authors have read and agreed to the published version of the manuscript.

Funding: This research received no external funding.

Institutional Review Board Statement: Not applicable.

Informed Consent Statement: Not applicable.

Data Availability Statement: The data presented in this study are available in the tables of this article.

Conflicts of Interest: The authors declare no conflict of interest.

References

1. Kim, M.W.; Koh, I.J.; Kim, J.H.; Jung, J.J.; In, Y. Efficacy and Safety of a Novel Three-Step Medial Release Technique in Varus Total Knee Arthroplasty. *J. Arthroplast.* **2015**, *30*, 1542–1547. [CrossRef] [PubMed]
2. Shetty, G.M.; Mullaji, A.; Khalifa, A.A.; Ray, A. Windswept Deformities—An Indication to Individualise Valgus Correction Angle during Total Knee Arthroplasty. *J. Orthop.* **2017**, *14*, 70–72. [CrossRef] [PubMed]
3. Babu, S.; Vaish, A.; Vaishya, R. Windswept Deformities of the Knee Are Challenging to Manage. *Knee Surg. Relat. Res.* **2020**, *32*, 46. [CrossRef] [PubMed]
4. Ranawat, A.S.; Ranawat, C.S.; Elkus, M.; Rasquinha, V.J.; Rossi, R.; Babhulkar, S. Total Knee Arthroplasty for Severe Valgus Deformity. *JBJS* **2005**, *87*, 14.

5. Alesi, D.; Meena, A.; Fratini, S.; Rinaldi, V.G.; Cammisa, E.; Lullini, G.; Vaccari, V.; Zaffagnini, S.; Marcheggiani Muccioli, G.M. Total Knee Arthroplasty in Valgus Knee Deformity: Is It Still a Challenge in 2021? *Musculoskelet. Surg.* **2021**, *106*, 1–8. [CrossRef] [PubMed]
6. Adravanti, P.; Vasta, S. Varus-Valgus Constrained Implants in Total Knee Arthroplasty: Indications and Technique. *Acta Bio-Med. Atenei Parm.* **2017**, *88*, 112–117.
7. Goyal, T.; Azam, M.Q.; Syed, A.; Paul, S. Simultaneous Single-Stage versus Two-Staged Bilateral Total Knee Arthroplasty: A Prospective Comparative Study. *Int. Orthop. (SICOT)* **2020**, *44*, 1305–1310. [CrossRef] [PubMed]
8. The Lundbeck Foundation Centre for Fast-Track Hip and Knee Replacement Collaborative Group; Lindberg-Larsen, M.; Pitter, F.T.; Husted, H.; Kehlet, H.; Jørgensen, C.C. Simultaneous vs Staged Bilateral Total Knee Arthroplasty: A Propensity-Matched Case–Control Study from Nine Fast-Track Centres. *Arch. Orthop. Trauma Surg.* **2019**, *139*, 709–716. [CrossRef] [PubMed]
9. Slim, K.; Nini, E.; Forestier, D.; Kwiatkowski, F.; Panis, Y.; Chipponi, J. Methodological Index for Non-Randomized Studies (Minors): Development and Validation of a New Instrument. *ANZ J. Surg.* **2003**, *73*, 712–716. [CrossRef] [PubMed]
10. Howell, S.M.; Shelton, T.J.; Gill, M.; Hull, M.L. A Cruciate-Retaining Implant Can Treat Both Knees of Most Windswept Deformities When Performed with Calipered Kinematically Aligned TKA. *Knee Surg. Sports Traumatol. Arthrosc.* **2021**, *29*, 437–445. [CrossRef] [PubMed]
11. Song, I.-S.; Jeon, J.-K.; Kim, J.-B. Total Knee Arthroplasty for Treating Valgus and Varus in the Knees of One Person. *Knee Surg. Relat. Res.* **2008**, *20*, 110–116.
12. Meding, J.B.; Anderson, A.R.; Ritter, M.A.; Faris, P.M.; Keating, E.M. Windswept Deformity in Bilateral Total Knee Arthroplasty. *J. Arthroplast.* **2000**, *15*, 562–566. [CrossRef] [PubMed]
13. Tanaka, T.; Hiranaka, T.; Okimura, K.; Fujishiro, T.; Okamoto, K. Bilateral Unicompartmental Knee Arthroplasty for Windswept Knee Osteoarthritis: A Report of 13 Cases. *Knee* **2020**, *27*, 1715–1720. [CrossRef] [PubMed]
14. Baldini, A.; Castellani, L.; Traverso, F.; Balatri, A.; Balato, G.; Franceschini, V. The Difficult Primary Total Knee Arthroplasty: A Review. *Bone Jt. J.* **2015**, *97-B*, 30–39. [CrossRef] [PubMed]
15. Peters, C.L.; Jimenez, C.; Erickson, J.; Anderson, M.B.; Pelt, C.E. Lessons Learned from Selective Soft-Tissue Release for Gap Balancing in Primary Total Knee Arthroplasty: An Analysis of 1216 Consecutive Total Knee Arthroplasties. *J. Bone Jt. Surg.* **2013**, *95*, e152. [CrossRef] [PubMed]
16. March, L.M.; Cross, M.; Tribe, K.L.; Lapsley, H.M.; Courtenay, B.G.; Cross, M.J.; Brooks, P.M. Two Knees or Not Two Knees? *Osteoarthr. Cartil.* **2004**, *12*, 400–408. [CrossRef] [PubMed]
17. Bohm, E.R.; Molodianovitsh, K.; Dragan, A.; Zhu, N.; Webster, G.; Masri, B.; Schemitsch, E.; Dunbar, M. Outcomes of Unilateral and Bilateral Total Knee Arthroplasty in 238,373 Patients. *Acta Orthop.* **2016**, *87*, 24–30. [CrossRef] [PubMed]
18. Richardson, S.S.; Kahlenberg, C.A.; Blevins, J.L.; Goodman, S.M.; Sculco, T.P.; Figgie, M.P.; Sculco, P.K. Complications Associated with Staged versus Simultaneous Bilateral Total Knee Arthroplasty: An Analysis of 7747 Patients. *Knee* **2019**, *26*, 1096–1101. [CrossRef] [PubMed]
19. Bin Sabir, A.; Faizan, M.; Ishtiaq; Jilani, L.Z.; Ahmed, S.; Shaan, Z.H. Limb Length Discrepancy after Total Knee Arthroplasty: Unilateral versus Bilateral, a Comparative Study at Tertiary Centre. *J. Clin. Orthop. Trauma* **2020**, *11*, S740–S745. [CrossRef] [PubMed]
20. Liu, L.; Liu, H.; Zhang, H.; Song, J.; Zhang, L. Bilateral Total Knee Arthroplasty: Simultaneous or Staged? A Systematic Review and Meta-Analysis. *Medicine* **2019**, *98*, e15931. [CrossRef] [PubMed]

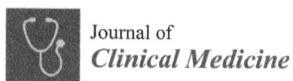

Journal of Clinical Medicine

Article

What Is the Inpatient Cost of Hip Replacement? A Time-Driven Activity Based Costing Pilot Study in an Italian Public Hospital

Andrea Fidanza [1,*], Irene Schettini [2,3], Gabriele Palozzi [2], Vasileios Mitrousias [3], Giandomenico Logroscino [1], Emilio Romanini [4] and Vittorio Calvisi [1]

[1] Mininvasive Orthopaedic Surgery, Department Life, Health and Environmental Sciences, University of L'Aquila, 67100 L'Aquila, Italy
[2] Department of Management and Law, Tor Vergata University of Rome, 00133 Roma, Italy
[3] Faculty of Medicine, School of Health Sciences, University of Thessaly, 41500 Larissa, Greece
[4] RomaPro Center for Hip and Knee Arthroplasty, Polo Sanitario San Feliciano, 00166 Rome, Italy
* Correspondence: andrea.fidanza@graduate.univaq.it

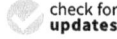

Citation: Fidanza, A.; Schettini, I.; Palozzi, G.; Mitrousias, V.; Logroscino, G.; Romanini, E.; Calvisi, V. What Is the Inpatient Cost of Hip Replacement? A Time-Driven Activity Based Costing Pilot Study in an Italian Public Hospital. *J. Clin. Med.* **2022**, *11*, 6928. https://doi.org/10.3390/jcm11236928

Academic Editors: Massimiliano Mosca, Alberto Grassi and Silvio Caravelli

Received: 25 October 2022
Accepted: 21 November 2022
Published: 24 November 2022

Publisher's Note: MDPI stays neutral with regard to jurisdictional claims in published maps and institutional affiliations.

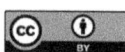

Copyright: © 2022 by the authors. Licensee MDPI, Basel, Switzerland. This article is an open access article distributed under the terms and conditions of the Creative Commons Attribution (CC BY) license (https:// creativecommons.org/licenses/by/ 4.0/).

Abstract: The emphasis on value-based payment models for primary total hip replacement (THA) results in a greater need for orthopaedic surgeons and hospitals to better understand actual costs and resource use. Time-Driven Activity-Based Costing (TDABC) is an innovative approach to measure expenses more accurately and address cost challenges. It estimates the quantity of time and the cost per unit of time of each resource (e.g., equipment and personnel) used across an episode of care. Our goal is to understand the true cost of a THA using the TDABC in an Italian public hospital and to comprehend how the adoption of this method might enhance the process of providing healthcare from an organizational and financial standpoint. During 2019, the main activities required for total hip replacement surgery, the operators involved, and the intraoperative consumables were identified. A process map was produced to identify the patient's concrete path during hospitalization and the length of stay was also recorded. The total inpatient cost of THA, net of all indirect costs normally included in a DRG-based reimbursement, was about EUR 6000. The observation of a total of 90 patients identified 2 main expense items: the prosthetic device alone represents 50.4% of the total cost, followed by the hospitalization, which constitutes 41.5%. TDABC has proven to be a precise method for determining the cost of the healthcare delivery process for THA, considering facilities, equipment, and staff employed. The process map made it possible to identify waste and redundancies. Surgeons should be aware that the choice of prosthetic device and that a lack of pre-planning for discharge can exponentially alter the hospital expenditure for a patient undergoing primary THA.

Keywords: TDABC; ABC; value-based health care; VBHC; hospital costs; costs and costs analysis; THA; outcomes; decreasing costs; optimization

1. Introduction

Osteoarthritis (OA) is one of the most common chronic degenerative diseases affecting a wide range of the population, as well as one of the most frequent causes of disability in the elderly. Symptomatic osteoarthritis is estimated to affect, in Italy alone, at least 4 million people, with a public annual cost of approximately EUR 6.5 billion [1,2]. Total hip arthroplasty (THA) is considered the best solution for the treatment of patients with severe hip osteoarthritis [3].

In 2019, 118,673 hip replacement surgeries were performed in Italy, and this number is increasing at a rate of approximately 2.7% per year: in 2017 and 2018, the number of surgeries were 112,375 and 115,308, respectively [4,5]. This pattern is in line with the Organization for Economic Co-operation and Development (OECD) data, which reveals a significant rise in THAs for the majority of OECD nations [6]. In the pre-COVID period, the reimbursement by the Italian National Health System related to arthroplasty surgery was about EUR 1,625,853,413 [7]. Due to its significant effect on healthcare system costs and the high frequency and demand for this surgical procedure, many authors have defined THA complications as a real health emergency [8,9]. This is also the reason for an increasing interest in understanding the real cost related to this procedure.

In fact, using resources for acquiring important information for the entire activity of healthcare organizations is crucial in the era of value-based healthcare. Tools for management accounting might be regarded helpful for information gathering in the context of healthcare, in order to accomplish this purpose. The costs of medical treatments calculated using Activity Based Costing (ABC) tend to have more accuracy in the computation of resource consumption than standard cost accounting systems, among other techniques of cost calculation or reimbursement, such as Diagnosis-Related Groups (DRG) [10]. Furthermore, the capacity to precisely identify expenses at the level of the treatment process and manage the complexities associated with accounting in the healthcare sector make the Time-Driven Activity-Based Costing (TDABC) [11,12] the most effective and straightforward instrument, even when compared to the traditional ABC. TDABC is an innovative approach used to measure costs more accurately by estimating the amount of time and cost per unit of time each provider uses during a care episode. For example, if a staff member spends 30 min with a patient and that staff member's time cost is EUR 100 per hour, the cost of interacting with that patient is EUR 50.

In addition, the use of the TDABC method estimates the practical capacity (i.e., actual production time) of each element providing capacity (operator and equipment) and the average time required for each element to carry out the action, on the basis of observation, data collection, and questionnaires. The improved process consistency makes TDABC particularly appropriate for the surgical area [13].

This "bottom-up" accounting method makes it possible to identify transparent analyses of the entire care cycle by adding up the individual costs of all the resources used by a single patient [13].

Furthermore, this model allows to redesign the process in order to reduce costs, incorporate new activities in the care cycle, make changes and, above all, it allows to compare the best pathway and offer the patient the best available solution, identifying areas for improvement in terms of time, goods consumed, and the activities carried out.

Clinical management, including medical professionals and support employees, would greatly benefit from this development in healthcare since it would make it easier for them to quickly assess a treatment's efficacy and resources usage. TDABC's process mapping might reveal which processes offer the most value, if waste can be reduced, and whether resources are being underutilized from the standpoint of redesigning the delivered healthcare process to create high value for the patient. According to numerous authors [13–16], its use in orthopaedic surgery is very suited. The ability of an activity-based methodology to not only supply more information but also to provide better detail and higher timeliness of the same, constituting a legitimate support to the decision-making process, is another point on which all of these authors agree. Furthermore, the use of this technique lowers the percentage of unspecified allocated overhead costs, and process mapping makes it easier to oversee every step of the process efficiently, taking corrective action as needed [17]. The resources used and the actions performed are precisely specified, ensuring that the cost analysis is accurate and complete [18].

A recent systematic review concluded that TDABC can help overcome a key challenge associated with current cost accounting methods and should be gradually incorporated into functional systems [12].

Additionally, the information gathered and the methods used to identify expenses improve the transparency in the business management that enable, as shown by the research by Demeere N. et al. [19], an internal examination aimed at establishing a reference benchmark and creating value.

The goal of this pilot study is to understand the true cost of a total hip replacement using the TDABC in an Italian public hospital and to comprehend how the adoption of this method might enhance the process of providing healthcare from an organizational and financial standpoint.

2. Materials and Methods

2.1. Study Design

During 2019 a prospective experimental case study [20,21] was conducted in a public hospital in central Italy. The orthopaedic department under observation is made up of 26 hospital beds, 7 orthopaedic and trauma surgeons, and 4 residents; it is part of a regional HUB and performs about 1600 orthopaedic surgeries per year.

Using the TDABC, details regarding all the activities, consumables, and participating healthcare professionals were gathered. Seven steps have been methodologically introduced, as is specifically mandatory for the use of this tool [12], and they are identified by the increasing number in brackets of the following paragraphs.

All procedures were performed in accordance with ethical standards, and the study protocol was approved by the Internal Review Board of authors' affiliated Institution (authorization number 22/2022).

2.2. Study Participants

(1) Inclusion criteria: patients 60–80 years old, suffering from primary hip arthritis with indication for THA. Patients with concomitant femoral neck fractures, cemented prostheses, intraoperative fractures, or systemic complications (such as cardiopulmonary diseases, which would have increased standard surgical times) were excluded.

2.3. Measurement

To comprehend how patients move through the care cycle and quantify the usage of human resources by activity, a process map for primary hip replacement was created from the entrance in the operating room to the exit (2).

Direct observation, interviews, and multidisciplinary care plan validation sessions with frontline personnel were used to build process maps with time estimates for each stage. The necessary resources for each process step (such as staff and consumables like implants) were noted (3).

We calculated the overall expenses over a patient's cycle of care after estimating the cost of providing each service based on the time needed for each resource type (4).

The questions performed to the healthcare staff are listed in the Appendix A (Table A1).

2.4. Costs Analysis of Hip Arthroplasty

(5) The average price stated by the regional fee schedules as compensation for services rendered in pre-hospitalization was used as a reference point to determine the cost of pre-hospitalization exams [22]. The cost of the majority of consumer goods used throughout the entire therapeutic process was provided by the Director of hospital's pharmacy by filling out a pre-set table based on the information needs derived from the process maps; the cost of the prosthetic device was obtained by extracting the price from the purchase of regional tender. The hourly cost of an active operating room used for major hip surgery, net of material, and labour costs, was derived from the literature [23], as well as the average cost of a day of hospitalization [24]. (6) Comparing the average monthly pay of the operators with the actual amount of time spent delivering the health service, the capacity cost rate [11], defined as practical capacity of each active operator, was determined. This method was used for all the operators present, taking into account the different remuneration (7). It is important to point out that in the Italian system, the salary for clinical staff in a public hospital is regulated nationally on a monthly basis. There is no difference pay based on the procedures carried out; rather, it is dependent on the total number of hours worked each month and the operators' seniority.

Finally, to define the total cost of hip arthroplasty, from the admission to the patient's discharge, all the calculated expenses (pre-operative tests + hospitalization + theatre + general consumer goods + prosthesis + staff employed) were added up.

3. Results

Ninety patients who met our inclusion criteria were included in this study. The cementless prosthetic implant was the same for each patient and the surgical team was the same for all operations. The average of actions and time spent on these patients made up the process map shown in Figure 1: this diagram outlines the arthroplasty operating day including anaesthesia preparation, surgical preparation, and surgery. From the moment the patient enters the pre-operative room until the last radiographic control following the surgery, the estimated time for the intervention is, on average, 90 min.

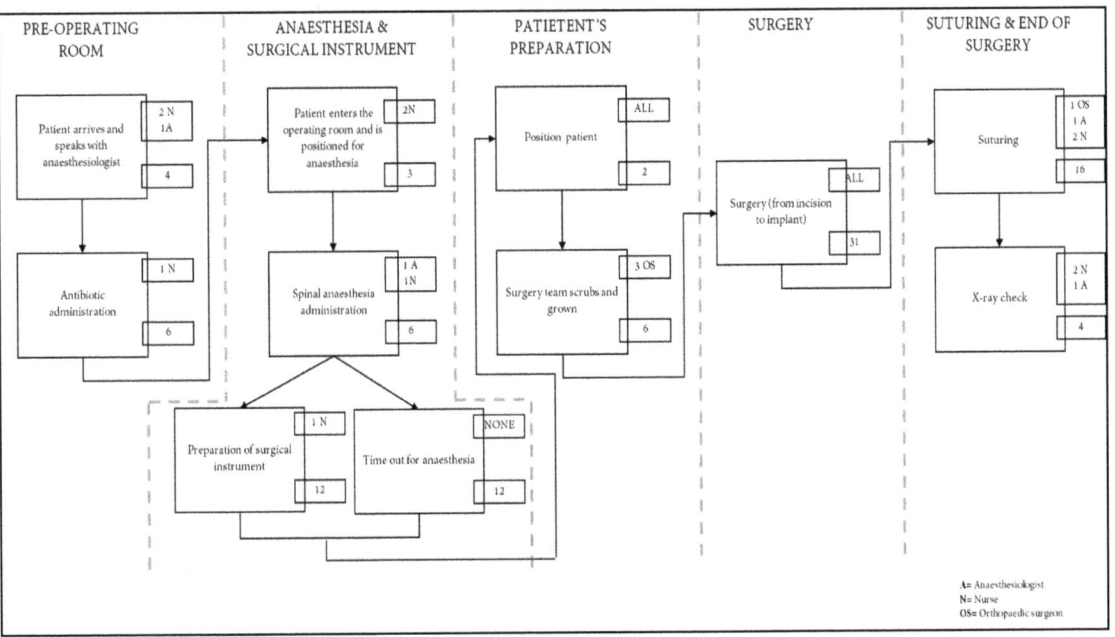

Figure 1. Process map of THA. The large boxes represent activities with arrows indicating sequence. The personnel ID is in the upper smaller boxes (see legend) while the numbers in the smaller boxes correspond to minutes used per activity.

The healthcare delivery process of THA in the hospital analysed involved seven healthcare professions, in particular:

- Three orthopaedic surgeons (one involved for 55 min and two involved for 39 min);
- One anaesthesiologist (involved all the time);
- One nurse dedicated to the anaesthesiologist (involved all the time);
- One surgical nurse (involved 85 min);
- One general nurse (involved 85 min).

The pre-operative tests, including blood tests, chest X-ray, pelvic X-ray, ECG, and anaesthesia evaluation reached a total cost of EUR 90.29 per patient, according to the regional fee.

The total cost related to the personnel involved in the THA implantation procedure is EUR 201.34 and it is shown in detail in Table 1. Considering the average of the wages specified in the Italian National Labour Contract for operators with that level of experience, 36 h per week were calculated for nurses, and 38 h per week for doctors.

Table 1. The cost refers to the total minutes spent by each health worker during the procedure.

Helthcare Professional	Monthly Pay	Total Time Spent	Total Cost
Orthopaedic Surgeons (x 2)	EUR 5330	39 min for each surgeon	EUR 45.59
Orthopaedic surgeon (x 1)	EUR 5330	55 min	EUR 32.14
Anaesthesiologist	EUR 6000	90 min	EUR 59.21
Nurses (x 2)	EUR 2052	85 min for each nurse	EUR 40.80
Nurse (x 1)	EUR 2052	90 min	EUR 21.60
TOTAL COST			EUR 201.74

The cost of the consumables charged for each operation performed by healthcare professionals was grouped by stage, and it represents an expense of EUR 97.02 (Table 2).

Table 2. The grouped-by-stage cost of consumables charged for each operation performed by healthcare professionals.

Stage	Cost of Consumables
Pre-operating room	EUR 8.44
Anesthesia and surgical field	EUR 42.25
Position of patient	EUR 18.16
Surgery (prosthetic implant excluded)	EUR 13.01
Suture and dressing	EUR 15.16
TOTAL COST	EUR 97.02

The cost of each consumable item is listed in the Appendix A (Table A2).
The final cost of the implanted prosthetic device was EUR 3029.208 according to the regional tender, and it is analysed in Table 3.

Table 3. The total cost of prosthesis refers to the specific components used.

	Purchase Prices of Prostheses	
1.	Cup	EUR 786.60
2.	Insert	EUR 425.60
3.	Head	EUR 280.25
4.	Stem	EUR 1420.25
	Total without VAT	EUR 2912.70
	VAT	EUR 4%
	TOTAL COST	EUR 3029.21

The cost of an active operating room used for major hip surgeries, minus material and labour expenses, was calculated by Cinquini et al. [23], who estimated an hourly cost of EUR 90 for the theatre. By multiplying the hourly cost by the amount of time spent in the operating room for the procedure (90 min), a cost of EUR 135 was obtained.

The average inpatient stay was 3.7 days. On 2007, the Italian Ministry of Economy and Finance estimated the average cost of hospitalization to be EUR 674 per day [24]. The final cost of hospitalization was calculated by multiplying the average daily cost of a day by the number of days spent in the hospital by the patient, resulting in EUR 2493.80.

The total cost of THA from pre-operative tests to discharge is EUR 6002.06. It is presented in detail in Table 4.

Table 4. The sum of all cost items calculated by the TDABC approach.

Inpatient Total Cost of Tha	
1. Pre-operative tests	EUR 90.29
2. Hospitalization	EUR 2493.80
3. Operating room	EUR 135.00
4. Consumables	EUR 97.02
5. Prosthesis	EUR 3029.21
6. Personnel	EUR 201.74
FINAL COST	EUR 6002.06

4. Discussion

The world health system is facing an unprecedented period of change and crisis. The ongoing war in Eastern Europe and the post-COVID crisis have also caused an increase in national healthcare spending, predictably far greater than inflation. This unsustainable health care expenditure has increased the demand for providing high quality care while reducing the costs of delivering these outcomes. The main finding of this pilot study is that the TDABC methodology can also be applied in an Italian public hospital and provides a complete and detailed description of the patient's path, of the staff involved, and an accurate understanding of the operation costs.

The value of health care, defined by health outcomes achieved for every dollar spent [25], can be improved if costs and outcomes are measured in sufficient detail to assess the impact of changes in care systems and processes [26,27]. It is not just economic stuff, since knowing organizational and clinical details can allow healthcare professionals to redesign care processes with a patient-centred view, thus providing the best possible care using resources efficiently.

An accurate understanding of costs is important for the effective implementation of cost saving strategies. Elective orthopaedic surgeries are often standardized and in order to increase the efficiency of such surgical procedures it is essential to develop process maps for each step of care in the total joint replacement. In this way, we will be able to identify redundancies and welfare inefficiencies, whose financial impact was not previously detectable due to the lack of detailed analysis of the processes obtained with traditional accounting methods. On the other hand, the times and consumables used are certainly different, depending on the surgeon's background, on the adhesion of the operating team to the most recent evidence-based scientific literature, or to guidelines. It is crucial to point out that regardless of the structure or volume of surgeons, standardization is associated with better processes and outcomes for patients undergoing THA and thus process mapping can also help improve procedures, increase productivity, and raise the number of hip replacement surgeries performed. The mapping of the clinical path, in fact, allows us to understand the connections between the activities, operators, roles, and responsibilities of the care delivery cycle. In addition, this allows service providers to have a better awareness of the costs related to certain services and allows them to evaluate the effects of changes to support systems and procedures.

The TDABC has been described by a number of authors as a managerial tool that promotes collaboration between medical professionals and support staff by outlining every step of the value-creation process [17–19]. In our experience, the total composition of the cost of a hospitalized patient to undergo THA has two major economic items: the component that has the greatest impact on this value is the cost of the prosthetic device, which alone represents 50.4% (about EUR 3000) of the total cost, followed by costs relating to hospitalization, which constitute 41.5% (about EUR 2500).

Our results agree with the literature showing that the largest and most common direct cost is the purchase price of the implant [28]. This is a common finding both in the literature on hip and knee arthroplasty [29], and in shoulder prostheses [30]. Robinson et al. showed that the average cost of the implant per case can range from USD 2392 to USD 12,651 for total hip replacement procedures [31].

Haas et al. [32] recently noted that hospitals using a joint committee of hospital administrators and surgeons to negotiate prices with vendors paid 17% less for implants than institutions without a joint purchasing committee.

Therefore, with a view to improving the efficiency or comparing costs with other institutes and methodologies, these data highlight the importance of rationalizing purchases and, where possible, reducing hospital stays.

While directly decreasing medication and personnel costs may not be feasible, indirectly lowering costs by reducing length of stay must be an area for improvement. It is proven that the common reasons why patients need to stay an extra day in hospital after joint replacement are outdated customs, unscientific fears and, at best, problems related to pain and social support, all potentially responsive to initiatives of quality improvement [33]. Strategies to reduce length of stay after THA have to start the first moment surgery is considered, ensuring adequate postoperative social support and setting realistic expectations about pain management [30].

Finally, to achieve higher-value care for patients undergoing THA, TDABC costs must be linked to patient experience, quality of life, and functional outcomes, which is the object of our future research. Nevertheless, this study is an important step toward introducing clarity into the cost conundrum of THA and will hopefully stimulate further research into this increasingly important topic.

Obviously, this study has limitations. First of all, as a pilot experiment it is a small-scale preliminary observational study undertaken to decide how and whether to start a large-scale project, which could aim at collecting data from multiple institutes in order to integrate and compare the results obtained in a public hospital with those obtainable in a private or university hospital. Secondly, it is important to underline that TDABC does not contain all expenses calculations usually included in a DRG-based reimbursement: it is a method to determine the cost of the process. The object cost is the healthcare delivery process of total hip replacement in the hospital. From this perspective, it may appear that the TDABC process does not fully account for all indirect and THA-related costs (such as administrative, research, or sterile treatment), nor time spent caring for the patient outside the hospital, such as medication, rehabilitation, and social support, but it does account for facilities, equipment, information technology, and most other traditional "overhead" costs [34]. In addition, our exclusion criteria reflect the assumption that surgery and postoperative recovery are without complications, which obviously would add costs to both staff and medications, blood transfusions, any new surgeries, and, in any case, a longer length of stay, which would certainly amplify the costs.

5. Conclusions

Time-Driven Activity-Based Costing provides an accurate assessment of costs in the field of hip replacement. The implementation of this methodology gives us more precise and detailed expense advice, a clear path of the patient, and information on the times and staff involved in each activity.

A careful choice of the prosthetic device among the wide range of offers on the market and a premeditated planning of the discharge can drastically reduce the hospital costs of a THA, without cutting staff or medications.

Author Contributions: Conceptualization, A.F. and I.S.; methodology, A.F., G.P., V.M. and I.S.; clinical investigations, A.F., G.L., E.R. and V.C.; economic investigations, G.P. and I.S.; data curation, A.F., G.P., V.M. and I.S.; writing—original draft preparation, A.F. and I.S.; writing—review and editing, G.L., E.R. and V.C.; supervision, V.C. All authors have read and agreed to the published version of the manuscript.

Funding: This research received no external funding.

Institutional Review Board Statement: The study was conducted in accordance with the Declaration of Helsinki and approved by the Institutional Review Board of University of L'Aquila (Italy) protocol code 22/2022 on 24 May 2022.

Informed Consent Statement: Informed consent was obtained from all subjects involved in the study.

Conflicts of Interest: The authors declare no conflict of interest.

Appendix A

Table A1. Questions submitted to the clinical staff.

1.	How many operators are engaged during the surgery?
2.	How long is the procedure?
3.	What is the patient's path through the operating unit?
4.	What is the timing of each stage of surgery?
5.	Are all operators present at each stage?
6.	What are the tasks of each individual operator in each phase?
7.	What consumables are needed?

Table A2. Unit costs consumables. Due to the low cost of the single element, cents were kept in.

	Unit Cost	Cost by Quantity
Pre operating room:		
Cannula	0.3416 EUR	0.3416 EUR
Betadine	0.99 EUR	0.99 EUR
Patch (9 mt roll)	0.28 EUR	0.005612 EUR
Saline solution 0.5 lt	0.37 EUR	1.122 EUR
Antibiotic:		
- Cefamezin	0.87 EUR	0.869 EUR
- Amicasil	0.55 EUR	0.55 EUR
Anti-allergic prophylaxis:		
- Flebocortid 1 g	3.25 EUR	3.245 EUR
- Trimeton	0.99 EUR	0.99 EUR
Needle	0.01 EUR	0.03 EUR
ECG Electrodes	0.10 EUR	0.2928 EUR
Washing:		
- Sponges	0.38 EUR	1.891 EUR
- Caps	0.02 EUR	0.1952 EUR
- Face mask	0.05 EUR	0.3416 EUR
Anesthesiologist:		
Sterile dressing (3 pack)	0.46 EUR	0.9272 EUR
Latex gloves	0.20 EUR	1.7568 EUR
Spinal needle	0.85 EUR	0.854 EUR
Syringe	0.02 EUR	0.0488 EUR
Chirocaine	8.80 EUR	8.8 EUR
Dressing	0.28 EUR	0.2806 EUR

Table A2. *Cont.*

	Unit Cost	Cost by Quantity
Surgeons/Nurse:		
Nurse Scrub	5.25 EUR	5.246 EUR
Surgeons scrubs	5.25 EUR	15.738 EUR
Hip prosthesis disposable kit	24.34 EUR	24.339 EUR
Aspirator/Hoses	0.76 EUR	0.7564 EUR
Electrosurgery equipment	3.12 EUR	3.1232 EUR
Scalpel blade	0.06 EUR	0.122 EUR
Disinfection pads (pack of 10)	0.05 EUR	0.0976 EUR
Oprafol	8.91 EUR	8.906 EUR
Drainage	4.39 EUR	4.392 EUR
Silkam 0	1.10 EUR	2.196 EUR
Safil1	2.81 EUR	5.612 EUR
Vicryl 2	1.10 EUR	2.196 EUR
Absorbent dressing.	0.73 EUR	0.732 EUR
Specific patch (10 mt roll)	1.71 EUR	0.03416 EUR

References

1. Veronese, N.; Cereda, E.; Maggi, S.; Luchini, C.; Solmi, M.; Smith, T.; Denkinger, M.; Hurley, M.; Thompson, T.; Manzato, E. Osteoarthritis and Mortality: A Prospective Cohort Study and Systematic Review with Meta-Analysis. *Semin. Arthritis Rheum.* **2016**, *46*, 160–167. [CrossRef] [PubMed]
2. Fidanza, A.; Leonardi, E.; Migliore, E.; Calvisi, V.; Indelli, P.F. Isolation, Cell Culture and Characterization of Autologous Mesenchymal Stem Cells from Adipose Tissue and Bone Marrow Older Donors: An Alternative Approach of Cell Therapy in the Orthopaedics. *G. Ital. Di Ortop. E Traumatol.* **2022**, *48*, 82–92.
3. Ghirardelli, S.; Touloupakis, G.; Antonini, G.; Violante, B.; Fidanza, A.; Indelli, P.F. Debridement, Antibiotic, Pearls, Irrigation and Retention of the Implant and Other Local Strategies on Hip Periprosthetic Joint Infections. *Minerva* **2022**, *73*, 409–415. [CrossRef]
4. Torre, M.; Carrani, E.; Luzi, I.; Ceccarelli, S.; Laricchiuta, P. Registro Italiano ArtroProtesi. *Rep. Annu.* **2018**, *57*, 132–133.
5. Torre, M.; Ceccarelli, S.; Carrani, E. *Il Registro Italiano ArtroProtesi: Uno Strumento per Potenziarela Sicurezza Dei Pazienti*; Bollettino Epidemiologico Nazionale; ISS Istituto Superiore di Sanità: Rome, Italy, 2019.
6. OECD. Hip and knee replacement. In *Health at a Glance 2021: OECD Indicators*; OECD Publishing: Paris, France, 2021.
7. Ministero della Salute. Rapporto Annuale sull'Attività di Ricovero Ospedaliero (Dati SDO 2019). Available online: https://www.salute.gov.it/portale/documentazione/p6_2_2_1.jsp?lingua=italiano&id=3002 (accessed on 8 April 2022).
8. Parisi, T.J.; Konopka, J.F.; Bedair, H.S. What Is the Long-Term Economic Societal Effect of Periprosthetic Infections after THA? A Markov Analysis. *Clin. Orthop. Relat. Res.* **2017**, *475*, 1891–1900. [CrossRef]
9. Ghirardelli, S.; Fidanza, A.; Prati, P.; Iannotti, F.; Indelli, P.F. Debridement, Antibiotic Pearls, and Retention of the Implant in the Treatment of Infected Total Hip Arthroplasty. *HIP Int.* **2020**, *30*, 34–41. [CrossRef]
10. Agyar, E.; Ayten, E.; Mehmet, B.; Murat, U. A Practical Application of Activity Based Costing in an Urology Department. In Proceedings of the 7th Global Conference on Business and Economics, Rome, Italy, 13–14 October 2007.
11. Kaplan, R.S.; Porter, M.E. How to Solve the Cost Crisis in Health Care. *Harv. Bus. Rev.* **2011**, *89*, 46–52.
12. Keel, G.; Savage, C.; Rafiq, M.; Mazzocato, P. Time-Driven Activity-Based Costing in Health Care: A Systematic Review of the Literature. *Health Policy* **2017**, *121*, 755–763. [CrossRef]
13. Akhavan, S.; Ward, L.; Bozic, K.J. Time-Driven Activity-Based Costing More Accurately Reflects Costs in Arthroplasty Surgery. *Clin. Orthop. Relat. Res.* **2016**, *474*, 8–15. [CrossRef]
14. DiGioia, A.M., III; Greenhouse, P.K.; Giarrusso, M.L.; Kress, J.M. Determining the True Cost to Deliver Total Hip and Knee Arthroplasty over the Full Cycle of Care: Preparing for Bundling and Reference-Based Pricing. *J. Arthroplast.* **2016**, *31*, 1–6. [CrossRef]
15. Palsis, J.A.; Brehmer, T.S.; Pellegrini, V.D.; Drew, J.M.; Sachs, B.L. The Cost of Joint Replacement: Comparing Two Approaches to Evaluating Costs of Total Hip and Knee Arthroplasty. *JBJS* **2018**, *100*, 326–333. [CrossRef]

16. Schettini, I.; Palozzi, G.; Chirico, A. Mapping the Service Process to Enhance Healthcare Cost-Effectiveness: Findings from the Time-Driven Activity-Based Costing Application on Orthopaedic Surgery. In *Service Design Practices for Healthcare Innovation: Paradigms, Principles, Prospects*; Pfannstiel, M.A., Brehmer, N., Rasche, C., Eds.; Springer International Publishing: Cham, Switzerland, 2022; pp. 235–251. ISBN 978-3-030-87273-1.
17. Dombrée, M.; Crott, R.; Lawson, G.; Janne, P.; Castiaux, A.; Krug, B. Cost Comparison of Open Approach, Transoral Laser Microsurgery and Transoral Robotic Surgery for Partial and Total Laryngectomies. *Eur. Arch. Otorhinolaryngol.* **2014**, *271*, 2825–2834. [CrossRef]
18. Baratti, D.; Scivales, A.; Balestra, M.R.; Ponzi, P.; Di Stasi, F.; Kusamura, S.; Laterza, B.; Deraco, M. Cost Analysis of the Combined Procedure of Cytoreductive Surgery and Hyperthermic Intraperitoneal Chemotherapy (HIPEC). *Eur. J. Surg. Oncol. (EJSO)* **2010**, *36*, 463–469. [CrossRef] [PubMed]
19. Demeere, N.; Stouthuysen, K.; Roodhooft, F. Time-Driven Activity-Based Costing in an Outpatient Clinic Environment: Development, Relevance and Managerial Impact. *Health Policy* **2009**, *92*, 296–304. [CrossRef] [PubMed]
20. Yin, R.K. *Case Study Research and Applications: Design and Methods*; Sage Publications: Thousand Oaks, CA, USA, 2017.
21. Scapens, R.W. Doing Case Study Research. In *The Real Life Guide to Accounting Research*; Elsevier: Amsterdam, The Netherlands, 2004; pp. 257–279.
22. Available online: https://sanita.regione.abruzzo.it/canale-assistenza-territoriale/catalogo-prestazioni (accessed on 11 November 2022).
23. di Lino Cinquini, P.M.V.; Pitzalis, A.; Campanale, C. *Titolo: Il Costo Dell'intervento Chirurgico in Laparoscopia con l'Activity Based Costing*; Associazione Italiana Economia Sanitaria: Milan, Italy, 2003; pp. 1–23.
24. Italia Ministero dell'Economia e delle Finanze; Commissione Tecnica per la Finanza Pubblica. *Libro Verde Sulla Spesa Pubblica. Spendere Meglio: Alcune Prime Indicazioni*; Ministero dell'Economia e delle Finanze: Roma, Italy, 2007; pp. 36–57.
25. Porter, M.E. What Is Value in Health Care. *N. Engl. J. Med.* **2010**, *363*, 2477–2481. [CrossRef]
26. Porter, M.E. A Strategy for Health Care Reform-Toward a Value-Based System. *N. Engl. J. Med.* **2009**, *361*, 109–112. [CrossRef] [PubMed]
27. Porter, M.E.; Teisberg, E.O. *Redefining Health Care: Creating Value-Based Competition on Results*; Harvard Business Press: Boston, MA, USA, 2006.
28. Pathak, S.; Snyder, D.; Kroshus, T.; Keswani, A.; Jayakumar, P.; Esposito, K.; Koenig, K.; Jevsevar, D.; Bozic, K.; Moucha, C. What Are the Uses and Limitations of Time-Driven Activity-Based Costing in Total Joint Replacement? *Clin. Orthop. Relat. Res.* **2019**, *477*, 2071–2081. [CrossRef]
29. Navathe, A.S.; Troxel, A.B.; Liao, J.M.; Nan, N.; Zhu, J.; Zhong, W.; Emanuel, E.J. Cost of Joint Replacement Using Bundled Payment Models. *JAMA Intern. Med.* **2017**, *177*, 214–222. [CrossRef]
30. Menendez, M.E.; Lawler, S.M.; Shaker, J.; Bassoff, N.W.; Warner, J.J.P.; Jawa, A. Time-Driven Activity-Based Costing to Identify Patients Incurring High Inpatient Cost for Total Shoulder Arthroplasty. *J. Bone Joint Surg. Am.* **2018**, *100*, 2050–2056. [CrossRef] [PubMed]
31. Robinson, J.C.; Pozen, A.; Tseng, S.; Bozic, K.J. Variability in Costs Associated with Total Hip and Knee Replacement Implants. *JBJS* **2012**, *94*, 1693–1698. [CrossRef]
32. Haas, D.A.; Bozic, K.J.; DiGioia, A.M.; Song, Z.; Kaplan, R.S. Drivers of the Variation in Prosthetic Implant Purchase Prices for Total Knee and Total Hip Arthroplasties. *J. Arthroplast.* **2017**, *32*, 347–350. [CrossRef] [PubMed]
33. Menendez, M.E.; Baker, D.K.; Fryberger, C.T.; Ponce, B.A. Predictors of Extended Length of Stay after Elective Shoulder Arthroplasty. *J. Shoulder Elbow. Surg.* **2015**, *24*, 1527–1533. [CrossRef] [PubMed]
34. Koolmees, D.; Bernstein, D.N.; Makhni, E.C. Time-Driven Activity-Based Costing Provides a Lower and More Accurate Assessment of Costs in the Field of Orthopaedic Surgery Compared With Traditional Accounting Methods. *Arthroscopy* **2021**, *37*, 1620–1627. [CrossRef] [PubMed]

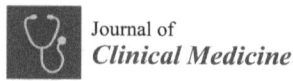

Article

Could Short Stems THA Be a Good Bone-Saving Option Even in Obese Patients?

Michela Saracco [1,2], Andrea Fidanza [3,*], Stefano Necozione [4], Giulio Maccauro [1] and Giandomenico Logroscino [3]

1. "A. Gemelli" IRCCS University Hospital Foundation, Catholic University of Sacred Heart, 00168 Rome, Italy
2. Department of Orthopaedics, ASL Napoli 2 Nord, 80027 Naples, Italy
3. Department Life, Health and Environmental Sciences—Mininvasive Orthopaedic Surgery, University of L'Aquila, 67100 L'Aquila, Italy
4. Department Life, Health and Environmental Sciences—Unit of Epidemiolody, University of L'Aquila, 67100 L'Aquila, Italy
* Correspondence: andrea.fidanza@graduate.univaq.it

Abstract: Short femoral stems, with preservation of the femoral bone stock, are commonly used in recent years for hip replacement in younger and more active patients. Obesity is increasingly spreading even in the younger population. The aim of this case-series study is to evaluate short stems compared to traditional hip prostheses in the obese population. A total of 77 consecutive patients with a BMI greater than or equal to 30 Kg/m^2 were enrolled in this prospective study and were divided into two groups: 49 patients have been implanted with short stems while 28 patients were implanted with traditional stems. All the patients were treated for primary osteoarthritis or avascular necrosis and all the stems were implanted by the same surgeon using a posterior approach. Clinical (Harris Hip Score—HHS, Western Ontario and McMaster Universities Osteoarthritis Index—WOMAC, visual analogue scale—VAS, 12-item Short Form Health Survey—SF-12) and radiographic outcomes were recorded. Radiological evaluations were carried out by three different blinded surgeons. A statistical analysis was performed (chi-square, t-test, Wilcoxon Rank Sum Test, 2-factor ANOVA). At a mean follow-up of 42.6 months both groups showed a marked improvement in pain and in the clinical scores between pre- and post-surgical procedures ($p < 0.05$) with no significant differences between the two groups at last follow-up ($p > 0.05$). The radiological evaluations, with high concordance correlation between the three blinded surgeons (ICC consistently >0.80), showed good positioning and osseointegration in all cases, with no significant differences in the restoration of the joint geometry and complications. No revisions were recorded during the follow-up period. In conclusion, short stems appear to be a good option for bone preservation even in obese patients, showing comparable results to traditional implants.

Keywords: osteoarthritis; obesity; mini-invasive THA; short stems; stemless hip prostheses; total hip arthroplasty; THA

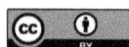

Citation: Saracco, M.; Fidanza, A.; Necozione, S.; Maccauro, G.; Logroscino, G. Could Short Stems THA Be a Good Bone-Saving Option Even in Obese Patients?. J. Clin. Med. 2022, 11, 7114. https://doi.org/10.3390/jcm11237114

Academic Editor: Lorenzo Drago

Received: 25 October 2022
Accepted: 26 November 2022
Published: 30 November 2022

Publisher's Note: MDPI stays neutral with regard to jurisdictional claims in published maps and institutional affiliations.

Copyright: © 2022 by the authors. Licensee MDPI, Basel, Switzerland. This article is an open access article distributed under the terms and conditions of the Creative Commons Attribution (CC BY) license (https://creativecommons.org/licenses/by/4.0/).

1. Introduction

Obesity is a significant and disabling disease, which affects a significant portion of the population due to poor habits and sedentary lifestyle, particularly in the most developed countries. The prevalence of obesity is increasing, and worldwide, 1.9 billion are overweight while 650 million are obese (WHO, 2016). Italy follows this trend, with about 4 million obese people and an increase of almost 30% in the last 3 decades. Previous studies estimated that 2–4% of the total health expenditure in Europe is attributed to obesity, and this is projected to double by 2050 [1]. Obesity is known to be a significant risk factor for the development of osteoarthritis (OA), often severe and of early onset, affecting the hip and knee. IL-1, TNF-α and IL-6 may cause OA indirectly by regulating the release of adiponectin and leptin from adipocytes, summarizing the relationship between obesity and inflammation [2]. Therefore, the demand for hip prostheses in young and obese patients is growing sharply. This implies executive difficulties but also doubts in choosing the most correct and safe implant, also considering the young age and the increased risk of revision due to long life expectancies. [3]

Over the last two decades, several conservative femoral prostheses have been designed for use particularly in young patients with high-activity requests. "Short stems" have been designed to be less invasive than conventional stems. Traditional femoral stems have provided successful long-term results. However, long femoral stems may have consequences related to stress shielding, thigh pain and cortical hypertrophy. Additionally, surgeons should always consider future revision, especially for young patients, because revision surgery of long stems is more invasive and require a significantly higher sacrifice of the residual bone stock. Short stems allow the preservation of more bone for future revisions and consequently are less invasive in case of revision surgery, with clear advantages and benefits for the patient and the surgeon.

The goals of short, conservative stems include saving of the trochanteric bone stock; a more physiological load in the proximal femur reduces the risk of stress shielding and avoiding the impingement of the tip of long stems with the femoral cortex with consequent thigh pain. Biomechanical studies showed that these metaphyseal-fitting stems exhibit good fixation, achieving durable bone ingrowth. Many papers on normal weight patients and short stems have been published [4–7]. Very little information is reported regarding whether short femoral stems in overweight patients offer the same reliability as in normal weight patients. [8] In particular, there are questions about the risk of increased subsidence and the fact that excessive weight can interfere with osseointegration. [9]

The purpose of this case-series is to compare two groups of obese patients, treated with traditional stems and short stems, respectively, in order to analyse the reliability and safety of the latter, not only in normal weight but even in obese patients.

2. Materials and Methods

We retrospectively studied a total of 77 patients who underwent primary total hip arthroplasty (THA) for end-stage hip OA. The inclusion criteria were: age between 35 and 85 years old, primary and monolateral THA and body mass index (BMI) greater than or equal to 30 Kg/m^2. The same surgeon performed all the arthroplasties with a posterior approach with external rotator reconstruction. The indications were primary OA and avascular necrosis (AVN). The exclusion criteria were: bilateral procedures, revision surgery (aseptic loosening, periprosthetic infections or fractures), cemented stems, inflammatory diseases (i.e., rheumatoid arthritis) and/or neurological diseases (i.e., stroke, degenerative diseases). The cohort was divided into 2 groups. The study group (SS) included 48 patients who were implanted with a short metaphyseal-fitting femoral stem, belonging to III A group (subcapital osteotomy) and III B group (standard osteotomy) according to Feven and Shimmin [10], coated or not with hydroxyapatite (HA) and cementless (i.e., SMF-S&N, GTS-Zimmer Biomet, Minima-Lima, Nanos-S&N, Proxima-DePuy-J&J, Pulchra-Adler Ortho, Parva-Adler Ortho, Fitmore- Zimmer Biomet). The mean age was 63 years (43–84 years old, SD: 10.05). The mean BMI was 33.5 Kg/m^2 (30.1–41.3, SD: 3.07) with a mean body weight of 92.3 kg (75–113 Kg, SD: 10.39). The control group (TS) included 28 patients who were implanted with traditional femoral stems belonging to type IV (traditional stems) coated or not with HA, and cementless (i.e., ABG-Stryker, Synergy-S&N, Mercurius-Adler Ortho, Hydra-Adler Ortho, Corail-DePuy-J&J). In this control group, the mean age was 67 years (50–85 years, SD: 10.03). The mean BMI was 34.7 Kg/m^2 (30–44.5 Kg, SD: 4.68) with a mean body weight of 96 kg (67–130 kg, SD: 17.89) (Table 1).

Table 1. Demographics of our sample and implanted devices. The case study group includes 48 patients undergoing THA with short stems. The control group includes 28 patients who underwent THA with standard traditional stems.

	Short Stems (SS)	Traditional Stems (TS)
AGE, years	63 (43–84) ± 10.05	67 (50–88) ± 10.03
BMI, Kg/m^2	33.5 (30.1–41.3) ± 3.07	34.7 (29.8–44.5) ± 4.68
WEIGHT, Kg	92.3 (75–113) ± 10.39	95.9 (67–130) ± 17.89
FOLLOW-UP, months	38 (3–120) ± 25.98	47.3 (12–168) ± 43.15
PARVA, Adler	20 (40%)	-
PROXIMA, DePuy-J&J	7 (16%)	-
MINIMA, Lima	7 (16%)	-
FITMORE, Zimmer Biomet	4 (10%)	-
PULCHRA, Adler	3 (6%)	-
SMF, S&N	3 (6%)	-
GTS, Zimmer Biomet	2 (3%)	-
NANOS, S&N	2 (3%)	-
ABG, Stryker	-	9 (59%)
SYNERGY, S&N	-	6 (17%)
MERCURIUS, Adler	-	5 (12%)
HYDRA, Adler	-	4 (6%)
CORAIL, DePuy-J&J	-	4 (6%)

For all the cases, baseline subjective and objective evaluations were recorded (Harris Hip Score—HHS, Western Ontario and McMaster Universities Osteoarthritis Index—WOMAC, visual analogue scale—VAS, 12-item Short Form Health Survey—SF-12 p). HHS is an objective and reproducible assessment method, based on the examination of two main parameters: pain and functional capacity of the hip. The secondary parameters examined are range of motion and the presence/absence of deformity. [11] WOMAC is a validated tool for measuring the symptoms and physical disability of patients suffering from hip and knee osteoarthritis. It is a self-administered questionnaire that probes clinically significant symptoms related to pain, stiffness and physical function. The questionnaire consists of 24 questions (5 on pain, 2 on stiffness and 17 on physical function) [12]. The VAS system allows the recording of the pain symptom, asking the patient to indicate a point on a straight line. Its extremes correspond to: zero pain–maximum possible pain. The SF-12 questionnaire represents a reduced version of the SF-36: it allows an estimation of physical (p) and mental (M) health perceived by the patient [13].

The 2 groups were compared in terms of preoperative and postoperative HHS, VAS, WOMAC and SF-12 scores.

Low-molecular-weight heparin was administered during the first 5 weeks after surgery, starting from 6 h after the procedure. In addition, 2 g of cefazolin was administered at anaesthesia induction and tranexamic acid was used intraoperatively for bleeding control.

The variables age, BMI, weight and follow-up are expressed on average (min–max) ± Standard Deviation. For each implanted device the percentage is shown in brackets.

For all the patients, anteroposterior (AP) pelvis radiographs were taken after the procedure and at the last follow-up visit, and all the measurements were taken by three of the authors in a blind fashion and random order using AXIOVISION 4.8.2 software (Carl Zeiss Microimaging GmbH). The post-operative pelvis X-rays were calibrated for size using the diameter of the prosthetic head or alternatively of the metal back, extracted from the operator registers. Firstly, off-set was evaluated by measuring the distance between the center of rotation of the femoral head and a line dissecting the long axis of the femur. Cervical-diaphyseal angle was evaluated as the angle between a line dissecting the long axis of the femur and a line dissecting the femur neck axis. Leg length discrepancy >1 cm was considered significant. We also evaluated the presence of subsidence on the last radiograph. Finally, we measured the cup inclination (the angle between a line dissecting the acetabular equator and the trans-ischiatic line, correctly included between 35° and 55°) and the linear polyethylene wear (Figure 1).

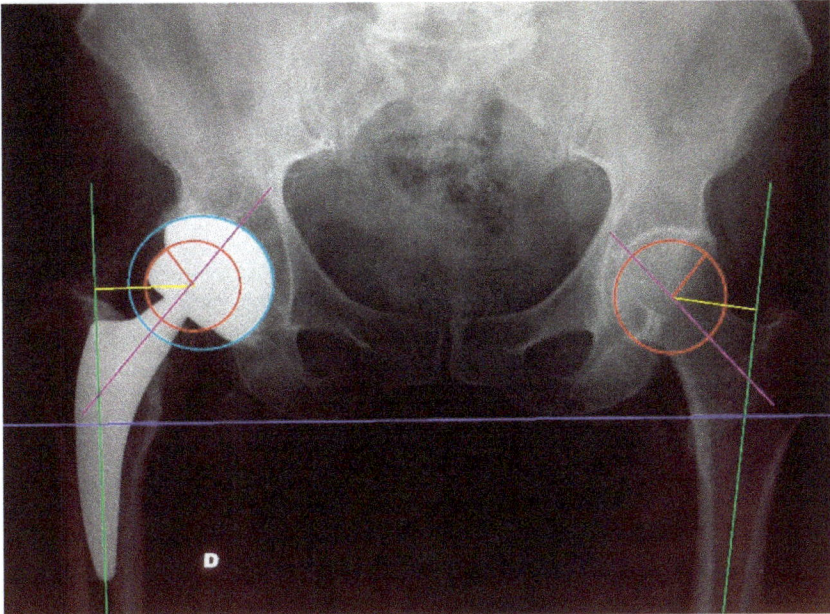

Figure 1. X-ray evaluation of joint geometry restoration.

Stress-shielding, spot-welds, cortical hypertrophy and femoral osteolysis were graded on the radiographs at the final follow-up according to the classification of Engh, dividing the interface between the bone and the stem of the hip prosthesis into the seven zones of Gruen [14,15]. Short stem radiological outcome was assessed according to a modified Gruen zoning system, eliminating zone three and five [4,16,17]. We also evaluated the metal-back osseointegration according to the classification of Hodgkinson, dividing the interface between the bone and the metal-back into the three zones of Charnley–De Lee [18,19]. Periprosthetic heterotopic ossifications were evaluated by the classification of Brooker (from one to four) [20].

Statistical Analysis

The distribution of the variables was tested by applying the Shapiro–Wilk test. The statistical tests performed to evaluate the initial demographic differences between the two groups were: *t-test* for normally distributed variables (age and weight), *Wilcoxon rank sum test* for non-normally distributed variables (BMI), *chi-squared test* for dichotomous variables and *Fisher's exact test*, as appropriate (follow-up).

In order to study the trend of clinical outcomes, time per techniques interaction was calculated with *2-factor ANOVA using the repeated statement*.

Finally, to more directly interpret the differences between the two groups at baseline and at the last follow-up, *unpaired T-test* (HHS, SF-12) and *Wilcoxon rank sum test* for nonparametric data (VAS, WOMAC) were performed.

For the analyses, a statistical confidence level of 95% was selected. A p value < 0.05 determined significance.

3. Results

No differences were found between the demographic data of the two groups; they appeared homogeneous for age ($p = 0.10$), weight ($p = 0.44$) and BMI ($p = 0.63$). The mean follow-up was 38 months (3–120 months, SD: 25.98) for the SS Group and 47.3 months (12–168 months, SD: 43.15) for the TS Group ($p = 0.77$).

All the implanted stems were well osseointegrated and positioned at the last follow-up. In both groups there was a marked improvement in all the parameters compared to the preoperative conditions. The difference between pre- and post-surgery was statistically significant for all the clinical scores evaluated (*2-factor ANOVA using the repeated statement*), and there were no significant differences between the two groups at last follow-up (*unpaired T-test* and *Wilcoxon rank sum test*). The statistical values of each analysed variable are shown below and represented in the graphs of Figure 2.

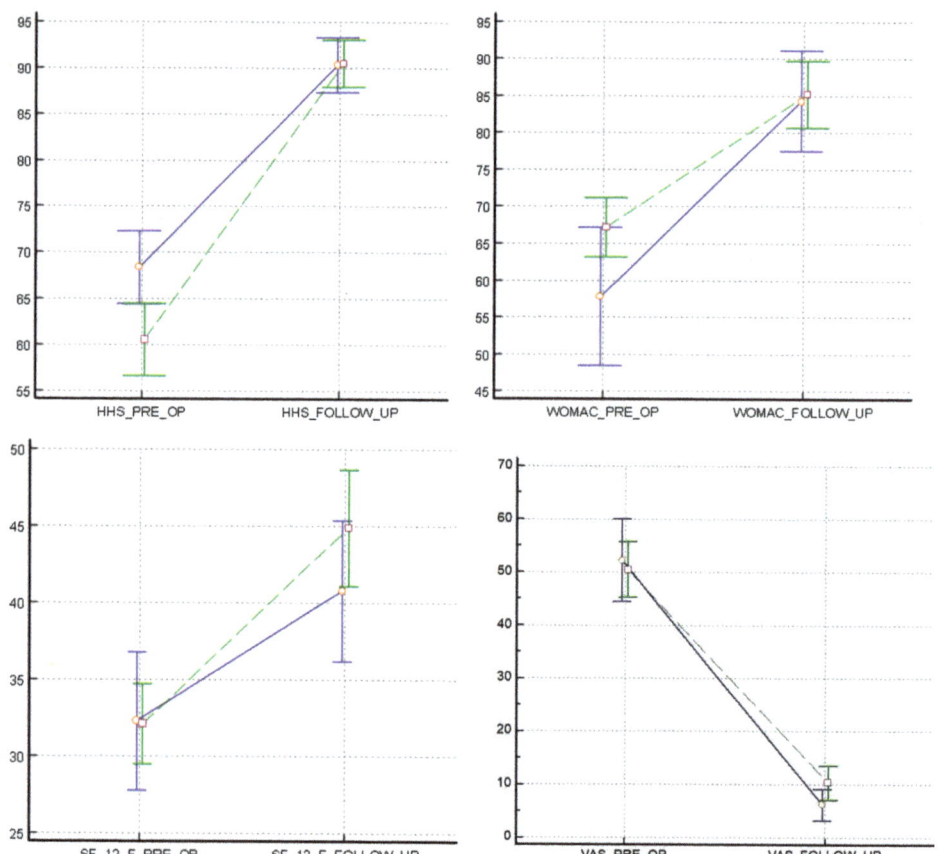

Figure 2. Trends in clinical scales before and after surgery in the two groups (SS—dashed green line vs TS—solid blue line). x: clinical scale evaluated; y: scores recorded. HHS: Harris Hip Score; WOMAC: Western Ontario and McMaster Universities Osteoarthritis Index; SF-12: 12-item Short Form Health Survey; VAS: Visual Analogue Scale.

Pain was significantly reduced in both groups, VAS (SS vs. TS) decreased from 49.8 to 9.2 and from 51.3 to 5.4 ($p < 0.001$), with no significant differences between the two groups at last follow-up ($p = 0.099$).

HHS SS increased from 60.5 to 90.4—TS from 68.4 to 90.3 (p <0.001) without statistical differences at the last control (p = 0.94). WOMAC also increased after the surgery in both groups: SS from 67.1 to 85.2—TS from 57.7 to 84.3 (p <0.001) with no differences at last follow-up (p = 0.816). SF-12 p increased in group SS from 32.1 to 44.9 SS and from 32.3 to 40.8 in group ST (p <0.001), with a final p = 0.16.

The radiological evaluations showed high concordance correlation between the three blinded surgeons (intraclass correlation coefficient (ICC) consistently >0.80) and no significant difference between the two groups in the ability to restore proper articular geometry. The average value of the C-D angle of the side undergoing arthroplasty with long stem was 136.4°, while that of the contralateral was 133.1° with a statistically insignificant difference (p: 0.41); the same can be said for short stems (SS 136.6° vs 135.1°; p: 0.51). As for the offset, it was on average 40.9 mm in long stems and 35.5 mm in the contralateral, with an insignificant difference given that the p value is equal to 0.18; on the other hand, considering the short stems, the average value was 38.3 mm, with the contralateral 36.3 mm (p: 0.27). No significant difference was found in hypermetria between the two groups: SS + 2.2 mm. vs ST + 2.9 mm. (p value: 0.85)

Even the subsidence values did not differ much and were still less than 1 cm, the value considered clinically significant. The radiographic parameter which showed a significant difference between the two groups was the cup inclination. The average inclination values were 43.9° for patients with short stems (min: 29.39°; max: 59.86 °) and 55.2° for long stems (min: 39.8°; max: 70.84°) (p: 0.010).

In two patients with long stems, areas of acetabular osteolysis were identified, in one patient in Chanley–De Lee zone one, while in the other was in zone three; areas of osteolysis were also found in two subjects with short stems, but in zones one and two (p: 0.16). Osteolysis of the femur was found in two patients in the SS group, one in zone two of Gruen and the other in zone six, and in three cases in the TS group, one in zone one and two in zone two (p: 0.25). A total of seven patients with long stems and 15 patients with short stems had radiographical signs of heterotopic ossifications (p: 0.39), without any clinical significance. Cortical hypertrophy was present in three patients with traditional stems, one in zone two of Gruen and two in zone three, and in six patients with short stems, in the area two of Gruen (p> 0.05). Stress-shielding was found in 11 patients with traditional stems in the zone one of Gruen, and in three of them also in zone two; a reduction in bone density was recorded in 14 patients with short stems, however in zone one of the Gruen scale, with only one patient also presenting it in zone seven.

A pedestal was observed in three long stems, and it was incomplete. No pedestals were observed in the short stems group. The spot-welds were recorded in five patients with long stems and in 15 with short stems, involving zones three and five of Gruen. Of the 77 patients studied, 10 complications were recorded: a neurological damage (one in TS), dislocations (two in SS, two in TS), infection (one in TS) and intra-operative periprosthetic fractures (one in SS, three in TS). Two fractures were metaphyseal cracks (two SS and one TS) type B1 by of the Vancouver classification and were solved by cerclages, while two other fractures occurred in the TS Group and were both A1 type that required cerclage stabilization in one case (undisplaced fracture) and ORIF (open reduction and internal fixation) with a proximal hooked plate in the other case (displaced fracture). No revision of the implant was required during the follow-up period due to implant failure, therefore, the Kaplan–Meier analysis showed a survival rate of 100% for both groups.

4. Discussion

The main finding of this study is that short stems, as well as traditional stems, guarantee good outcomes in THA even in overweight/obese patients. It is believed that obesity is a risk factor for osteoarthritis leading to joint replacement surgery and that body weight also affects the severity of the disease [21–23]. Regarding the clinical benefits of hip replacement, no significant difference between non-obese and obese people is reported in the literature since these patients seem to have great benefits regardless of their BMI [24–26]. In a study conducted by Jackson et al. it was found that the non-obese group had a significantly higher postoperative HHS and a greater range of motion. The researchers believe that the main reason for the difference in the range of motion is linked to the apposition of soft tissue that occurs in extreme positions, with an impact on the results of functionality and activity, but overall satisfaction after surgery was comparable or higher in in the obese patients. The greater satisfaction of obese patients is possibly explained by the fact that they start with a lower score but after surgery they will obtain a score similar to non-obese patients so that the greater difference between the preoperative and the last follow up scores leads them to a more relevant satisfaction. In addition, radiological analysis of the acetabular and femoral components did not show significant differences in the two groups [27]. Consequently, avoiding hip replacement surgery for obese patients is not justified [28]. Obese patients are often significantly younger than non-obese patients and, thanks to the good functional results of hip replacements, the indications have been extended to patients of lower age and the techniques have followed the trend for minimally invasive and bone preservation surgery [23,24]. Due to the promising biomechanics of short stems, added to the growing prevalence of obesity in the general population, it is necessary to evaluate the impact of BMI on this type of prosthesis. In our study, patients showed excellent values of HHS, VAS, WOMAC and SF-12 scales that confirm the data already present in the literature about patient satisfaction, improvement in physical activity and quality of life [29–32].

Pirard and De Lint, Todkar and Bosker et al. found no influence of the BMI on component positioning [33–35], while Callanan et al. and Elson et al. highlighted an association between BMI and cup mal-positioning [36,37]. In the majority of cases, only the posterior approach is used since it allows excellent exposure [38]. Few data are available on the lateral or anterolateral approach regarding cup positioning. Brodt et al. have seen how in direct lateral approach the anteversion of the cup is related to the patient's BMI and age, assuming that the cause is the greater traction exerted by the retractors on the surrounding tissues [39]. In our study we also found a major tendency to cup malposition in the TS group. On the other hand, joint geometry was correctly restored in both groups.

Currently, there is conflicting evidence that obesity has a negative impact on the survival of the hip prostheses. In a large analysis, Culliford et al. showed that BMI has a low but statistically significant association with revision risk [40]. The reason for the increase in the rate of early failure due to aseptic loosening/osteolysis in the obese may be related to the higher mechanical stresses on the bone-implant interface and the reaction forces of the joint proportional to the body weight. Recent studies have shown that BMI has no statistically significant influence on the subsidence of uncemented short stem prostheses. Only one study has shown that body weight over 75 kg has a significant impact on subsidence and therefore on the stability of the prostheses, while there is no correlation with BMI [3,41]. To date, only few studies have focused on the relationship between BMI and functional results of short stem implants. The study by Freitag et al. analysed the relationship between BMI and functional results of short-stemmed THA, demonstrating the absence of correlation between obesity and subsidence [42]. A case-control study of the functional outcomes of Metha B-Braun prostheses demonstrated that the postoperative clinical improvement is similar in obese versus non-obese patients [8]. Hungerford et al. studied the influence of obesity on the placement and outcome of minimally invasive anterior implants and reported that there is no statistically significant difference between obese and the non-obese groups [9].

Indeed, no statistically significant difference was found in our study regarding subsidence, which is less than 2 mm in both groups. This evidence further supports that the stability of implants is not influenced by obesity. Furthermore, both groups showed few cases of osteolysis and no significant differences were found on leg length discrepancy. No statistically significant differences were found on osseointegration, with excellent results in both groups. Regarding the incidence of heterotopic ossifications, Andrew et al. noted that there is no statistically significant difference between the obese and the non-obese [43]. We found heterotopic ossifications in both groups without any significant functional limitation or clinical relevance.

Although the literature on the post-operative risk of thromboembolic events documents an increasing risk in obesity, this is not consistently replicated in the orthopaedic literature [44–46]. Similarly, it has been empirically shown that the risk of dislocation increases with extreme excursions of the joint angle and fat tissues around the hip [47]. Paradoxically, however, obese patients have structural and functional limitations that tend to reduce the excursion of the hip during walking and daily life activities. In our study, few patients reported this complication.

The association between obesity and wound infections is reported in the current literature, including orthopaedic procedures [48,49]. In a recent large-scale study, an association between BMI and infection after THA was initially reported. However, when the influence of coexisting diseases such as diabetes mellitus was no longer taken into account, obesity was no longer an independent risk factor for infection [50]. Dowsey and Choong demonstrated the existence of a significantly higher incidence of acute periprosthetic infection after primary hip arthroplasty in obese and super-obese patients compared to non-obese patients [51–53]. There is also an increased risk of wound dehiscence due to increased surface tension, as well as hematoma formation correlated with prolonged wound drainage [54–56]. In our study, previous or active periprosthetic infection was a criterion for the exclusion of patients and we recorded only one case of post-surgical superficial wound infection. Since obesity is a known risk factor for wound complications and regardless of the surgical approach, it is essential to identify the best surgical approach in patients with high BMI to limit the risks related to surgery [57,58]. Previous studies suggested that the risk for obese patients is relatively higher following a direct anterior approach when compared to a posterolateral approach (particularly BMI ≥ 40 kg/m^2) [59]. Consequently, in obese patients, the choice of a posterolateral approach is therefore advisable, and for this reason it was chosen for all the patients in our study.

5. Conclusions

The results of this study demonstrate that short stems in total hip arthroplasty are a valid option in obese patients in whom, until now, traditional long-stem prostheses have been commonly implanted. Short stems were showed to be able to withstand overload, allowing excellent osseointegration and implant stability. Considering that obese patients have an early onset of osteoarthritis and undergo earlier to THA, and that they are more greatly subjected to the risk of failure or complications, short stem implants preserving bone may represent an advantage in case of revision surgery and in long life-expectancy patients. Due to the limitations of our study, no definitive judgment can be made; however, this study may represent the basis for future studies with a larger sample and longer follow-up to provide more solid statistical evidence.

Author Contributions: Conceptualization, M.S. and G.L; methodology, M.S.; formal analysis, S.N.; investigation, S.N.; data curation, M.S. and A.F.; writing—original draft preparation, M.S.; writing—review and editing, M.S. and A.F., G.L.; supervision, G.M. and G.L.; project administration, M.S. All authors have read and agreed to the published version of the manuscript.

Funding: This research received no external funding.

Institutional Review Board Statement: The study was approved by the ethical committee of Fondazione Policlinico Gemelli (Rome, Italy) (reference number:16188/19 ID:2534).

Informed Consent Statement: Informed consent was obtained from all subjects involved in the study.

Conflicts of Interest: The authors declare no conflict of interest.

References

1. D'Errico, M.; Pavlova, M.; Spandonaro, F. The economic burden of obesity in Italy: A cost-of-illness study. *Eur. J. Health Econ.* **2022**, *23*, 177–192. [CrossRef] [PubMed]
2. Wang, T.; He, C. Pro-inflammatory cytokines: The link between obesity and osteoarthritis. *Cytokine Growth Factor Rev.* **2018**, *44*, 38–50. [CrossRef] [PubMed]
3. Stihsen, C.; Radl, R.; Keshmiri, A.; Rehak, P.; Windhager, R. Subsidence of a cementless femoral component influenced by body 339 weight and body mass index. *Int. Orthop.* **2012**, *36*, 941–947. [CrossRef] [PubMed]
4. Anderl, C.; Steinmair, M.; Hochreiter, J. Bone Preservation in Total Hip Arthroplasty. *J. Arthroplast.* **2022**, *37*, 1118–1123. [CrossRef]
5. Logroscino, G.; Ciriello, V.; D'Antonio, E.; De, T.V.; Piciocco, P.; Magliocchetti, L.G.; Santori, F.S.; Albanese, C.V. Bone integration of new stemless hip implants (proxima vs. nanos). A DXA study: Preliminary results. *Int. J. Immunopathol. Pharmacol.* **2011**, *24*, 113–116. [CrossRef]
6. Rometsch, E.; Bos, P.K.; Koes, B.W. Survival of short hip stems with a "modern", trochanter-sparing design—A systematic literature review. *Hip Int.* **2012**, *22*, 344–354. [CrossRef]
7. Banerjee, S.; Pivec, R.; Issa, K.; Harwin, S.F.; Mont, M.A.; Khanuja, H.S. Outcomes of short stems in total hip arthroplasty. *Orthopedics* **2013**, *36*, 700–707. [CrossRef]
8. Chammaï, Y.; Brax, M. Medium-term comparison of results in obese patients and non-obese hip prostheses 345 with Metha® short stem. *Eur. J. Orthop. Surg. Traumatol.* **2015**, *25*, 503–508. [CrossRef]
9. Hungerford, M.W.; Schuh, R.; O'Reilly, M.P.; Jones, L.C. Outcome of minimally invasive hip replacement in obese, 347 overweight, and nonobese patients. *J. Surg. Orthop. Adv.* **2014**, *23*, 68–74. [CrossRef]
10. Feyen, H.; Shimmin, A.J. Is the length of the femoral component important in primary total hip replacement? *Bone Jt. J.* **2014**, *96*, 442–448. [CrossRef]
11. Harris, W.H. Traumatic arthritis of the hip after dislocation and acetabular fractures: Treatment by mold arthroplasty. An end-result study using a new method of result evaluation. *J. Bone Jt. Surg. Am.* **1969**, *51*, 737–755. [CrossRef]
12. Bellamy, N.; Buchanan, W.W.; Goldsmith, C.H.; Campbell, J.; Stitt, L.W. Validation study of WOMAC: A health status instrument for measuring clinically important patient relevant outcomes to antirheumatic drug therapy in patients with osteoarthritis of the hip or knee. *J. Rheumatol.* **1988**, *15*, 1833–1840. [PubMed]
13. Busija, L.; Pausenberger, E.; Haines, T.P.; Haymes, S.; Buchbinder, R.; Osborne, R.H. Adult measures of general health and health-related quality of life: Medical Outcomes Study Short Form 36-Item (SF-36) and Short Form 12-Item (SF-12) Health Surveys, Nottingham Health Profile (NHP), Sickness Impact Profile (SIP), Medical Outcomes Study Short Form 6D (SF-6D), Health Utilities Index Mark 3 (HUI3), Quality of Well-Being Scale (QWB), and Assessment of Quality of Life (AQoL). *Arthritis Care Res.* **2011**, *63* (Suppl. 11), S383–S412. [CrossRef]
14. Engh, C.A.; Massin, P.; Suthers, K.E. Roentgenographic assessment of the biologic fixation of porous-surfaced femoral components. *Clin. Orthop. Relat. Res.* **1990**, *257*, 107–128. [CrossRef]
15. Gruen, T.; McNeice, G.; Amstutz, H.C. "Model of failure" of cemented stem-type femoral components. A radiographic analysis of loosening. *Clin. Orthop. Relat. Res.* **1979**, *141*, 17–27. [CrossRef]
16. Albanese, C.V.; Santori, F.S.; Pavan, L.; Learmonth, I.D.; Passariello, R. Periprosthetic DXA after total hip arthroplasty with short vs. ultra-short custom-made femoral stems: 37 patients followed for 3 years. *Acta Orthop.* **2009**, *80*, 291–297. [CrossRef]
17. Logroscino, G.; Donati, F.; Campana, V.; Saracco, M. Stemless hip arthroplasty versus traditional implants: A comparative observational study at 30 months follow-up. *Hip Int.* **2018**, *28* (Suppl. 2), 21–27. [CrossRef]
18. Hodgkinson, J.P.; Shelley, P.; Wroblewski, B.M. The correlation between the roentgenographic appearance and operative findings at the bone-cement junction of the socket in Chanley lower friction arthroplasties. *Clin. Orthop. Relat. Res.* **1988**, *228*, 105–109. [CrossRef]
19. DeLee, J.G.; Charnley, J. Radiological demarcation of cemented sockets in total hip replacement. *Clin. Orthop. Relat. Res.* **1976**, *121*, 20–32. [CrossRef]
20. Brooker, A.F.; Bowerman, J.W. Ectopic ossification following total hip replacement. *J. Bone Jt. Surg. Am.* **1973**, *55*, 1629–1632. [CrossRef]
21. Lementowski, P.W.; Zelicof, S.B. Obesity and osteoarthritis. *Am. J. Orthop.* **2008**, *37*, 148–151. [PubMed]
22. Wendelboe, A.M.; Hegmann, K.T.; Biggs, J.J.; Cox, C.M.; Portmann, A.J.; Gildea, J.H.; Gren, L.H.; Lyon, J.L. Relationships between body mass indices and surgical replacements of knee and hip joints. *Am. J. Prev. Med.* **2003**, *25*, 290–295. [PubMed]
23. Muehleman, C.; Margulis, A.; Bae, W.C.; Masuda, K. Relationship between knee and ankle degeneration in a population of organ donors. *BMC Med.* **2010**, *8*, 48. [CrossRef] [PubMed]
24. Horan, F. Obesity and joint replacement. *J. Bone Jt. Surg.* **2006**, *88*, 1269–1271. [CrossRef] [PubMed]
25. McLaughlin, J.R.; Lee, K.R. The outcome of total hip replacement in obese and nonobese patients at 10- to 18-years. *J. Bone Jt. Surg.* **2006**, *88*, 1286–1292. [CrossRef]
26. Jiganti, J.J.; Goldstein, W.M.; Williams, C.S. A comparison of the perioperative morbidity in total joint arthroplasty in the obese and nonobese patient. *Clin. Orthop.* **1993**, *289*, 175–179. [CrossRef]
27. Jackson, M.P.; Sexton, S.A.; Yeung, E.; Walter, W.L.; Walter, W.K.; Zicat, B.A. The effect of obesity on the mid-term survival and clinical outcome of cementless total hip replacement. *J. Bone Jt. Surg. Br.* **2009**, *91*, 1296–1300. [CrossRef]

28. Michalka, P.K.; Khan, R.J.; Scaddan, M.C.; Haebich, S.; Chirodian, N.; Wimhurst, J.A. The influence of obesity on early outcomes in primary hip arthroplasty. *J. Arthroplast.* **2012**, *27*, 391–396.
29. Kim, Y.; Morshed, S.; Joseph, T.; Bozic, K.; Ries, M.D. Clinical impact of obesity on stability following revision total hip arthroplasty. *Clin. Orthop.* **2006**, *453*, 142–146. [CrossRef]
30. Pipino, F.; Keller, A. Tissue-sparing surgery: 25 years experience with femoral neck preserving hip arthroplasty. *J. Orthop. Traumatol.* **2006**, *7*, 36–41. [CrossRef]
31. Lübbeke, A.; Stern, R.; Garavaglia, G.; Zurcher, L.; Hoffmeyer, P. Differences in outcomes of obese women and men undergoing primary total hip arthroplasty. *Arthritis Rheum* **2007**, *57*, 327–334. [CrossRef] [PubMed]
32. Ibrahim, T.; Hobson, S.; Beiri, A.; Esler, C.N. No influence of body mass index on early outcome following total hip arthroplasty. *Int. Orthop.* **2005**, *29*, 359–361. [CrossRef] [PubMed]
33. Pirard, E.; De Lint, J.A. Anteversion of the acetabular component in obese patients. *Hip Int.* **2007**, *17*, 99–103. [CrossRef] [PubMed]
34. Todkar, M. Obesity does not necessarily affect the accuracy of acetabular cup implantation in total hip replacement. *Acta Orthop. Belg.* **2008**, *74*, 206–209. [PubMed]
35. Bosker, B.H.; Verheyen, C.C.P.M.; Horstmann, W.G.; Tulp, N.J.A. Poor accuracy of freehand cup positioning during total hip arthroplasty. *Arch. Orthop. Trauma Surg.* **2007**, *127*, 375–379. [CrossRef] [PubMed]
36. Callanan, M.C.; Jarrett, B.; Bragdon, C.R.; Zurakowski, D.; Rubash, H.E.; Freiberg, A.A.; Malchau, H. The John Charnley Award: Risk factors for cup malpositioning: Quality improvement through a joint registry at a tertiary hospital. *Clin. Orthop. Relat. Res.* **2011**, *469*, 319–329. [CrossRef]
37. Elson, L.C.; Barr, C.J.; Chandran, S.E.; Hansen, V.J.; Malchau, H.; Kwon, Y.M. Are morbidly obese patients undergoing total hip arthroplasty at an increased risk for component malpositioning? *J. Arthroplast.* **2013**, *28*, 41–44. [CrossRef]
38. Tai, S.M.; Imbuldeniya, A.M.; Munir, S.; Walter, W.L.; Walter, W.K.; Zicat, B.A. The effect of obesity on the clinical, functional and radiological outcome of cementless total hip replacement: A case-matched study with a minimum 10-year follow-up. *J. Arthroplast.* **2014**, *29*, 1758–1762. [CrossRef]
39. Brodt, S.; Jacob, B.; Windisch, C.; Seeger, J.; Matziolis, G. Morbidly Obese Patients Undergoing Reduced Cup Anteversion Through a Direct LateralApproach. *J. Bone Jt. Surg. Am.* **2016**, *98*, 729–734. [CrossRef]
40. Culliford, D.; Maskell, J.; Judge, A.; Arden, N.K.; COAST Study Group. A population-based survival analysis describing the association of body mass Index on time to revision for total hip and knee replacements: Results from the UK general practice research database. *BMJ Open* **2013**, *3*, e003614. [CrossRef]
41. Braud, P.; Freeman, M.A. The effect of retention of the femoral neck and of cement upon the stability of proximal femoral prosthesis. *J. Arthroplast.* **1990**, *5*, S5–S10. [CrossRef] [PubMed]
42. Freitag, T.; Kappe, T.; Fuchs, M.; Jung, S.; Reichel, H.; Bieger, R. Migration pattern of a femoral short-stem prosthesis: A 2-year ERBA-FCA-study. *Arch. Orthop. Trauma Surg.* **2014**, *134*, 1003–1008. [CrossRef] [PubMed]
43. Andrew, J.G.; Palan, J.; Kurup, H.V.; Gibson, P.; Murray, D.W.; Beard, D.J. Obesity in total hip replacement. *J. Bone Jt. Surg. Br.* **2008**, *90*, 424–429. [CrossRef] [PubMed]
44. Wattanakit, K.; Lutsey, P.L.; Bell, E.J.; Gornik, H.; Cushman, M.; Heckbert, S.R.; Heckbert, S.R.; Folsom, A.R. Association between cardiovascular disease risk factors and occurrence of venous thromboembolism. A time-dependent analysis. *Thromb. Haemost.* **2012**, *108*, 508–515. [CrossRef] [PubMed]
45. Friedman, R.J.; Hess, S.; Berkowitz, S.D.; Homering, M. Complication rates after hip or knee arthroplasty in morbidly obese patients. *Clin. Orthop. Relat. Res.* **2013**, *471*, 3358–3366. [CrossRef] [PubMed]
46. Fidanza, A.; Schettini, I.; Palozzi, G.; Mitrousias, V.; Logroscino, G.; Romanini, E.; Calvisi, V. What Is the Inpatient Cost of Hip Replacement? A Time-Driven Activity Based Costing Pilot Study in an Italian Public Hospital. *J. Clin. Med.* **2022**, *11*, 6928. [CrossRef]
47. Nadzadi, M.E.; Pedersen, D.R.; Yack, H.J.; Callaghan, J.J.; Brown, T.D. Kinematics, kinetics, and finite element analysis of commonplace maneuvers at risk for total hip dislocation. *J. Biomech.* **2003**, *36*, 577–591. [CrossRef]
48. Liu, W.; Wahafu, T.; Cheng, M.; Cheng, T.; Zhang, Y.; Zhang, X. The influence of obesity on primary total hip arthroplasty outcomes: A meta-analysis of prospective cohort studies. *Orthop. Traumatol. Surg. Res.* **2015**, *101*, 289–296. [CrossRef]
49. Elkins, J.M.; Stroud, N.J.; Rudert, M.J.; Tochigi, Y.; Pedersen, D.R.; Ellis, B.J.; Callaghan, J.J.; Weiss, J.A.; Brown, T.D. The capsule's contribution to total hip construct stability: A finite element analysis. *J. Orthop. Res.* **2011**, *29*, 1642–1648. [CrossRef]
50. Pulido, L.; Ghanem, E.; Joshi, A.; Purtill, J.J.; Parvizi, J. Periprosthetic joint infection: The incidence, timing, and predisposing factors. *Clin. Orthop. Relat. Res.* **2008**, *466*, 1710–1715. [CrossRef]
51. Iannotti, F.; Prati, P.; Fidanza, A.; Iorio, R.; Ferretti, A.; Pèrez Prieto, D.; Kort, N.; Violante, B.; Pipino, G.; Schiavone Panni, A.; et al. Prevention of Periprosthetic Joint Infection (PJI): A Clinical Practice Protocol in High-Risk Patients. *Trop. Med. Infect. Dis.* **2020**, *5*, 186. [CrossRef] [PubMed]
52. Moran, M.; Walmsley, P.; Gray, A.; Brenkel, I.J. Does body mass index affect the early outcome of primary total hip arthroplasty? *J. Arthroplast.* **2005**, *20*, 866–869. [CrossRef] [PubMed]
53. Dowsey, M.M.; Choong, P.F. Obesity is a major risk factor for prosthetic infection after primary hip arthroplasty. *Clin. Orthop. Relat Res.* **2008**, *466*, 153–158. [CrossRef] [PubMed]
54. Zmistowski, B.; Tetreault, M.W.; Alijanipour, P.; Chen, A.F.; Della Valle, C.J.; Parvizi, J. Recurrent periprosthetic joint infection: Persistent or new infection? *J. Arthroplast.* **2013**, *28*, 1486–1489. [CrossRef]

55. Patel, V.P.; Walsh, M.; Sehgal, B.; Preston, C.; DeWal, H.; Di Cesare, P.E. Factors associated with prolonged wound drainage after primary total hip and knee arthroplasty. *J. Bone Jt. Surg.* **2007**, *89*, 33–38. [CrossRef]
56. Cordero-Ampuero, J.; De Dios, M. What are the risk factors for infection in hemiarthroplasties and total hip arthroplasties? *Clin. Orthop. Relat. Res.* **2010**, *468*, 3268–3277. [CrossRef]
57. Baek, S.H. Identification and preoperative optimization of risk factors to prevent periprosthetic joint infection. *World J. Orthop.* **2014**, *5*, 362–367. [CrossRef]
58. Belmont, P.J., Jr.; Goodman, G.P.; Hamilton, W.; Waterman, B.R.; Bader, J.O.; Schoenfeld, A.J. Morbidity and mortality in the thirty-day period following total hip arthroplasty: Risk factors and incidence. *J. Arthroplast.* **2014**, *29*, 2025–2030. [CrossRef]
59. Watts, C.D.; Houdek, M.T.; Wagner, E.R.; Sculco, P.K.; Chalmers, B.P.; Taunton, M.J. High Risk of Wound Complications Following Direct Anterior Total Hip Arthroplasty in Obese Patients. *J. Arthroplast.* **2015**, *30*, 2296–2298. [CrossRef]

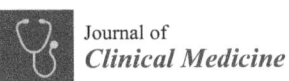

Article

A 20-Year Retrospective Study of Children and Adolescents Treated by the Three-in-One Procedure for Patellar Realignment

Giovanni Trisolino [1,*], Alessandro Depaoli [1], Giovanni Gallone [1], Marco Ramella [1], Eleonora Olivotto [2], Paola Zarantonello [1], Stefano Stallone [3], Valentina Persiani [4], Giacomo Casadei [1] and Gino Rocca [1]

1. Pediatric Orthopedics and Traumatology, IRCSS—Istituto Ortopedico Rizzoli, 40136 Bologna, Italy
2. RAMSES Laboratory, RIT Department, IRCSS—Istituto Ortopedico Rizzoli, 40136 Bologna, Italy
3. Department of Trauma and Orthopedic Surgery, Maggiore Hospital, 40133 Bologna, Italy
4. Unit of Orthopedics and Traumatology, IRCCS—Policlinico Sant'Orsola-Malpighi, 40137 Bologna, Italy
* Correspondence: giovanni.trisolino@ior.it; Tel.: +39-051-636-6484

Abstract: Background: Patellar instability is the most common disorder of the knee during childhood and adolescence. Surgical treatment significantly reduces the rate of redislocation, but the underlying pathologies and pattern of instability may affect the results. We aimed to report the clinical and functional outcomes of the three-in-one procedure for patellar realignment in a cohort of skeletally immature patients with or without syndromes and various patterns of chronic patellar instability. Methods: We retrospectively investigated 126 skeletally immature patients (168 knees) affected by idiopathic or syndromic patellar instability, who underwent patella realignment through a three-in-one procedure. We classified the instability according to the score proposed by Parikh and Lykissas. Results: Patellar dislocation was idiopathic in 71 patients (94 knees; 56.0%) and syndromic in 55 (74 knees; 44.0%). The mean age at surgery was 11.5 years (range 4–18) and was significantly lower in syndromic patients. Syndromic patients also exhibited more severe clinical pattern at presentation, based on the Parikh and Lykissas score. The mean follow-up was 5.3 years (range 1.0–15.4). Redislocation occurred in 19 cases, with 10 cases requiring further realignment. The Parikh and Lykissas score and the presence of congenital ligamentous laxity were independent predictors of failure. A total of 22 knees in 18 patients required additional surgical procedures. The post-operative Kujala score was significantly lower in patients with syndromic patellar instability. Conclusions: The type of instability and the presence of underlying syndromes negatively affect the rate of redislocation and the clinical and functional outcome following patellar realignment through the three-in-one procedure. We recommend the consideration of alternative surgical strategies, especially in children with severe syndromic patellar dislocation.

Keywords: patellar instability; pediatric; three-in-one procedure; green procedure; Roux-Goldthwait; syndrome; congenital ligamentous laxity; neurologic; obligatory patella dislocation; fixed patella dislocation

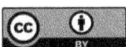

Citation: Trisolino, G.; Depaoli, A.; Gallone, G.; Ramella, M.; Olivotto, E.; Zarantonello, P.; Stallone, S.; Persiani, V.; Casadei, G.; Rocca, G. A 20-Year Retrospective Study of Children and Adolescents Treated by the Three-in-One Procedure for Patellar Realignment. *J. Clin. Med.* **2023**, *12*, 702. https://doi.org/10.3390/jcm12020702

Academic Editor: Christian Carulli

Received: 11 September 2022
Revised: 8 January 2023
Accepted: 10 January 2023
Published: 16 January 2023

Copyright: © 2023 by the authors. Licensee MDPI, Basel, Switzerland. This article is an open access article distributed under the terms and conditions of the Creative Commons Attribution (CC BY) license (https://creativecommons.org/licenses/by/4.0/).

1. Introduction

Patellar instability is one of the most common disorders of the knee during childhood and adolescence [1,2]. It includes several different conditions, such as acute dislocations, subluxations, recurrent instability, and congenital dislocations [3,4]. The etiology is multifactorial involving trauma, congenital bone abnormalities, neuromuscular impairment, and ligamentous laxity [5,6].

Patellar dislocation in children and adolescents is more challenging because of the heterogeneity of the clinical patterns at presentation, the skeletal immaturity, and the frequency of associated conditions. Several classification systems have been proposed for enabling surgeons to recommend specific treatment options and for allowing comparison among different conditions and treatments [5,7–11]. Recently, Parikh and Lykissas proposed a comprehensive classification system which classified patella instability into four types based on increasing severity and complexity of required treatment (see Table 1) [4]. While type 1 and type 2 dislocations are commonly seen in adolescents and young adults, type 3 obligatory (habitual) and type 4 congenital (fixed) dislocations are less frequent. In fact, type 3 and 4 dislocations are generally encountered in young children and are the most demanding patterns, due to the potential underlying etiologies and complex anatomic pathology. These dislocations can be associated with neuromuscular diseases (i.e., cerebral palsy), congenital deformities (nail–patella syndrome, amyoplasia, congenital limb defects), and collagen disorders due to chromosomic or genetic pathologies (Down syndrome, Elhers–Danlos syndrome, etc.). Patients with congenital or obligatory dislocation may present with knee malalignment, which may be either primary, contributing to the patellar dislocation mechanism, or secondary to the malpositioned extensor mechanism. Flexion contracture and limping are also typical findings [12].

Table 1. Classification of patellar instability according to Parikh and Lykissas [4].

Parikh and Lykissas Classification Type/Subtype	Description
Type 1	First patellar dislocation
A	With osteochondral fracture
B	Without osteochondral fracture
Type 2	Recurrent patellar instability
A	Recurrent patellar subluxation
B	Recurrent (>2) patellar dislocation
Type 3	Dislocatable patella
A	Passive patellar dislocation
B	Habitual patellar dislocation in flexion or extension
Type 4	Dislocated patella
A	Reducible
B	Irreducible

Although conservative management is generally indicated in acute lesions without osteochondral defects, surgical treatment is recommended in the case of recurrent patellar instability, osteochondral fractures with loose bodies, and failed non-operative measures [13–16]. There is a consensus that the surgical results may be affected by the type of dislocation and the presence of underlying pathologies [4,13,17]. However, the impact of these factors has not been clearly quantified.

Therefore, the aim of the present study is to report the mid- to long-term results of a cohort of children and adolescents affected by various types of patellar instability, with or without underlying pathologies, that underwent patellar realignment through a three-in-one surgical procedure. Our question is if the type of patellar instability and the associated conditions may affect the post-operative results.

2. Materials and Methods

2.1. Study Design

The present study is a retrospective analysis of a cohort of skeletally immature patients affected by patellar instability, undergoing patellar realignment through a three-in-one procedure. Our unit is a tertiary referral department for pediatric orthopedics, which treats approximately 20–30 cases of patellar instability per year. The hospital's electronic medical records (charts and radiograms) were used to collect data retrospectively. Skeletally immature patients with still-open physes who underwent the three-in-one procedure were included in the study. Conservative treatment and other surgical treatments (such as isolated lateral release, MPFL reconstruction, isolated proximal or distal realignment,

Langenskiöld or Stanisavljevic techniques) were considered exclusion criteria. The investigation was conducted by independent observers who were not involved in the treatment of the patients.

2.2. Baseline Variables

Clinical baseline variables included age, sex, body mass index (BMI) percentile adjusted for sex and age, history of trauma, comorbidities, and previous operations. From an etiologic point of view, the patella dislocation was classified as idiopathic or syndromic. The latter encompasses patients with neuromuscular disorders (e.g., cerebral palsy), connective tissue disorders (e.g., Ehlers–Danlos syndrome), or other syndromes with abnormalities of the lower limb (e.g., longitudinal defects of the lower limb, amyoplasia, etc.).

The pattern of patellar instability was classified according to the Parikh and Lykissas score by two of the authors (G.T. and S.S.) who independently read medical records: Type 1 means first-time patellar dislocation, type 2 means second or subsequent patellar dislocation or continued symptoms after an initial instability episode, type 3 is a habitually dislocatable (actively or passively) patella, and type 4 is a permanently dislocated (reducible or fixed) patella (see Table 1).

The radiographic baseline variables included patellar height evaluated according to the Caton–Deschamps methods, patellar congruence, patellar tilt, Tibial Tuberosity-Trochlear Groove distance (TT-TG), and Hip–Knee–Ankle (HKA) angle [18–23].

2.3. Surgical Technique

In all the cases, we performed a three-in-one procedure (See Figure 1A–G). The surgical technique was already described elsewhere [24]. Briefly, a long lateral parapatellar incision was used, extending 2 cm from the supero-lateral pole of the patella, to 2–3 cm below the tibial tuberosity. A quadricepsplasty, including an extensive lateral retinacular release (leaving the synovium intact, when possible) and a dissection of the vastus medialis obliquus from the quadriceps tendon was performed, according to Green [25]. Afterward, the vastus medialis complex was transferred distally and laterally to the anterior surface of the patella. The patellar tendon was split longitudinally and the lateral half was detached from its distal insertion and passed medially, beneath its intact medial half, and then sutured in a pouch of periosteum, under the insertion of the pes anserinus [24,26]. The knee was held at about 30° of flexion during the operation, to avoid excessive tension to the patellar tendon.

2.4. Post-Operative Management and Follow-Up

The leg was immobilized in an above-the-knee cast with 30° of knee flexion for a 4-week period. Then, a period of 12–20 weeks of physical therapy and the use of a patellar bracing were recommended.

The rate of recurrent instability, the rate of reoperation, and the rate of additional surgical procedures were reported. An Italian validated version of the Kujala Anterior Knee Pain Scale (AKPS) Score [27,28], was administered to each patient at the last evaluation at follow-up or with a self-filled form. For non-cooperating patients (e.g., young children and syndromic patients), parents were asked to answer the questions. The final score was rated as good/excellent (AKPS ≥ 85), fair (AKPS 65–84), and poor (AKPS < 65) [29].

2.5. Data Analysis

Patients were assigned a numerical code, and their data were entered into Excel (Microsoft, Redmond, WA, USA) and SPSS (version 22.0; SPSS, Chicago, IL, USA). Continuous data were expressed as mean ± standard deviation (SD) and range, whereas categorical and ordinal data were expressed as raw numbers and proportions with a 95% confidence interval (C.I.). Normality was tested using the χ^2 test for categorical variables and the Kolmogorov–Smirnov test for continuous variables. Differences between groups were analyzed using the Fisher's exact test for categorical variables and the Student's t-test (normal data) or the Mann–Whitney U test (skewed data) for continuous variables. The Spearman's rank test was used for correlations. Exploratory univariate analyses with General Linear Models were performed to assess the impact of the baseline variables on the outcome. Unconditional logistic regression with Wald backward selection was then used to adjust for variables identified in univariate analysis to be significantly different between the outcomes. The survival free from redislocation was calculated using the method of Kaplan and Meyer, and we conducted Cox proportional hazards modeling entering variables found to be significantly related to the survival time free from redislocation. A p-value of <0.05 was considered to be statistically significant, and all reported p-values were 2-sided.

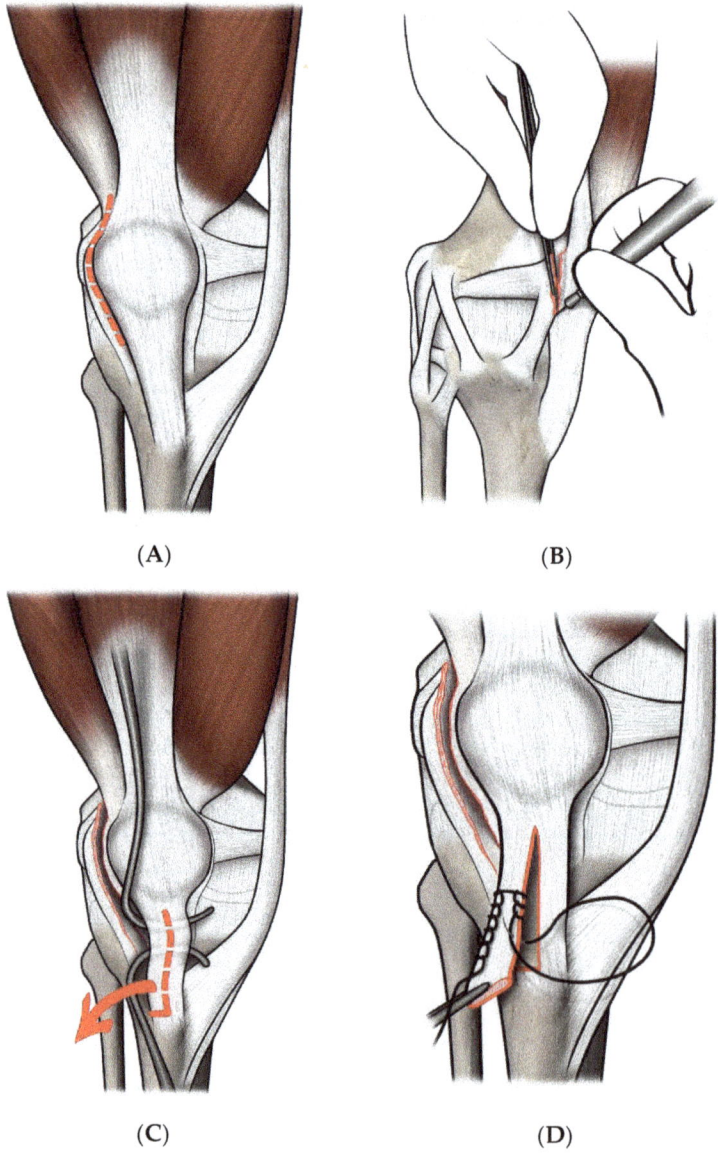

Figure 1. *Cont.*

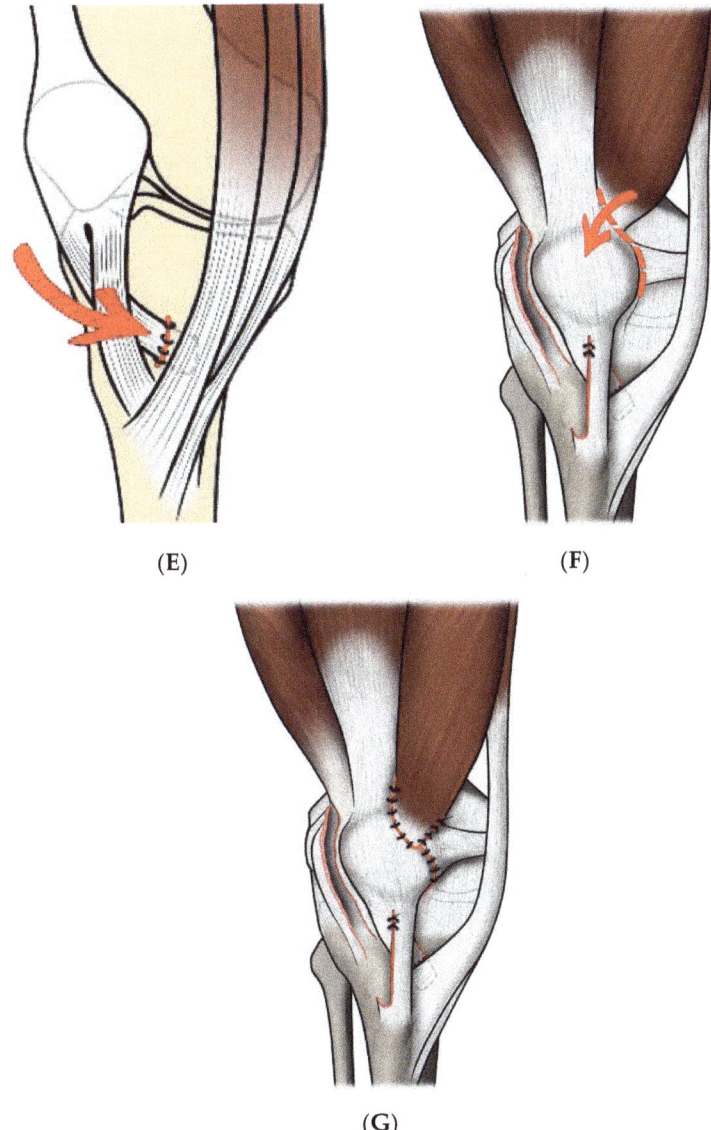

Figure 1. (**A**) lateral parapatellar incision; (**B**) extensive lateral retinacular release; (**C**) the patellar tendon was split longitudinally (red arrow); (**D**) the lateral half was detached from its distal insertion and passed medially; (**E**) the lateral half was sutured in a pouch of periosteum, under the pes anserinus (red arrow); (**F**) the vastus medialis obliquus was detached from the quadriceps tendon, and the medial capsule was dissected; (**G**) the vastus medialis obliquus and the medial capsule were transferred distally and laterally to the anterior surface of the patella (red arrow).

3. Results

3.1. Demographics and Clinical/Radiographic Parameters at Baseline

From May 2004 to July 2020, 126 patients (168 knees) underwent the three-in-one procedure for patella realignment. Demographic, clinical, and radiographic baseline data are reported in Table 2.

Table 2. Demographic and radiographic baseline data.

Baseline Variable	Measurement	Value
Patients/Knees	Number (male/females)	126/168 (46/80)
Age at treatment (years)	Mean ± SD (range)	11.5 ± 3.7 (4.1–17.6)
BMI (kg/m^2)	Mean ± SD (range)	20.2 ± 4.3 (11.2–38.1)
BMI (percentile)	Median (IQR)	74.5 (37.0–93.0)
Caton–Deschamps ratio	Mean ± SD (range)	1.4 ± 0.4 (0.6–2.6)
Congruence angle (°)	Mean ± SD (range)	39.1 ± 32.5 (2.6–128.4)
Patellar tilt (°)	Mean ± SD (range)	26.1 ± 25.5 (0–127.3)
Sulcus angle (°)	Mean ± SD (range)	149.0 ± 15.8 (111–180)
TT-TG distance (mm)	Mean ± SD (range)	14.1 ± 8.1 (5–20.6)
HKA angle	Mean ± SD (range)	7.6 ± 8.5 (−10.4 varus–+41.0 valgus)

SD = standard deviation; BMI = body mass index; TT-TG = tibial tuberosity–trochlear groove; HKA angle = hip–knee–ankle angle; IQR = interquartile range.

The patellar dislocation was idiopathic in 71 patients (94 knees; 56.0%) and syndromic in 55 (74 knees; 44.0%). Among the idiopathic patients, a history of trauma was reported in 12 cases. Among the syndromic children, thirty had congenital ligamentous laxity (fourteen Down syndrome, four Elhers–Danlos syndrome, four multiple epiphyseal dysplasia/spondyloepiphyseal dysplasia, two DiGeorge syndrome, one Jacobsen syndrome, one Prune belly syndrome, one Marfan syndrome, one type I osteogenesis imperfecta, one Prader–Willi syndrome, one Coffin–Siris syndrome), eight had neuromuscular disorders (seven cerebral palsy, one muscular dystrophy), and eighteen had congenital deformities of the lower limb (five amyoplasia congenita, two torsional malalignment, two sequelae of tibial and femoral bone infection during infancy, one Sotos syndrome, one Moebius syndrome, one VACTERL syndrome, one nail–patella syndrome, one congenital pseudarthrosis of tibia in NF1, three tibial hemimelia).

As expected, syndromic patients had a lower age at surgery (mean difference = 2.4 years; 95% C.I.: 1.3–3.5 years; p-value = 0.0001, see Table 3) and more severe clinical pattern at presentation (p-value = 0.0001, see Figure 2 for details).

Table 3. Differences in baseline clinical and radiographic variables between idiopathic and syndromic cases.

Baseline Variable	Group	N	Mean ± SD	p-Value
Age at treatment (years)	Idiopathic	94	12.6 ± 3.5	0.0001 *
	Syndromic	74	10.2 ± 3.6	
BMI	Idiopathic	91	21.1 ± 4.4	0.002 *
	Syndromic	67	19.0 ± 4.0	
Caton–Deschamps ratio	Idiopathic	47	1.4 ± 0.6	0.649
	Syndromic	40	1.4 ± 0.4	
Congruence angle (°)	Idiopathic	46	34.89 ± 29.9	0.172
	Syndromic	34	44.9 ± 35.4	
Patellar tilt (°)	Idiopathic	45	18.4 ± 11.7	0.001 *
	Syndromic	33	36.6 ± 34..3	
Sulcus angle (°)	Idiopathic	47	148.7 ± 14.3	0.848
	Syndromic	34	149.4 ± 17.9	
TT-TG distance (mm)	Idiopathic	20	12.4 ± 5.5	0.884
	Syndromic	13	12.7 ± 6.5	
HKA angle (°)	Idiopathic	33	7.5 ± 7.0	0.943
	Syndromic	36	7.7 ± 9.8	

HKA angle = hip–knee–ankle angle; N = number of knees; SD = standard deviation. *: difference between groups were statistically significant (p-value < 0.05).

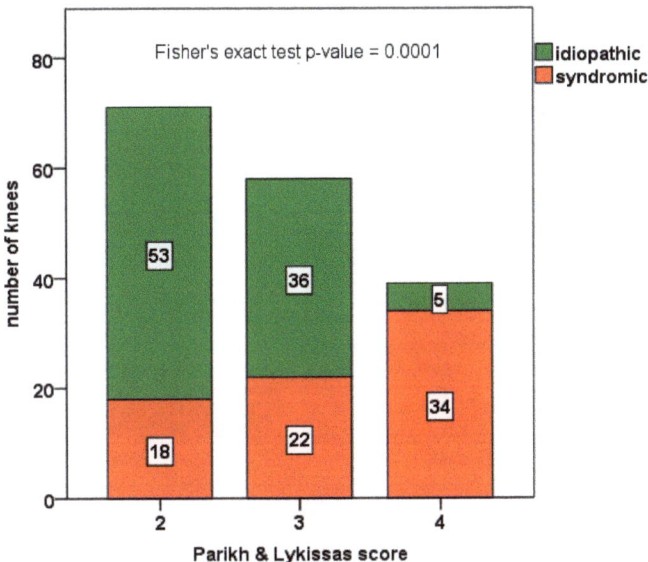

Figure 2. Distribution of idiopathic (depicted in green) and syndromic knees with patellar instability (depicted in red) in groups by Parikh and Lykissas score. Fisher's exact test *p*-value = 0.0001.

With the available radiographic imaging, only patellar tilt was significantly different between idiopathic and syndromic patients (see Table 3).

3.2. Complications and Rate of Redislocation

A total of 14 patients (20 knees; 11.9%) did not return for follow-up visits and were unavailable to phone or email interview. For the remaining patients, the mean follow-up averaged 5.3 ± 3.1 (1–15.4) years and was significantly higher in syndromic patients (*p*-value = 0.0001). We did not report any infection and/or wound healing problem. Recurrent dislocation was observed in 19 knees (12.8%; 95% C.I.: 7.9–19.3%), with 14 cases (9.5%; 95% C.I.: 5.3–15.3%) receiving further realignment procedures. Patients with redislocation had a lower age at surgery (mean difference 2.0 years, 95% C.I.: 0.2–3.8, *p*-value 0.0303) and higher grade of severity according to the Parikh and Lykissas score (Mann–Whitney U test *p*-value 0.007). In particular, the rate of recurrent instability was 5.2% in type 2 of the Parikh and Lykissas score, 13.2% in type 3, and 24.3% in type 4.

The rate of recurrent instability was also higher in syndromic cases compared with idiopathic cases (19.1% vs. 7.5%, *p*-value = 0.031), especially in children with congenital ligamentous laxity (see Figure 3). However, in a logistic regression model including age at surgery, Parikh and Lykissas score, and congenital ligamentous laxity, children with congenital ligamentous laxity showed a five-fold increased risk for redislocation, compared to the rest of the cohort (OR 5.4, 95% C.I. 2.0–15.0, *p*-value 0.001, see Figure 3).

3.3. Survival Free from Redislocation

The overall cumulative 5-year survival rate free from redislocation was 87.0% (95% C.I.: 83.5—90.5%), while the 10-year survival rate was 70.6% (95% C.I.: 63.1—78.1%). The log-rank test confirmed that significant differences existed in the survival curves between children with syndromic congenital ligamentous laxity compared to the rest of the cohort (10-year survival: 51.6% vs. 86.4%; *p* = 0.018, see Figure 4).

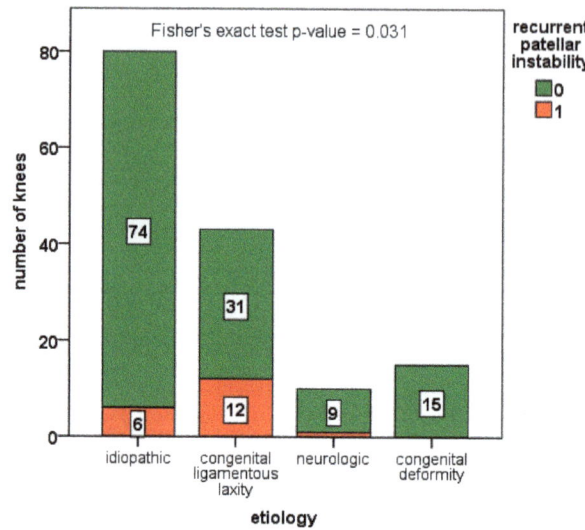

Figure 3. Number of redislocations (depicted in red) among the different subgroups of patients, based on etiology.

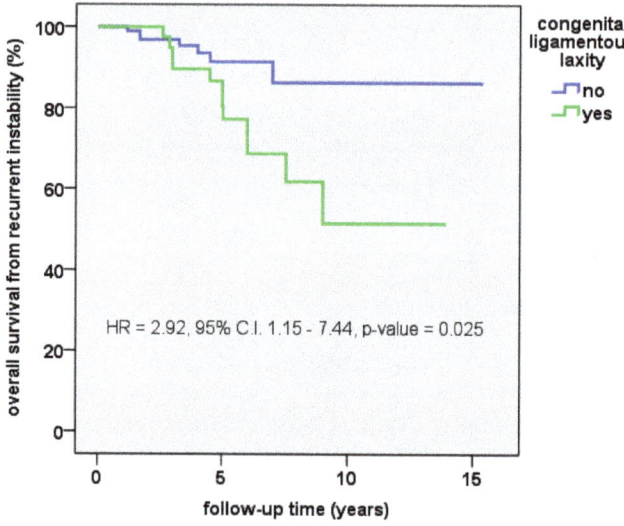

Figure 4. Kaplan–Meyer survival curve free from recurrent instability in children with and without syndromic congenital ligamentous laxity. HR = hazard ratio; C.I. = confidence interval.

With the numbers available, none of the other pre-operative variables significantly affected the survival rate free from redislocation.

3.4. Additional Surgical Procedures

A total of 22 knees (13.1%) in 18 patients underwent additional staged surgical procedures (ten femoral and/or tibial osteotomies, three hamstring lengthenings, four femoral medial hemiepiphysiodesis, one limb lengthening, one controlateral femur shortening osteotomy, one subtalar arthroeresis, one fixation of osteochondral fragment, and one open reduction and fixation with K-wire of knee subluxation in DiGeorge syndrome). The proportion of additional surgical procedures was significantly higher in syndromic children (23.0% vs. 5.3%; *p*-value = 0.001, see Figure 5) and correlated with Parikh and Lykissas score (5.6% in grade 2, 10.3% in grade 3, 30.8% in grade 4; *p*-value = 0.001).

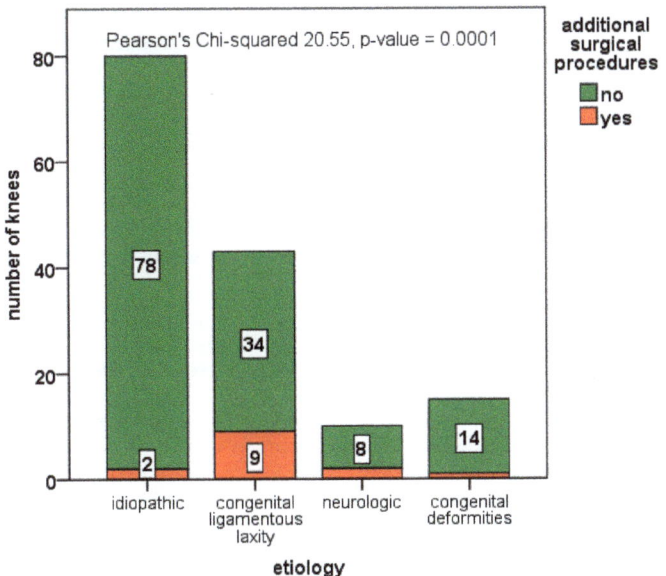

Figure 5. Number of additional surgical procedures (depicted in red) among the different subgroups of patients, based on etiology.

3.5. Clinical and Functional Outcomes

At the latest follow-up, The AKPS score was available in 136 knees and averaged 86.4 ± 16.3 points (28–100); overall, 85 knees had good/excellent results (62.5%), 38 had fair results (27.9%), and 13 had poor results (9.6%). Syndromic patients had significantly lower scores compared to idiopathic patients (mean difference = 9.1 points; 95% C.I.: 3.7–14.1; *p*-value = 0.001, see Table 4). Among the patients who did not return the AKPS, one patient developed avascular necrosis of the patella, with severe chondral damage, early onset osteoarthritis, and poor outcome. Another patient refused to participate to the survey, since he was leg amputated due to congenital pseudarthrosis of the tibia in NF1.

Table 4. Post-operative variables.

Post-Operative Variable	Group	N	Mean ± SD	*p*-Value
Follow-up time (years)	Idiopathic	79	4.2 ± 2.6	0.0001 *
	Syndromic	68	6.5 ± 3.3	
Kujala AKPS score	Idiopathic	74	90.5 ± 13.1	0.001 *
	Syndromic	62	81.4 ± 18.3	

N = number of knees; SD = standard deviation; AKPS = anterior knee pain scale. *: difference between groups were statistically significant (*p*-value < 0.05).

4. Discussion

Many papers in the current literature faced with the management of patellar dislocation in a pediatric population and several surgical techniques have been described to realign the patella in skeletally immature patients [6,30]. Currently, there is evidence that surgical treatment is superior to conservative treatment in reducing the recurrence of the dislocation [13–16,31]. In particular, the combination of proximal and distal procedures has demonstrated high effectiveness in preventing relapse [14,32]. However, there is still poor evidence about the superiority of any technique of patellar realignment over the others [33].

Pagliazzi et al. reported a meta-analysis of 10 RCTs and 510 patients, demonstrating that surgical treatment significantly reduces the rate of redislocation at short (9% vs. 21%; Risk Ratio for redislocation = 0.40 in favor of surgery) and medium follow-up (21% vs. 30% Risk Ratio for redislocation = 0.58 in favor of surgery) and improves clinical and functional outcomes compared to nonoperative treatment [16]. However, in the subgroup analysis on the adolescent population, the authors noticed a slight increase in the pooled rate of redislocation (23% in the surgical group, 31% in the non-surgical group), concluding that, although trends were similar, the higher redislocation rate in adolescents, together with the variability of the clinical outcome, suggests large heterogeneity of this peculiar population.

Another systematic review including retrospective case series and non-randomized studies reported results from 21 studies and overall 448 knees in pediatric patients treated with various surgical procedures. The authors reported a cumulative rate of redislocation of 13.8%, consistent with our results [34]. The authors also confirmed the large variation of results among studies (from 0% to 82%), while excluding syndromic cases from analysis, and no superiority of a specific technique over the others.

The main issue of these systematic reviews is that the most valuable RCTs and prospective studies were tailored on homogeneous populations, with inconsistent applicability to the broad spectrum of patients with patellar instability [14]. Children with high-grade patellar instability and underlying conditions, such as neuromuscular disorders, collagen disorders, and congenital deformities, were generally excluded from these studies, and only sparse case series dealt with these rare conditions [24,35,36]. Therefore, a gap in knowledge exists about the role of congenital pathologies in affecting the surgical results of these complex cases, that, on the other hand, are not so uncommon in highly specialized referral centers for pediatric orthopedics.

Different from sports medicine and adult knee services, in our experience, children with idiopathic and syndromic patellar dislocation were almost equally represented, since our unit is a tertiary referral center for pediatric orthopedics and rare bone diseases. This peculiarity allows us to deal with the entire spectrum of patellar instability, but it lowers the consistency of our information about prognosis. To stratify these heterogeneous cohorts of patients, comprehensive and reliable classification tools are required. We used a recent classification system proposed by Parikh and Lykissas. Despite the fact that several scores were proposed in the past for classifying patellar instability in children [5,7–11], the system proposed by Parikh and Lykissas seems to be comprehensive, reliable, and simple to adopt, since it was based only on the clinical history and patient examination, not requiring specific manual or instrumental tests. We demonstrated that this classification can accurately predict the risk of redislocation after patellar realignment in children; therefore, we recommend this classification both for research purposes (data standardization) and in clinical practice (for decision making).

We also quantified the risk of recurrent dislocation for children with congenital disorders and syndromes. We found that, compared to idiopathic cases, syndromic patients have more than twice the risk of recurrent dislocation. In particular, children with congenital collagen disorders have a five-fold increased risk of redislocation, and it is conceivable that almost 50% of cases will relapse within ten years after surgery. Other sparse series and case reports regarding recurrent, obligatory, and fixed patella dislocation in syndromic children and adolescents treated with various techniques showed a rate of residual instability and redislocation ranging from 0 to 100% [24,35,37–39]. These case series also reported results about different techniques, such as the four-in-one procedure [35,40], the Langenskiöld procedure [41,42], and the Stanisavljevic procedure [37,38,43], which are considered the treatment of choice in congenital obligatory or fixed patellar dislocation. However, due to the rarity of these conditions, no evidence is available about the superiority of each technique over the others.

The use of the three-in-one procedure in skeletally immature patients has been previously reported in the literature. Myers et al. described 42 knees in 37 children undergoing the three-in-one procedure to treat recurrent patella dislocation. Among them, 11 patients had congenital ligamentous laxity [44]. The authors reported a redislocation rate of 9.5% at 2 to 7 years of follow-up, good or excellent clinical outcomes in 76%, and no association between redislocation and congenital ligamentous laxity. They also reported a deterioration of results over time, which is consistent with our findings. In fact, based on the Kaplan–Meyer analysis, we estimated an 86.6% survival rate free from redislocation at 5 years of follow-up, but only 70.9% at 10 years and even lower in the subgroup with congenital ligamentous laxity (51%). Bettuzzi et al. reported results from six children (10 knees) with patella instability and Down syndrome treated by the three-in-one procedure [24]. They reported no redislocation and overall improved symptoms and function at 8.7 years of follow-up. Oliva et al. reported results from a cohort of 25 children with unilateral recurrent patellar dislocation (at least two documented dislocations) undergoing the three-in-one procedure [45]. The authors selected only children without major knee deformities (such as genu valgum, increased Q-angle, patella alta, torsional deformities, patellar and trochlear dysplasia) and did not mention syndromic case management. The authors reported only one case of redislocation (4%) and general improvement of clinical and functional outcomes, although they noticed permanent side-to-side differences in isokinetic strength and thigh diameter, despite subjective success of the procedure. Malecki et al. compared 31 knees undergoing the three-in-one procedure and 32 knees receiving MPFL reconstruction by the adductor magnus tendon [46]. The authors did not report significant differences between groups regarding the rate of redislocation and functional results, although they found a significant difference in pain complaints, favoring the MPFL group.

The need for additional procedures for achieving a stable patella and restoring knee function and alignment is another matter of concern. In our experience, only 13% of patients underwent additional staged procedures for improving knee alignment. This could explain the high number of redislocations, especially in syndromic patients with irreducible patellar dislocation. Although bony procedures, such as trochleoplasty or transposition of the anterior tibial tuberosity, are generally contraindicated in such young patients, the restoration of the knee axis through epiphysiodesis or sparing-physis osteotomies is sometimes required for correcting severe genu valgum, knee flexion, or femoral torsion, especially in children with congenital deformities or neurologic disorders. Alternatively, other surgical procedures, such as the Langenskiöld or the Stanisavljevic procedures, should be considered for these severe conditions. For this purpose, meticulous pre-operative planning is required. The recent advancement in the field of computer-aided surgical simulation, virtual surgical planning, and motion analysis will provide us with innovative digital solutions for increasing the rate of successful and durable long-term outcomes even in extreme cases [47,48].

Limitations

The strengths of our study include the large number of cases, the use of a comprehensive, reliable, and simple classification of pediatric patellar instability, the homogeneity of surgical treatment, and the heterogeneity of the population, which allowed us to investigate the role of rare conditions as potential risk factors for treatment failure.

However, our study has limitations. First, the retrospective design limits the amount of data that could be obtained by medical records and the significance of the results. For instance, radiographic imaging was insufficient to investigate the role of radiographic parameters as predictors of redislocation and criteria for alternative surgical treatments. Second, the procedures were performed by 13 different surgeons, the indication to surgery and the choice of the procedure was made according to the treating surgeon's experience and preference, and no established criteria or algorithms for surgical decision making were used. Third, we merged multiple pathologic conditions into single subgroups; this could have introduced selection bias. Moreover, we cannot exclude with absolute certainty that some "idiopathic" patient could not have underlying undiagnosed collagen disorders or other syndromes. Fourth, the Parikh and Lykissas score was applied retrospectively, and its reliability is questionable. In particular, we decided not to consider A and B subtypes in type 3 and type 4 patellar dislocation. However, subtypes could be very different entities of patellar instability with possibly different prognosis. Finally, the Kujala AKPS was obtained only at follow-up, and no comparison with the pre-operative status was possible. This is essential to understand how effective the surgical treatment is in improving symptoms and function, especially in syndromic patients, when the surgical choice may be debatable.

5. Conclusions

The three-in-one procedure can be still considered a suitable treatment option for patella realignment in skeletally immature patients. However, the etiology and the type of patellar instability must be strictly considered in surgical decision making, and alternative techniques and strategies must be recommended, as the three-in-one procedure could be ineffective in the most severe patterns of dislocation.

Author Contributions: Conceptualization, G.T.; methodology, G.T., E.O. and S.S.; software, G.T., A.D., G.C. and M.R.; formal analysis, G.T. and A.D.; investigation, G.G., P.Z., V.P., S.S., G.C., M.R. and A.D.; resources, G.T.; data curation, A.D.; writing—original draft preparation, G.T.; writing—review and editing, G.T., A.D. and M.R.; visualization, A.D. and M.R.; supervision, G.T. and G.R.; project administration, E.O.; funding acquisition, G.T. and G.R. All authors have read and agreed to the published version of the manuscript.

Funding: The work reported in this publication was funded by the Italian Ministry of Health, RCR-2022-23682299 project, under the The Italian Musculoskeletal Apparatus Network RAMS.

Institutional Review Board Statement: The study was conducted in accordance with the Declaration of Helsinki and approved by the Local Ethics Committee "AREA VASTA EMILIA CENTRO" (protocol code: 0013161; date of approval 29 December 2017).

Informed Consent Statement: Written informed consent was obtained from all subjects involved in the study to publish this paper.

Data Availability Statement: The datasets generated during and/or analyzed during the current study are available from the corresponding author on reasonable request.

Acknowledgments: Dedicated to the memory of Stefano Stilli, who continues to inspire us with his example and dedication to the students, young doctors, and researchers he served over the course of his career. We would like to thank Maria Pia Cumani for her artwork and illustrations of this manuscript.

Conflicts of Interest: The authors declare no conflict of interest.

References

1. Gravesen, K.S.; Kallemose, T.; Blønd, L.; Troelsen, A.; Barfod, K.W. High incidence of acute and recurrent patellar dislocations: A retrospective nationwide epidemiological study involving 24.154 primary dislocations. *Knee Surg. Sports Traumatol. Arthrosc.* **2017**, *26*, 1204–1209. [CrossRef] [PubMed]
2. Sanders, T.L.; Pareek, A.; Hewett, T.E.; Stuart, M.J.; Dahm, D.L.; Krych, A.J. High rate of recurrent patellar dislocation in skeletally immature patients: A long-term population-based study. *Knee Surg. Sports Traumatol. Arthrosc.* **2017**, *26*, 1037–1043. [CrossRef] [PubMed]
3. A Arendt, E.; Fithian, D.C.; Cohen, E. Current concepts of lateral patella dislocation. *Clin. Sports Med.* **2002**, *21*, 499–519. [CrossRef] [PubMed]
4. Parikh, S.N.; Lykissas, M.G. Classification of Lateral Patellar Instability in Children and Adolescents. *Orthop. Clin. N. Am.* **2016**, *47*, 145–152. [CrossRef] [PubMed]
5. DeJour, H.; Walch, G.; Nove-Josserand, L.; Guier, C. Factors of patellar instability: An anatomic radiographic study. *Knee Surg. Sports Traumatol. Arthrosc.* **1994**, *2*, 19–26. [CrossRef]
6. Schlichte, L.M.; Sidharthan, S.; Green, D.W.; Parikh, S.N. Pediatric Management of Recurrent Patellar Instability. *Sports Med. Arthrosc. Rev.* **2019**, *27*, 171–180. [CrossRef] [PubMed]
7. Dugdale, T.W.; Renshaw, T.S. Instability of the patellofemoral joint in Down syndrome. *J. Bone Jt. Surg.* **1986**, *68*, 405–413. [CrossRef]

8. Chotel, F.; Bérard, J.; Raux, S. Patellar instability in children and adolescents. *Orthop. Traumatol. Surg. Res.* **2014**, *100*, S125–S137. [CrossRef]
9. Hiemstra, L.A.; Kerslake, S.; LaFave, M.; Heard, S.M.; Buchko, G.M.L. Introduction of a classification system for patients with patellofemoral instability (WARPS and STAID). *Knee Surg. Sports Traumatol. Arthrosc.* **2013**, *22*, 2776–2782. [CrossRef]
10. Sillanpää, P.J.; Salonen, E.; Pihlajamäki, H.; Mäenpää, H.M. Medial patellofemoral ligament avulsion injury at the patella: Classification and clinical outcome. *Knee Surg. Sports Traumatol. Arthrosc.* **2014**, *22*, 2414–2418. [CrossRef]
11. Garin, C.; Chaker, M.; Dohin, B.; Kohler, R. Permanent, habitual dislocation and recurrent dislocation of the patella in children: Surgical management by patellar ligamentous transfer in 50 knees. *Rev. Chir. Orthop. Reparatrice Appar. Mot.* **2007**, *93*, 690–700. [CrossRef] [PubMed]
12. Herring, J. *Tachdjian's Pediatric Orthopaedics: From the Texas Scottish Rite Hospital for Children*, 6th ed.; Elsevier: Amsterdam, The Netherlands, 2020.
13. Bitar, A.C.; Demange, M.; D'Elia, C.O.; Camanho, G.L. Traumatic patellar dislocation: Nonoperative treatment compared with MPFL reconstruction using patellar tendon. *Am. J. Sports Med.* **2011**, *40*, 114–122. [CrossRef] [PubMed]
14. Smith, T.; Donell, S.; Song, F.; Hing, C. Surgical versus non-surgical interventions for treating patellar dislocation. *Cochrane Database Syst. Rev.* **2015**, *2*, CD008106. [CrossRef] [PubMed]
15. Nwachukwu, B.U.; So, C.; Schairer, W.W.; Green, D.W.; Dodwell, E.R. Surgical versus conservative management of acute patellar dislocation in children and adolescents: A systematic review. *Knee Surg. Sports Traumatol. Arthrosc.* **2015**, *24*, 760–767. [CrossRef]
16. Pagliazzi, G.; Napoli, F.; Previtali, D.; Filardo, G.; Zaffagnini, S.; Candrian, C. A Meta-analysis of Surgical Versus Nonsurgical Treatment of Primary Patella Dislocation. *Arthrosc. J. Arthrosc. Relat. Surg.* **2019**, *35*, 2469–2481. [CrossRef] [PubMed]
17. Beasley, L.S.; Vidal, A.F. Traumatic patellar dislocation in children and adolescents: Treatment update and literature review. *Curr. Opin. Pediatr.* **2004**, *16*, 29–36. [CrossRef]
18. Pookarnjanamorakot, C.; Jaovisidha, S.; Apiyasawat, P. The patellar tilt angle: Correlation of MRI evaluation with anterior knee pain. *J. Med. Assoc. Thail.* **1998**, *81*, 958–963.
19. Grelsamer, R.P.; Weinstein, C.H.; Gould, J.; Dubey, A. Patellar tilt: The physical examination correlates with MR imaging. *Knee* **2008**, *15*, 3–8. [CrossRef]
20. Diederichs, G.; Issever, A.S.; Scheffler, S. MR Imaging of Patellar Instability: Injury Patterns and Assessment of Risk Factors. *Radiographics* **2010**, *30*, 961–981. [CrossRef]
21. Steensen, R.N.; Bentley, J.C.; Trinh, T.Q.; Backes, J.R.; Wiltfong, R.E. The prevalence and combined prevalences of anatomic factors associated with recurrent patellar dislocation: A magnetic resonance imaging study. *Am. J. Sports Med.* **2015**, *43*, 921–927. [CrossRef]
22. Franco, B.A.F.M.; Sadigursky, D.; Daltro, G.D.C. Patellar position in patients with patellofemoral syndrome as characterized by anatomo-radiographic study. *Rev. Bras. Ortop.* **2018**, *53*, 410. [CrossRef] [PubMed]
23. Vairo, G.L.; Moya-Angeler, J.; Siorta, M.A.; Anderson, A.H.; Sherbondy, P. Tibial Tubercle-Trochlear Groove Distance Is a Reliable and Accurate Indicator of Patellofemoral Instability. *Clin. Orthop. Relat. Res.* **2019**, *477*, 1450. [CrossRef] [PubMed]
24. Bettuzzi, C.; Lampasi, M.; Magnani, M.; Donzelli, O. Surgical treatment of patellar dislocation in children with Down syndrome: A 3- to 11-year follow-up study. *Knee Surg. Sports Traumatol. Arthrosc.* **2008**, *17*, 334–340. [CrossRef] [PubMed]
25. Green, W.T. Recurrent dislocation of patella—Its surgical correction in growing child. *J. Bone Jt. Surg. Am. Vol.* **1965**, *8*, 1670.
26. Fondren, F.B.; Goldner, J.L.; Bassett, F.H., 3rd. Recurrent dislocation of the patella treated by the modified Roux-Goldthwait procedure. A prospective study of forty-seven knees. *J. Bone Jt. Surg.* **1985**, *67*, 993–1005. [CrossRef]
27. Kujala, U.M.; Jaakkola, L.H.; Koskinen, S.K.; Taimela, S.; Hurme, M.; Nelimarkka, O. Scoring of patellofemoral disorders. *Arthrosc. J. Arthrosc. Relat. Surg.* **1993**, *9*, 159–163. [CrossRef]
28. Cerciello, S.; Corona, K.; Morris, B.J.; Visonà, E.; Maccauro, G.; Maffulli, N.; Ronga, M. Cross-cultural adaptation and validation of the Italian versions of the Kujala, Larsen, Lysholm and Fulkerson scores in patients with patellofemoral disorders. *J. Orthop. Traumatol.* **2018**, *19*, 18. [CrossRef]
29. Sillanpää, P.J.; Mäenpää, H.M.; Mattila, V.M.; Visuri, T.; Pihlajamäki, H. Arthroscopic surgery for primary traumatic patellar dislocation: A prospective, nonrandomized study comparing patients treated with and without acute arthroscopic stabilization with a median 7-year follow-up. *Am. J. Sports Med.* **2008**, *36*, 2301–2309. [CrossRef]
30. Vavken, P.; Wimmer, M.D.; Camathias, C.; Quidde, J.; Valderrabano, V.; Pagenstert, G. Treating Patella Instability in Skeletally Immature Patients. *Arthrosc. J. Arthrosc. Relat. Surg.* **2013**, *29*, 1410–1422. [CrossRef]
31. Zhang, K.; Jiang, H.; Li, J.; Fu, W. Comparison Between Surgical and Nonsurgical Treatment for Primary Patellar Dislocations in Adolescents: A Systematic Review and Meta-analysis of Comparative Studies. *Orthop. J. Sports Med.* **2020**, *8*, 2325967120946446. [CrossRef]
32. Longo, U.G.; Rizzello, G.; Ciuffreda, M.; Loppini, M.; Baldari, A.; Maffulli, N.; Denaro, V. Elmslie-Trillat, Maquet, Fulkerson, Roux Goldthwait, and Other Distal Realignment Procedures for the Management of Patellar Dislocation: Systematic Review and Quantitative Synthesis of the Literature. *Arthrosc. J. Arthrosc. Relat. Surg.* **2016**, *32*, 929–943. [CrossRef] [PubMed]
33. Murray, I.R.; LaPrade, C.M.; Pullen, W.M.; Sherman, S.L. Medial Patellofemoral Ligament Repair or Medial Advancement: Is There a Role? *Clin. Sports Med.* **2022**, *41*, 157–169. [CrossRef] [PubMed]

34. Wilkens, O.E.; Hannink, G.; van de Groes, S.A.W. Recurrent patellofemoral instability rates after MPFL reconstruction techniques are in the range of instability rates after other soft tissue realignment techniques. *Knee Surg. Sports Traumatol. Arthrosc.* **2019**, *28*, 1919–1931. [CrossRef] [PubMed]
35. Joo, S.Y.; Park, K.B.; Kim, B.R.; Park, H.W.; Kim, H.W. The 'four-in-one' procedure for habitual dislocation of the patella in children: Early results in patients with severe generalised ligamentous laxity and aplasis of the trochlear groove. *J. Bone Jt. Surg.* **2007**, *89*, 1645–1649. [CrossRef]
36. Ruzzini, L.; Donati, F.; Russo, R.; Costici, P.F. Modified Roux-Goldthwait Procedure for Management of Patellar Dislocation in Skeletally Immature Patients with Down Syndrome. *Indian J. Orthop.* **2019**, *53*, 122–127. [CrossRef]
37. Camathias, C.; Rutz, E.; Götze, M.; Brunner, R.; Vavken, P.; Gaston, M.S. Poor outcome at 7.5 years after Stanisavljevic quadriceps transposition for patello-femoral instability. *Arch. Orthop. Trauma Surg.* **2014**, *134*, 473–478. [CrossRef]
38. Sever, R.; Fishkin, M.; Hemo, Y.; Wientroub, S.; Yaniv, M. Surgical Treatment of Congenital and Obligatory Dislocation of the Patella in Children. *J. Pediatr. Orthop.* **2019**, *39*, 436–440. [CrossRef]
39. Imerci, A.; McDonald, T.C.; Rogers, K.J.; Thacker, M.M.; Atanda, A. Outcomes of medial patellofemoral ligament reconstruction and tibial tubercle osteotomy in syndromic adolescents with patellar dislocation. *J. Clin. Orthop. Trauma* **2022**, *25*, 101770. [CrossRef]
40. Hire, J.M.; Parikh, S.N. 4-in-1 Quadricepsplasty for Fixed and Habitual Dislocation of Patella. *Arthrosc. Tech.* **2022**, *11*, e537–e544. [CrossRef]
41. Ramos, O.; Burke, C.; Lewis, M.; Morrison, M.J.; Paley, D.; Nelson, S.C. Modified Langenskiöld procedure for chronic, recurrent, and congenital patellar dislocation. *J. Child. Orthop.* **2020**, *14*, 318–329. [CrossRef]
42. Mo, Y.; Jing, Y.; Wang, D.; Paley, D.; Ning, B. Modified Langenskiöld procedure for congenital patella dislocations in pediatric patients. *BMC Musculoskelet. Disord.* **2022**, *23*, 241. [CrossRef] [PubMed]
43. Marumo, K.; Fujii, K.; Tanaka, T.; Takeuchi, H.; Saito, H.; Koyano, Y. Surgical management of congenital permanent dislocation of the patella in nail patella syndrome by Stanisavljevic procedure. *J. Orthop. Sci.* **1999**, *4*, 446–449. [CrossRef] [PubMed]
44. Myers, P.; Williams, A.; Dodds, R.; Bülow, J. The three-in-one proximal and distal soft tissue patellar realignment procedure. Results, and its place in the management of patellofemoral instability. *Am. J. Sports Med.* **1999**, *27*, 575–579. [CrossRef] [PubMed]
45. Oliva, F.; Ronga, M.; Longo, U.G.; Testa, V.; Capasso, G.; Maffulli, N. The 3-in-1 Procedure for Recurrent Dislocation of the Patella in Skeletally Immature Children and Adolescents. *Am. J. Sports Med.* **2009**, *37*, 1814–1820. [CrossRef]
46. Malecki, K.; Fabis, J.; Flont, P.; Lipczyk, Z.; Niedzielski, K. Preliminary results of two surgical techniques in the treatment of recurrent patellar dislocation: Medial patellofemoral ligament reconstruction versus combined technique of vastus medialis advancement, capsular plasty and Roux-Goldthwait procedure in treatment of recurrent patellar dislocation. *Int. Orthop.* **2016**, *40*, 1869–1874. [CrossRef]
47. Frizziero, L.; Santi, G.; Liverani, A.; Napolitano, F.; Papaleo, P.; Maredi, E.; Gennaro, G.; Zarantonello, P.; Stallone, S.; Stilli, S.; et al. Computer-Aided Surgical Simulation for Correcting Complex Limb Deformities in Children. *Appl. Sci.* **2020**, *10*, 5181. [CrossRef]
48. Frizziero, L.; Trisolino, G.; Santi, G.M.; Alessandri, G.; Agazzani, S.; Liverani, A.; Menozzi, G.C.; Di Gennaro, G.L.; Farella, G.M.G.; Abbruzzese, A.; et al. Computer-Aided Surgical Simulation through Digital Dynamic 3D Skeletal Segments for Correcting Torsional Deformities of the Lower Limbs in Children with Cerebral Palsy. *Appl. Sci.* **2022**, *12*, 7918. [CrossRef]

Disclaimer/Publisher's Note: The statements, opinions and data contained in all publications are solely those of the individual author(s) and contributor(s) and not of MDPI and/or the editor(s). MDPI and/or the editor(s) disclaim responsibility for any injury to people or property resulting from any ideas, methods, instructions or products referred to in the content.

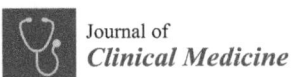

Article

Simultaneous Bilateral Total Hip Arthroplasty with Straight-Stems and Short-Stems: Does the Short One Do a Better Job?

Patrick Reinbacher [1], Andrzej Hecker [2,*], Joerg Friesenbichler [1], Maria Smolle [1], Lukas Leitner [1], Sebastian Klim [1], Alexander Draschl [1], Danijel Colovic [1], Kevin Brunnader [1], Andreas Leithner [1] and Werner Maurer-Ertl [1]

[1] Department of Orthopaedics & Traumatology, Medical University of Graz, Auenbruggerplatz 5, 8036 Graz, Austria
[2] Division of Plastic, Aesthetic and Reconstructive Surgery, Department of Surgery, Medical University of Graz, Auenbruggerplatz 5, 8036 Graz, Austria
* Correspondence: andrzej.hecker@medunigraz.at

Abstract: Background: Total hip arthroplasty (THA) is known to be the most successful orthopaedic surgery of the last century, but it is still struggling with controversies concerning one-stage bilateral THA. The current study aimed to compare the clinical outcome of patients with unilateral or simultaneous bilateral THA by using short-stem and straight-stem designs and focusing on operation time, blood loss, and length of hospital stay (LOS). Material and Methods: Between 2006 and 2018, 92 patients were enrolled in this study. Forty-six patients underwent a bilateral THA in one session, and forty-six matched patients underwent a unilateral THA. In each of the two groups (unilateral vs. bilateral), 23 patients received either a straight (unilateral: 10 females, 13 males, mean age 63; bilateral: 12 females, 11 males, mean age 53 years) or short stem (unilateral: 11 females, 12 males, mean age 60 years; bilateral: 12 females, 11 males, 53 mean age 62 years). The blood count was checked preoperatively as well as one and three days after surgery. Furthermore, the operation time and LOS were investigated. Results: Compared to THA with straight-stems, short-stem THA showed significantly less blood loss; there was no difference in the LOS of both groups. A significantly shorter operative time was only observed in the bilateral THA. Conclusion: The current study showed that simultaneous bilateral THA appears to be safe and reliable in patients without multiple comorbidities. In addition, short-stem THA appears to be beneficial in terms of clinical performance and outcome, and it appears to be superior to straight-stem THA, regardless of whether the patient underwent unilateral or simultaneous bilateral THA.

Keywords: total hip arthroplasty; short-stem; straight-stem; one-stage; bilateral

1. Introduction

Total hip arthroplasty (THA) is widely known as "the orthopaedic surgery of the last century". Furthermore, it is one of the safest and most cost-effective orthopaedic surgical procedures. Since the first hip replacements in the early 1960s, surgical techniques and implants have significantly improved. Furthermore, THA has developed from a geriatric surgery to a lifestyle surgery, with increasing numbers of operations being performed on younger and physically more active patients [1–4]. Therefore, the requirements for implant survival, durability, and functional outcomes in terms of daily activities and sports continue to increase. Primary unilateral THA is a very successful operation that improves patient quality of life and is associated with low complication rates. However, some previous studies have shown that patients undergoing unilateral THA may require contralateral surgery within 1–10 years [5–9]. In addition, if both hips are affected simultaneously, bilateral THA may be necessary and might also be of interest to younger patients with concerns about loss of work. The advantages of one-stage bilateral THA include that patients only need to undergo anaesthesia once and only have one hospital stay, resulting in a shorter length of hospital stay (LOS) as well as a reduction in cost compared with two-staged bilateral procedures [1,3,6,7,10–13].

On the other hand, several opposing studies have shown that one-stage bilateral THA poses greater risks to patients, such as higher transfusion rates due to increased blood loss, more adverse events, and suboptimal functional outcomes [6,9,10,12,14–16]. However, Donner et al. [5] have reported that patients with one-stage bilateral short-stem THA were highly satisfied with their sports and recreational activity at mid-term follow-up. Bilateral one-stage THA offers the advantage of the patient being prosthetically treated with respect to the replacement of both hip joints after one session if their physical health allows for it [17–20]. Furthermore, by having a shorter LOS, bilateral one-stage THA is beneficial in reducing overall hospital costs compared with two-stage bilateral THA [17–21]. Taking into account the advantages of one-stage bilateral THA as mentioned above, according to Micicoi et al., bilateral THA in one operative session is recommended for ASA 1 and 2 patients, aged under 80 years with disabling bilateral osteoarthritis [20].

Short-stem THA was introduced in the 1990s to preserve proximal femoral bone stock, prevent proximal stress shielding, guarantee better functional outcomes due to more physiologic biomechanical properties, and increase the survival rates of the implants [1,5,22]. Another advantage of short-stem THA is the more accessible application of minimally invasive approaches [3]. However, there is a large variety of different short-stem designs available on the market, and owing to their design, they are reduced in length and diaphyseal fixation compared with straight-stems, which has raised concerns regarding higher rates of aseptic loosening and, consequently, revision rates [23–26]. Moreover, short-stems have shown a tendency towards early distal migration, which might occur due to their mainly metaphyseal anchorage and smaller bone–implant interface [2,24,27,28]. Hauer et al. [2] reported low revision rates with satisfying results when comparing different types of short-stem devices in a comparative analysis of 52 studies. Schnurr et al. [29] published the revision rates of short-stem designs that were comparable to traditional cementless straight-stem designs. Therefore, with short-stems showing excellent short- to mid-term results, traceable early subsidence may be interpreted differently from straight-stems [28].

The current study aimed to report our clinical experience with simultaneous bilateral THA with two different stem designs by comparing a short-stem with a straight-stem. We focused on the transfusion rates, complications, LOS, and early readmission rates. Additionally, we compared the clinical findings of patients having simultaneous bilateral THA procedures with matched patients having unilateral THA procedures.

2. Materials and Methods

In this study, a retrospective comparative analysis was performed on 92 prospectively included patients. For this purpose, the institutional database was reviewed for patients who had received unilateral or simultaneous bilateral THA at the Medical University of Graz, Austria (Department of Orthopaedics & Traumatology) between 2006 and 2018. The present study was approved by the Ethics Committee of the Medical University of Graz, Austria (Ethical Committee No. 28-152 ex 15/16).

As per standard procedure, an anterolateral approach to the hip was performed by two experienced orthopaedic surgeons at a single university hospital. All patients received uncemented components. The cementless straight-stem (Corail® Hip System, DePuy International Ltd., Leeds, England, UK) was regularly used for more than 10 years at our department before the short-stem with mainly metaphyseal fixation (ANA.NOVA® Alpha Schaft® Proxy, ImplanTec GmbH, Moedling, Austria) was introduced in 2016. The characteristics of the two stems have been previously illustrated by our research group [30]. In general, the more symptomatic hip joint was operated on first in the case of bilateral THA, and no operations were aborted because of intraoperative complications. After completing the first hip, a sterile dressing was applied, and the second hip joint was prepared with the same instruments. An intraoperative cell saver was not used routinely, and no drains were used postoperatively. No tranexamic acid was used perioperatively. Full weight bearing using two crutches was allowed in all cases postoperatively, prophylaxis against deep vein thrombosis was administered for 6 weeks, and patients had to wear stockings against deep vein thrombosis (DVT). Usually, the patients were discharged home, and older patients or patients who could not go home were transferred to geriatric mobilisation units.

The patients' hospital records, rehabilitation discharge summaries, and follow-up office notes were used for the analysis. The data on blood loss were collected from the available hospital records, and the blood count was checked preoperatively as well as one day and three days post-operation. Furthermore, the clinical documents were reviewed to administer allogenic blood products. The operation time was documented and collected from the surgical reports. The length of stay (LOS) was also gathered from the clinical reports and were calculated from the day before the operation until the day of discharge. The major complications were death, pulmonary embolism (PE), DVT, cardiovascular and/or pulmonary complications, neurological complications, and complications associated with the implant needing revision surgery.

SPSS Statistics program 25 (SPSS Inc., Chicago, IL, USA) was used for the statistical analysis. The Shapiro–Wilk test was used to test the normality of the data. For the demographic data, a Student's t-test for independent samples was chosen to determine the statistical differences in the parametric data; in the non-parametric data, the Mann–Whitney U-test was used. A one-way ANOVA test was used to compare continuous datasets, and the Bonferroni post hoc test was subsequently used when the significant main effects were present. All of the statistical tests were two-tailed, and the differences were considered to be statistically significant when $p < 0.05$. A post hoc power analysis was calculated according to Hoenig and Heisey for the magnitude of differences in all compared parameters [31]. The selected sample size per group was sufficient for a statistical analysis.

3. Results

All demographic data between patient groups were quite similar; only the patients in the bilateral short-stem group were significantly older than the straight-stem group (Table 1). Furthermore, significant differences were observed for the follow-up due to the fact that the short-stem was introduced in 2016.

3.1. Straight-Stem Groups

Forty-six patients underwent THA between 2006 and 2017 and received a straight-stem design (Corail® Hip System, DePuy International Ltd., Leeds, England, UK). Meanwhile, 23 patients had a unilateral procedure, and 23 patients had a one-stage simultaneous bilateral THA. There were 11 male and 12 female patients with a mean age of 53 years at the time of operation (range, 25–88 years) in the simultaneous bilateral THA group. In the unilateral THA group, there were 12 male and 11 female patients, with a mean age of 63 years (range, 38–85 years).

3.2. Short-Stem Groups

Forty-six patients underwent THA between 2016 and 2018, receiving a short-stem THA (ANA.NOVA® Alpha Schaft® Proxy, ImplanTec GmbH, Moedling, Austria) with a novel implant design. These patients were also enclosed in an ongoing prospective clinical surveillance study. In the bilateral group, there were 11 male and 12 female patients, with an average age of 62 years (range, 38–78 years). In the unilateral short-stem group, there were 13 male and 10 female patients, with a mean age of 60 years (range, 46–72 years).

Table 1. Demographic and clinical data.

	Group I (Straight-Stem Bilateral)	Group III (Short-Stem Bilateral)	p-Value	Group II (Straight-Stem Unilateral)	Group IV (Short-Stem Unilateral)	p-Value
Age at OP, mean (range)	53 (25–88)	62 (38–78)	0.023 [a]	63 (38–85)	60 (46–72)	0.339 [a]
ASA score, mean (range)	2 (1–4)	2 (1–3)	0.750 [b]	3 (1–4)	2 (1–3)	0.152 [b]
BMI mean (range)	25 (17–39)	26 (18–36)	0.634 [a]	28 (24–49)	29 (17–36)	0.505 [a]
Operation time (min), mean (range)	115 (48–254)	68 (51–103)	<0.001 [c]	55 (38–82)	41 (27–56)	0.303 [c]
Hb (g/dL) preop., mean (range)	13.2 (9.5–15.6)	14.4 (11.1–16.6)	0.015 [c]	14.1 (12.0–16.5)	14.4 (12.3–16.3)	1.000 [c]
Hb (g/dL) day 1 postop., mean (range)	8.8 (5.5–11.1)	10 (7.4–13.1)	0.060 [c]	10.8 (7.9–14.7)	11.3 (9.4–13.7)	1.000 [c]
Hb (g/dL) day 3 postop., mean (range)	9.0 (7.3–11.5)	9.5 (7.4–11.4)	1.000 [c]	10.3 (5.7–13.5)	10.8 (8.1–12.9)	0.475 [c]
LOS (days), mean (range)	9 (5–17)	8 (4–11)	0.653 [c]	7 (4–13)	7 (4–10)	1.000 [c]
Follow-up (months), mean (range)	87 (29–164)	31 (24–49)	<0.001 [c]	103 (62–137)	49 (47–51)	<0.001 [c]

[a] Unpaired t-test, [b] Mann–Whitney U test, [c] one-way ANOVA test. OP: operation; ASA: American Society of Anesthesiologists; BMI: body mass index; Hb: hemaglobin; preop: preoperative; postop: postoperative; LOS: length of stay.

The bilateral short-stem group showed a significantly shorter operation time and less blood loss. The unilateral short-stem group showed no significantly shorter operation time but significantly less blood loss. However, no difference was found in the LOS when compared with straight-stem THA patients (Table 1).

Within the first three days after surgery, five patients in the bilateral and three patients in the unilateral straight-stem group received allogenic blood products (two units per patient) due to a lowered red blood count and suffered from clinical symptoms such as low blood pressure, dizziness, or reduced general condition. In the same time period, another three patients in the bilateral short-stem group also received blood products (two units per patient) for the same indications.

Overall, there was no history of myocardial infarction, deep vein thrombosis, pulmonary embolism, or death associated with the surgical procedure during follow-up. Furthermore, there was no postoperative readmission to the hospital in the short-term (30 days) for any medical or surgical reason for neither the straight-stem nor short-stem groups.

Two revisions had to be performed in the bilateral straight-stem group (overall complication rate: 2.1%), the first one being due to increased serum metal ions concentrations after the usage of a metal-on-metal bearing 57 months after implantation; the second one was due to a low-grade periprosthetic joint infection (PJI) with *Staphylococcus epidermidis* 32 months after the index procedure. The PJI was treated with a one-stage procedure and antibiotics; the patient is doing well 16 months after revision surgery. One patient from the straight-stem group died 32 months after index surgery due to chronic renal failure with dialysis.

4. Discussion

The current study revealed satisfying results with low complication rates in all implant groups and in both the bilateral and unilateral groups. Overall, patients with short-stem THA showed better clinical data with respect to operation time, blood loss, and LOS, although these differences were not statistically significant.

In the literature, there are still controversies regarding the advantages and disadvantages of one-stage or two-stage bilateral THA, and there are no actual recommendations from orthopaedic societies [1,4,6,8–12,14,29,32,33]. The decision and indication for the single-stage bilateral procedure and the selection of the appropriate patient remain the responsibility of the orthopaedic surgeon. Most studies reporting one-stage bilateral THA were performed in dedicated centres with similar effectiveness and morbidity for unilateral or two-stage bilateral THAs. Many previous studies have reported outcome and complication rates comparing one-stage and two-stage THA procedures; in a smaller number of studies, the surgical approach was also analysed as an influencing factor [3,12]. The current study's aim was to compare one-stage and two-stage THA procedures using different stem types regarding the outcome and complication rates.

The meta-analysis of Shao et al. [8] showed that one-stage bilateral THA had a lower risk of major systemic complications, less deep venous thrombosis, and shorter operative time compared with two-stage bilateral THA; Guo et al. [6] and Charity et al. [1] recently confirmed these observations as well. There were no major complications in the current series, which might be explained by the small number of patients enrolled. Furthermore, in most studies, patients receiving simultaneous bilateral THA are more so selected with respect to demographics and comorbidities. In all implant groups in the current series, the distribution of comorbidities was equal with respect to the ASA score (Table 1). Additionally, improvements in anticoagulation therapy have significantly reduced the rate of deep venous thrombosis and pulmonary embolism.

Aghayev et al. [32], Parvizi et al. [15], and other studies have related low complication and morbidity rates in one-stage bilateral THA with the higher numbers of patients included [1,6,12]. Stavrakis et al. [9] have reported that the overall risk for complications following bilateral THA was similar to that observed after unilateral procedures; on the other hand, higher rates of septic complications were reported in the bilateral group. As short stems offer the possibility of revision surgery with conventional straight stems, using short stems in bilateral THA could be clinically beneficial in the long term for surgical management, especially for patients under the age of 65 years, who are known to be at higher risk for surgical revision in the future [23,34–37]. However, there is a lack of long-term results regarding the effect of short-stems' observed early subsidence on implant survival [28]. Therefore, long-term studies are needed to assess the axial migration's impact on implant survival, as short stems seem to be a promising alternative to straight stems in simultaneous bilateral THA.

Previous studies have described the age at the time of surgery as an important factor influencing the outcome of one-stage bilateral procedures. However, in the current series, the mean age of patients receiving simultaneous bilateral THA using a short-stem device was significantly higher than the straight-stem group. Still, no higher complication rates were observed, which is novel when compared with the literature.

Short-stem THA procedures showed significantly shorter operation times in the bilateral group as well as the unilateral group. Several other studies comparing the operative time between one- and two-stage bilateral THA procedures have demonstrated that the one-stage bilateral procedure takes less surgical time than the two-stage procedure [1,3,6,8,12,15]. Moreover, it has been reported that using a conventional rather than a short stem is a significantly influential factor regarding longer operative time [38]. Furthermore, Surace et al. [39] have suggested a strong correlation between increased operative time and perioperative complications in primary short-stem THA. Additional factors such as the surgeon's experience and routine will also positively influence the theatre time and influence the use of gentler and bone-sparing operation techniques in short-stem designs. A shorter operation time might result in reduced blood loss, lower transfusion rates, and earlier postoperative mobilisation due to missing fatigue complications.

Parvizi et al. [4] found no statistically significant difference in the 90-day mortality between unilateral and bilateral THA in a prospective matched study, although the simultaneous bilateral THA group required more blood transfusions and showed lower haemoglobin concentrations upon discharge than the unilateral group. The current series also showed a low transfusion rate of 12% (11 out of 92 patients); eight transfusions had to be performed in the simultaneous bilateral groups, and three had to be performed in the unilateral straight-stem group. Nevertheless, no major cardiovascular complications or increased infection rates were observed in patients receiving allogenic blood products.

Besides functional outcome and complication rates following THA surgery, the postoperative hospital costs and LOS are important factors. Several studies have indicated shorter stays and lower costs in one-stage bilateral procedures than in the two-stage bilateral THA [3,6,8,10,13,15]. In the current series, the LOS was shorter in the bilateral short-stem group compared with the straight-stem group, although the difference was statistically insignificant. In the unilateral group, the LOS was equal, which contrasts the findings of Hauer et al., who have reported a significantly shorter LOS for the unilateral short-stem THA compared with the unilateral straight-stem THA—although the study was conducted in a younger study population—but without a significant difference in the return to work time, indicating that the stem design does not influence the recovery time [40]. Lorenze et al. [11] and Reuben et al. [13] reported a 25% cost savings in the simultaneous bilateral THA group because the majority of cost reduction can be attributed to the decreased overall LOS. Taking this into account, with a lower LOS for short-stem THA [40,41], total hospital costs can be even more reduced. Recently, Villa et al. [16] reported longer LOS in patients with simultaneous bilateral THA through a direct anterior approach (DAA), which was not proven by Kamath et al. [42] or Parcells et al. [43].

5. Limitations

One limitation of the current study is the small number of patients enrolled; on the other hand, we provided matched control groups for both implant types. Another limitation might be the different follow-ups concerning the determination of implant survival. Still, the shorter follow-up of the short-stem groups did not influence the outcome that evaluated the short-term readmission rate. Additionally, the surgical techniques and skills of the operating surgeons increased over time, which might be beneficial for operation time, re-transfusion rates, complications, LOS, and early readmission rates, which makes it more challenging to assess and compare the outcomes. Furthermore, no clinical scoring systems were available to quantify and report the functional results. Given the limitations mentioned above, our results should be mainly interpreted from a health economics point of view.

6. Conclusions

The current series showed that simultaneous bilateral THA operation appears safe and reliable in selected patients without multiple comorbidities. In addition, short-stem THA appears to be beneficial in terms of clinical performance and outcome over straight-stem THA, whether unilateral or simultaneous bilateral implantation. Nevertheless, further studies are necessary to confirm these observations.

Author Contributions: Conceptualisation: J.F. and W.M.-E.; methodology: J.F., W.M.-E., P.R. and L.L.; investigation: P.R., A.H., S.K., A.D., D.C., M.S., L.L. and K.B.; statistical analysis: A.H.; writing—draft preparation: P.R. and A.H.; writing—review and editing: J.F., A.D., A.L. and W.M.-E.; supervision: J.F. and W.M.-E. All authors have read and agreed to the published version of the manuscript.

Funding: This research received no external funding.

Institutional Review Board Statement: The study was conducted according to the guidelines of the Declaration of Helsinki and was approved by the Ethics Committee of Medical University Graz, Austria (protocol code 28–152 ex 15/16).

Informed Consent Statement: Informed consent was obtained from all subjects involved in the study.

Data Availability Statement: Detailed data supporting the results are available from the authors.

Conflicts of Interest: The authors declare no conflict of interest.

References

1. Charity, J.; Wyatt, M.C.; Jameson, S.; Whitehouse, S.L.; Wilson, M.J.; Gie, G.A. Is Single-Anaesthetic Bilateral Total Hip Replacement Using Cemented Stems Safe and Appropriate? A Review of Four Decades of Practice. *Hip Int.* **2019**, *29*, 468–474. [CrossRef]
2. Hauer, G.; Vielgut, I.; Amerstorfer, F.; Maurer-Ertl, W.; Leithner, A.; Sadoghi, P. Survival Rate of Short-Stem Hip Prostheses: A Comparative Analysis of Clinical Studies and National Arthroplasty Registers. *J. Arthroplasty* **2018**, *33*, 1800–1805. [CrossRef]
3. Malahias, M.-A.; Chulsomlee, K.; Thorey, F. Simultaneous Bilateral Minimally Invasive Total Hip Arthroplasty: A Comprehensive Review of the Literature. *Orthop. Rev.* **2018**, *10*, 7677. [CrossRef] [PubMed]
4. Parvizi, J.; Pour, A.E.; Peak, E.L.; Sharkey, P.F.; Hozack, W.J.; Rothman, R.H. One-Stage Bilateral Total Hip Arthroplasty Compared with Unilateral Total Hip Arthroplasty: A Prospective Study. *J. Arthroplasty* **2006**, *21*, 26–31. [CrossRef]
5. Donner, S.; Rehbein, P.; Schneider, M.; Pfeil, J.; Drees, P.; Kutzner, K.P. Return to Sports and Recreational Activity After Single-Stage Bilateral Short-Stem Total Hip Arthroplasty: 5-Year Results of a Prospective Observational Study. *Orthop. J. Sports Med.* **2019**, *7*, 2325967119872746. [CrossRef] [PubMed]
6. Guo, S.-J.; Shao, H.-Y.; Huang, Y.; Yang, D.-J.; Zheng, H.-L.; Zhou, Y.-X. Retrospective Cohort Study Comparing Complications, Readmission, Transfusion, and Length of Stay of Patients Undergoing Simultaneous and Staged Bilateral Total Hip Arthroplasty. *Orthop. Surg.* **2020**, *12*, 233–240. [CrossRef]
7. Morcos, M.W.; Hart, A.; Antoniou, J.; Huk, O.L.; Zukor, D.J.; Bergeron, S.G. No Difference in Major Complication and Readmission Rates Following Simultaneous Bilateral vs Unilateral Total Hip Arthroplasty. *J. Arthroplasty* **2018**, *33*, 2541–2545. [CrossRef]
8. Shao, H.; Chen, C.-L.; Maltenfort, M.G.; Restrepo, C.; Rothman, R.H.; Chen, A.F. Bilateral Total Hip Arthroplasty: 1-Stage or 2-Stage? A Meta-Analysis. *J. Arthroplasty* **2017**, *32*, 689–695. [CrossRef]
9. Stavrakis, A.I.; SooHoo, N.F.; Lieberman, J.R. Bilateral Total Hip Arthroplasty Has Similar Complication Rates to Unilateral Total Hip Arthroplasty. *J. Arthroplasty* **2015**, *30*, 1211–1214. [CrossRef]
10. Alfaro-Adrián, J.; Bayona, F.; Rech, J.A.; Murray, D.W. One- or Two-Stage Bilateral Total Hip Replacement. *J. Arthroplasty* **1999**, *14*, 439–445. [CrossRef]
11. Lorenze, M.; Huo, M.H.; Zatorski, L.E.; Keggi, K.J. A Comparison of the Cost Effectiveness of One-Stage versus Two-Stage Bilateral Total Hip Replacement. *Orthopedics* **1998**, *21*, 1249–1252. [CrossRef] [PubMed]
12. Partridge, T.C.J.; Charity, J.A.F.; Sandiford, N.A.; Baker, P.N.; Reed, M.R.; Jameson, S.S. Simultaneous or Staged Bilateral Total Hip Arthroplasty? An Analysis of Complications in 14,460 Patients Using National Data. *J. Arthroplasty* **2020**, *35*, 166–171. [CrossRef] [PubMed]
13. Reuben, J.D.; Meyers, S.J.; Cox, D.D.; Elliott, M.; Watson, M.; Shim, S.D. Cost Comparison between Bilateral Simultaneous, Staged, and Unilateral Total Joint Arthroplasty. *J. Arthroplasty* **1998**, *13*, 172–179. [CrossRef] [PubMed]
14. Berend, K.R.; Lombardi, A.V.; Adams, J.B. Simultaneous vs Staged Cementless Bilateral Total Hip Arthroplasty: Perioperative Risk Comparison. *J. Arthroplasty* **2007**, *22*, 111–115. [CrossRef] [PubMed]
15. Parvizi, J.; Tarity, T.D.; Sheikh, E.; Sharkey, P.F.; Hozack, W.J.; Rothman, R.H. Bilateral Total Hip Arthroplasty: One-Stage versus Two-Stage Procedures. *Clin. Orthop. Relat. Res.* **2006**, *453*, 137–141. [CrossRef]
16. Villa, J.M.; Pannu, T.S.; Higuera, C.A.; Suarez, J.C.; Patel, P.D.; Barsoum, W.K. Hospital Adverse Events and Perioperative Outcomes in Bilateral Direct Anterior Approach Total Hip Arthroplasty. *J. Arthroplasty* **2020**, *35*, 762–766. [CrossRef] [PubMed]
17. Muskus, M.; Rojas, J.; Gutiérrez, C.; Guio, J.; Bonilla, G.; Llinás, A. Bilateral Hip Arthroplasty: When Is It Safe to Operate the Second Hip? A Systematic Review. *Biomed. Res. Int.* **2018**, *2018*, 3150349. [CrossRef]
18. Inoue, D.; Grace, T.R.; Restrepo, C.; Hozack, W.J. Outcomes of Simultaneous Bilateral Total Hip Arthroplasty for 256 Selected Patients in a Single Surgeon's Practice. *Bone Joint J.* **2021**, *103-B*, 116–121. [CrossRef]
19. Ramezani, A.; Ghaseminejad Raeini, A.; Sharafi, A.; Sheikhvatan, M.; Mortazavi, S.M.J.; Shafiei, S.H. Simultaneous versus Staged Bilateral Total Hip Arthroplasty: A Systematic Review and Meta-Analysis. *J. Orthop. Surg. Res.* **2022**, *17*, 392. [CrossRef] [PubMed]
20. Micicoi, G.; Bernard de Dompsure, R.; Boileau, P.; Trojani, C. Comparative Study of Bilateral Total Hip Arthroplasty in One or Two Stages. *Orthop. Traumatol. Surg. Res.* **2022**, *108*, 103359. [CrossRef]
21. Pironti, P.; Ambrosanio, A.; Vismara, V.; Viganò, M.; Bucci, E.; Sirtori, P.; Peretti, G.M.; Mangiavini, L. One-Stage vs Two-Stage Bilateral THA in Lombardy: A Cost-Effectiveness Analysis. *Cost Eff. Resour. Alloc.* **2023**, *21*, 3. [CrossRef] [PubMed]
22. Mancino, F.; Di Matteo, V.; Mocini, F.; Cacciola, G.; Malerba, G.; Perisano, C.; De Martino, I. Survivorship and Clinical Outcomes of Proximal Femoral Replacement in Non-Neoplastic Primary and Revision Total Hip Arthroplasty: A Systematic Review. *BMC Musculoskelet. Disord.* **2021**, *22*, 933. [CrossRef] [PubMed]
23. Van Oldenrijk, J.; Molleman, J.; Klaver, M.; Poolman, R.W.; Haverkamp, D. Revision Rate after Short-Stem Total Hip Arthroplasty: A Systematic Review of 49 Studies. *Acta Orthop.* **2014**, *85*, 250–258. [CrossRef] [PubMed]
24. Kutzner, K.P. Calcar-Guided Short-Stem Total Hip Arthroplasty: Will It Be the Future Standard? Review and Perspectives. *World J. Orthop.* **2021**, *12*, 534–547. [CrossRef]
25. Falez, F.; Casella, F.; Papalia, M. Current Concepts, Classification, and Results in Short Stem Hip Arthroplasty. *Orthopedics* **2015**, *38*, S6–S13. [CrossRef] [PubMed]
26. Jerosch, J. Unterschiede zwischen verschiedenen Kurzschaftendoprothesen. *Orthopäde* **2014**, *43*, 783. [CrossRef]
27. Loppini, M.; Grappiolo, G. Uncemented Short Stems in Primary Total Hip Arthroplasty: The State of the Art. *EFORT Open Rev.* **2018**, *3*, 149–159. [CrossRef]

28. Reinbacher, P.; Smolle, M.A.; Friesenbichler, J.; Draschl, A.; Leithner, A.; Maurer-Ertl, W. Three-Year Migration Analysis of a New Metaphyseal Anchoring Short Femoral Stem in THA Using EBRA-FCA. *Sci. Rep.* **2022**, *12*, 17173. [CrossRef]
29. Schnurr, C.; Schellen, B.; Dargel, J.; Beckmann, J.; Eysel, P.; Steffen, R. Low Short-Stem Revision Rates: 1-11 Year Results From 1888 Total Hip Arthroplasties. *J. Arthroplasty* **2017**, *32*, 487–493. [CrossRef]
30. Maurer-Ertl, W.; Friesenbichler, J.; Pfann, M.; Maier, M.; Reinbacher, P.; Leithner, A.; Smolle, M.A. Restoration of Hip Geometry after Total Hip Arthroplasty: Retrospective Comparison of Two Short Stems and One Straight Stem. *BMC Musculoskelet. Disord.* **2022**, *23*, 1035. [CrossRef]
31. Hoenig, J.M.; Heisey, D.M. The Abuse of Power: The Pervasive Fallacy of Power Calculations for Data Analysis. *Am. Stat.* **2001**, *55*, 19–24. [CrossRef]
32. Aghayev, E.; Beck, A.; Staub, L.P.; Dietrich, D.; Melloh, M.; Orljanski, W.; Röder, C. Simultaneous Bilateral Hip Replacement Reveals Superior Outcome and Fewer Complications than Two-Stage Procedures: A Prospective Study Including 1819 Patients and 5801 Follow-Ups from a Total Joint Replacement Registry. *BMC Musculoskelet. Disord.* **2010**, *11*, 245. [CrossRef]
33. Tsiridis, E.; Pavlou, G.; Charity, J.; Tsiridis, E.; Gie, G.; West, R. The Safety and Efficacy of Bilateral Simultaneous Total Hip Replacement: An Analysis of 2063 Cases. *J. Bone Joint Surg. Br.* **2008**, *90*, 1005–1012. [CrossRef]
34. Kurtz, S.M.; Lau, E.; Ong, K.; Zhao, K.; Kelly, M.; Bozic, K.J. Future Young Patient Demand for Primary and Revision Joint Replacement: National Projections from 2010 to 2030. *Clin. Orthop. Relat Res.* **2009**, *467*, 2606–2612. [CrossRef]
35. Bayliss, L.E.; Culliford, D.; Monk, A.P.; Glyn-Jones, S.; Prieto-Alhambra, D.; Judge, A.; Cooper, C.; Carr, A.J.; Arden, N.K.; Beard, D.J.; et al. The Effect of Patient Age at Intervention on Risk of Implant Revision after Total Replacement of the Hip or Knee: A Population-Based Cohort Study. *Lancet* **2017**, *389*, 1424–1430. [CrossRef] [PubMed]
36. Liang, H.-D.; Yang, W.-Y.; Pan, J.-K.; Huang, H.-T.; Luo, M.-H.; Zeng, L.-F.; Liu, J. Are Short-Stem Prostheses Superior to Conventional Stem Prostheses in Primary Total Hip Arthroplasty? A Systematic Review and Meta-Analysis of Randomised Controlled Trials. *BMJ Open* **2018**, *8*, e021649. [CrossRef] [PubMed]
37. Yan, S.G.; Woiczinski, M.; Schmidutz, T.F.; Weber, P.; Paulus, A.C.; Steinbrück, A.; Jansson, V.; Schmidutz, F. Can the Metaphyseal Anchored Metha Short Stem Safely Be Revised with a Standard CLS Stem? A Biomechanical Analysis. *Int. Orthop.* **2017**, *41*, 2471–2477. [CrossRef]
38. Bredow, J.; Boese, C.K.; Flörkemeier, T.; Hellmich, M.; Eysel, P.; Windhagen, H.; Oppermann, J.; von Lewinski, G.; Budde, S. Factors Affecting Operative Time in Primary Total Hip Arthroplasty: A Retrospective Single Hospital Cohort Study of 7674 Cases. *Technol. Health Care* **2018**, *26*, 857–866. [CrossRef]
39. Surace, P.; Sultan, A.A.; George, J.; Samuel, L.T.; Khlopas, A.; Molloy, R.M.; Stearns, K.L.; Mont, M.A. The Association Between Operative Time and Short-Term Complications in Total Hip Arthroplasty: An Analysis of 89,802 Surgeries. *J. Arthroplasty* **2019**, *34*, 426–432. [CrossRef]
40. Hauer, G.; Smolle, M.; Zaussinger, S.; Friesenbichler, J.; Leithner, A.; Maurer-Ertl, W. Short-Stem Total Hip Arthroplasty Is Not Associated with an Earlier Return to Work Compared to a Straight-Stem Design. *Sci. Rep.* **2021**, *11*, 4968. [CrossRef] [PubMed]
41. Tahim, A.S.; Stokes, O.M.; Vedi, V. The Effect of Femoral Stem Length on Duration of Hospital Stay. *Hip Int.* **2012**, *22*, 56–61. [CrossRef] [PubMed]
42. Kamath, A.F.; Monteiro, E.L.; Spranger, A.; Impellizzeri, F.; Leunig, M. Simultaneous versus Staged Bilateral Direct Anterior Total Hip Arthroplasty: Are Early Patient-Centered Outcomes Equivalent? *Acta Orthop. Belg.* **2016**, *82*, 497–508.
43. Parcells, B.W.; Macknet, D.M.; Kayiaros, S.T. The Direct Anterior Approach for 1-Stage Bilateral Total Hip Arthroplasty: Early Outcome Analysis of a Single-Surgeon Case Series. *J. Arthroplasty* **2016**, *31*, 434–437. [CrossRef] [PubMed]

Disclaimer/Publisher's Note: The statements, opinions and data contained in all publications are solely those of the individual author(s) and contributor(s) and not of MDPI and/or the editor(s). MDPI and/or the editor(s) disclaim responsibility for any injury to people or property resulting from any ideas, methods, instructions or products referred to in the content.

Article

Elbow Arthroscopy for the Treatment of Radial Head Fractures: Surgical Technique and 10 Years of Follow Up Results Compared to Open Surgery

Enrico Guerra [1], Alessandro Marinelli [1], Fabio Tortorella [1], Michelle Dos Santos Flöter [2], Alice Ritali [1], Andrea Sessa [1], Giuseppe Carbone [1] and Marco Cavallo [1,*]

[1] Shoulder and Elbow Unit, IRCCS Istituto Ortopedico Rizzoli, 40136 Bologna, Italy
[2] Orthopedics and Traumatology Department, Kantonsspital St. Gallen, 9000 St. Gallen, Switzerland
* Correspondence: marco.cavallo@ior.it; Tel.: +39-051-636-6927

Abstract: Background: This study aimed to describe the ARIF (Arthroscopic Reduction Internal Fixation) technique for radial head fractures and to compare the results with ORIF (Open Reduction Internal Fixation) at mean 10 years. Methods: A total of 32 patients affected by Mason II or III fractures of the radial head who underwent ARIF or ORIF by screws fixation were retrospectively selected and evaluated. A total of 13 patients were treated (40.6%) by ARIF and 19 patients (59.4%) by ORIF. Mean follow-up was 10 years (7–15 years). All patients underwent MEPI and BMRS scores at follow-up, and statistical analysis was performed. Results: No statistical significance was reported in Surgical Time ($p = 0.805$) or BMRS ($p = 0.181$) values. Significative improvement was recorded in MEPI score ($p = 0.036$), and between ARIF (98.07, SD ± 4.34) and ORIF (91.57, SD ± 11.67). The ARIF group showed lower incidence of postoperative complications, especially regarding stiffness (15.4% with ORIF at 21.1%). Conclusions: The radial head ARIF surgical technique represents a reproducible and safe procedure. A long learning curve is required, but with proper experience, it represents a tool that might be beneficial for patients, as it allows a radial head fracture to be treated with minimal tissue damage, evaluation and treatment of the concomitant lesions, and with no limitation of the positioning of screws.

Keywords: elbow arthroscopy; radial head fracture; portals; radial head ARIF; elbow fractures

1. Introduction

Radial head fractures are a common occurrence, with a reported incidence of 2.5 per 10,000 per year [1]. These fractures are usually caused by a fall onto outstretched hand [2], and about 30% of cases include associated injuries. The radial head is important because it functions as the elbow's secondary stabilizer for valgus stresses as well as a primary stabilizer for axial loads, with the interosseus membrane as a secondary stabilizer [3]. Its shape has highly variable angles, dimensions and curvature [4], so even though improvements have been achieved in anatomical prosthesis design, preserving the native radial head when possible remains the gold standard. For the same reasons, it is important to avoid radial head resection as much as possible during surgeries [5].

The most common classification of radial head fractures was introduced by Mason, was then modified by Hotchkiss [6], and then further modified by Bromberg and Morrey [7]. Radial head fractures type 1, with a displacement inferior to 2 mm, are usually treated conservatively if there is not a mechanical block during pronation–supination movements. Controversies arise for type II, however, when a displacement between >2 mm and <5 mm occurs without mechanical block [8–10], because conservative treatment can be indicated even if a radial head deformity is present. Type II and III are classically treated with ORIF (Open Reduction Internal Fixation), partial resection of the radial head (when less than 30% of the articular surface is involved) or radial head prosthetic replacement [11,12].

Over recent years, advances in elbow arthroscopy instruments, surgeons' skills, and increased knowledge of local anatomy have all led to an increment improvement of radial head fractures fixation, [13] allowing fractures that would have been treated by ORIF [14] to be treated by ARIF.

Studies have shown that it can be technically challenge to arthroscopically expose the radial head to allow for appropriate screw placement. To obtain stable screw fixation, it is important not only to reach the desired radial head portion, but also to achieve an optimal Kirschner wires entry point and direction and to precisely direct cannulated screws [15,16]. Recent studies have shown how, with skilled use of a combination of anteromedial, anterolateral, and midlateral portals, it is possible to reach a 360° exposure of the radial head for arthroscopic fracture fixation [17]. Furthermore, the distalization of anteromedial and anterolateral portals is useful to obtain a biomechanical stronger fixation [17].

To our knowledge there are no current studies that compare radial head ARIF and ORIF. Therefore, the aim of this study was to describe the technique used to perform radial head ARIF and to compare the results after 10 years by analyzing patients who received ARIF to those who received ORIF.

We hypothesized that skilled surgeons who were trained on elbow arthroscopy would be able to perform ARIF of the radial head with a comparable surgical time, better early functional outcome, and a lower rate of postoperative complications than for ORIF.

2. Materials and Methods

A retrospective study was conducted on patients who underwent surgery between June 2007 and October 2015. All the procedures were performed by the same skilled surgeon (EG).

Patients who were eligible for the study were those who underwent arthroscopic or open field radial head fixation with screws and who did not have ligament injuries or coronoid associated fractures. Indications for surgery were: mechanical block in pronosupination movements; two-part fractures with displacement greater than 5 mm if involving head or greater than 4 mm if involving the neck; and fractures that had multiple fragments but were still treated with screw fixation. Patients treated with plate and screws fixation or radial head removal or replacement were excluded.

Patients' demographics are reported in Table 1.

Table 1. Patients' demographics.

Demographic Data of the Study Population	ORIF	ARIF	TOTAL
Patients (no.) (%)	19 (59.41)	13 (40.62)	32
Age (years)	43.31 (±11.03/15–61)	45.38 (±16.37/14–65)	44.16 (±13.57) (14–65)
Gender (M/F) (%)	12/7 (63.25/36.84)	5/8 (38.54/61.52)	17/15 (53.12/46.92)
Classification (Mason II/III) (no.) (%)	12/7 (63.2/436.83)	11/2 (84.63/15.42)	23/9 (71.93/28.12)

Legend: no.—number; M—Male; F—Female; ORIF—Open Reduction Internal Fixation; ARIF—Arthroscopic Reduction Internal Fixation.

2.1. Surgical Planning

Every patient underwent a pre-op CT scan with multiplanar 2D and 3D reconstructions to study the number, size, and dislocation of fracture fragments, as well as bone impaction and involvement of the 'safe zone'.

ARIF was performed in 13 cases where the pre-operative plan was to perform a screw fixation, and there was an absence of gross associated injuries or Fracture type Mason II and III without LCL at varus stress test under anesthesia. A total of 19 patients who underwent ARIF were compared to a group of patients who underwent ORIF with the same indications.

2.2. ARIF Surgical Technique Description

Elbow varus–valgus stability was tested with the patient supine under anesthesia (brachial plexus block or general anesthesia).

Patients were positioned in lateral decubitus with the affected arm supported by a dedicated holder, and a tourniquet was inflated at 250 mmHg. Joint landmarks were drawn on the skin. An articular lavage was performed by a spinal needle through the 'soft spot' in the posterolateral portion of the elbow.

Three standard anterior portals were routinely performed: anteromedial, anterolateral and proximal anterolateral. The pump maintained an intra-articular pressure in an interval between 30 and 40 mmHg.

2.2.1. 1st Step: Fracture Visualization and Reduction

The arthroscopic camera was inserted in the anteromedial portal with the shaver in the anterolateral; at the same time, an elevator kept the joint capsule open from the anterolateral proximal portal.

The hematoma was removed, and the fracture was visualized from both the anteromedial and anterolateral portal to confirm CT scans.

The fracture was then mobilized and reduced using two probes that were introduced from the anterolateral and proximal anterolateral portals along with pronation and supination movements. If necessary, a third probe could be inserted through the midlateral portal/soft spot to achieve and/or maintain the reduction. Some fractures can be difficult to reduce because the radial head fragment can be dislocated either through the anterior capsule or in the posterior aspect of the elbow. As no fractures with high dislocations were present in the cases in this series, no cases required the capsule to be opened, and none were converted into open field surgeries. This could occur because associated ligamentous or coronoid lesions are often present when the fragment is dislocated through the capsule or in the posterior aspect of the elbow, and these associated injuries were an exclusion criteria for the study.

Once reduction was achieved, the best position between pronation and supination to perform definitive fragment fixation was chosen, and the fragments were stabilized with temporary 1.4 mm K-wires.

2.2.2. 2nd Step: Working Position and Fixation

Using specimen studies, the elbow and wrist ESSKA committee showed that the entire radial head circumference is approachable for fixation, and that modified anteroinferior portals are more effective for performing a correct radial head fracture ARIF1 [17,18].

Fractures can be divided according to the position of the fragment in relation to the "safe zone" (i.e., the part of the radial head that does not have contact with the small sigmoid notch). Ideally, the radial head is divided into two halves in the neutral position: the lateral half (which includes the safe zone) and the medial half.

Fractures of the lateral half can be fixed from the anterolateral portal (*working position AL*) by placing the forearm in pronation and examining from the AM portal (Figure 1).

The retractor and the probe help to maintain the reduction and keep the workspace open. It may be useful to temporarily fix the fracture by using a K-wire either posteriorly (soft spot portal) or anterolaterally (anterolateral portal).

An accessory lateral portal from a more distal location could be useful for placing the screws parallel to the radial head surface. A small 5 mm cannula was needed to protect the soft tissues from the rotating tools (K-wire, drill, screwdriver) and to prevent the thin K-wire from bending or breaking. The K-wire was inserted through the cannula, and then the fixation procedure was performed (measurement, drilling, screw).

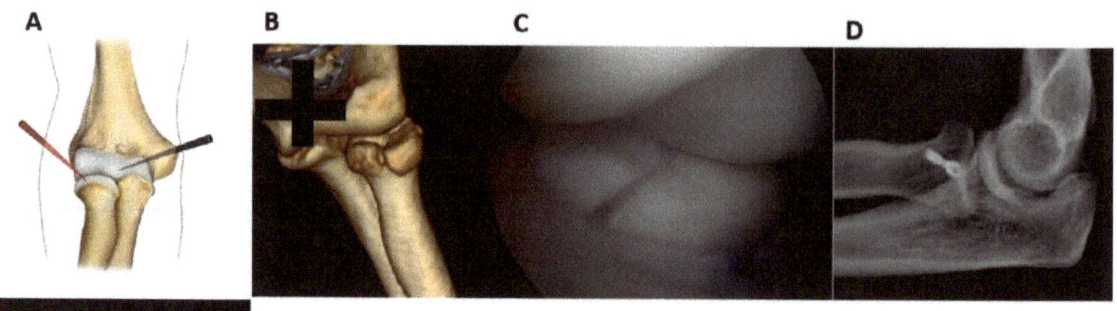

Figure 1. Fractures of the lateral half can be fixed from the anterolateral working position (**A**). (**B**): pre-operative 3D CT scan showing the fracture. (**C**): intraoperative image of fracture fixation. (**D**): Control x-ray.

Fractures of the lateral half could be alternatively fixed by working posteriorly (working position PL) as described by Rolla et al. [16] (Figure 2).

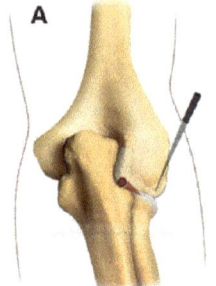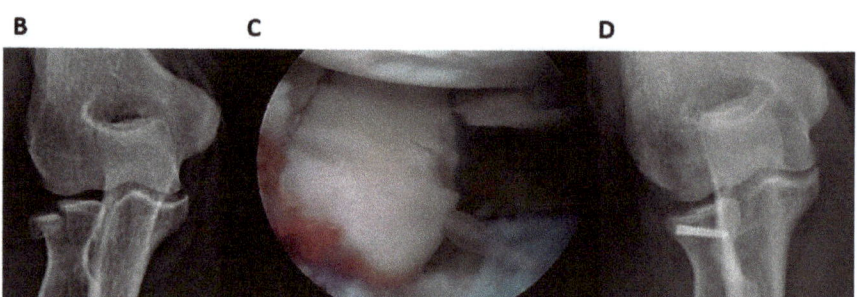

Figure 2. Fracture of lateral half of radial head that is fixed using the posterolateral working position; posterolateral and midlateral portals were created (**A**). From the superior view, the shaver and probe created the necessary space to reduce the fragment. (**B**): Pre-operative x-ray showing the fracture. (**C**): Intraoperative image of fracture fixation. (**D**): Control x-ray.

Posterolateral and midlateral portals were created. From the superior view, the shaver and probe created the necessary space to reduce the fragment. The fixation technique was then completed by following the steps previously described.

For medial half fractures, it was helpful to change the view (working position AM, Figure 3).

While viewing from the anterolateral portal, the cannula was inserted through the anteromedial portal. The procedure for the fixation was the same, and no other accessory portals were needed.

Following these considerations, the three working positions can be summarized as in Table 2.

All fractures were fixed using headless cannulated screws (Micro Acutrak screws, Acumed) with lengths varying from 14 mm to 26 mm.

Evaluating the appropriate length of the screws is difficult because the sensation of the second cortex cannot be determined while drilling the K-wire into place, and x-ray evaluation is dangerous because pronosupination movements can bend the K-wires. Therefore, the Authors recommend measurements during pre-operative CT scans to determine the diameter of radial head, as the screw's length should never exceed that value. The Authors inserted the first screw in the largest fragment until the sensation of a stable fixation was reached; the K-wire was then removed, the stability of the fragment was rechecked, and then x-rays were performed. If the fracture was reduced and stable, then other fragments (if present) were treated using the same procedure.

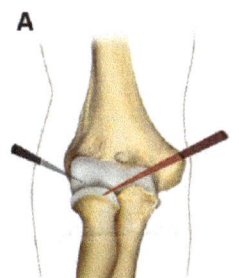 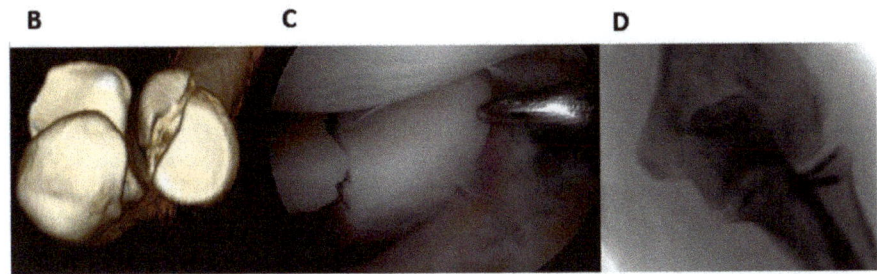

Figure 3. For the medial half fractures, the working position AM was more appropriate; the field was viewed from the anterolateral portal and the cannula was inserted through the anteromedial portal (**A**). (**B**): Pre-operative 3D CT scan showing the fracture. (**C**): Intraoperative image of fracture fixation. (**D**): Control x-ray.

Table 2. Description of arthroscopic working position to address fixation of radial head fragments.

Working Position	Direction of Screws Insetion	Camera Portal Position	Probe/Elevator Portal Position	Portal of Screws Insertion
PL	Posterolateral	Posterolateral	Midlateral portal (soft spot)	Direct radial head accessory
AL	Anterolateral	Anteromedial	Anterolateral Ant lat proximal Midlateral	Direct radial head accessory
AM	Anteromedial	Anterolateral	Ant lat proximal Midlateral	Anteromedial

The rehabilitation program began the day after surgery with gentle self-assisted active movements. A sling was positioned to protect the elbow from valgus stresses for three weeks, and manual activities were forbidden for two months.

2.3. Follow-Up and Functional Evaluation

All patients underwent x-rays and clinical examination at 1, 3, 6, and 12 months after surgery, and at the final follow-up. Functional evaluation was performed using the Mayo Elbow Performance Index (MEPI) and the Broberg and Morrey Rating System (BMRS) [19–21].

2.4. Statistical Analysis

Statistical evaluation was performed using the IBM SSPS Statistics Software Version 23 (IBM, Armonk, NY, USA) for MAC. The independent t-test and the Chi-squared test were performed to compare both ARIF and ORIF subjects using the variables Surgery Duration, Functional Outcome Scores (MEPI and BMRS), and Complications rate. A p value < 0.05 was considered significative.

3. Results

A total of 32 subjects (15 females and 17 males) were selected for the study using radiological criteria (standard AP and lateral x-ray views and CT scan of the elbow with 2D and 3D reconstruction) to classify the radial head fractures, according to Mason.

Between June 2007 and October 2015, 13 patients were treated with ARIF and 19 patients with ORIF.

Patients' age ranged from 14 to 65 years (mean of 44.16 years) and the time between trauma and surgery ranged from 2 to 64 days (mean of 8.1 days).

A total of 13 subjects were treated with ARIF. The patients were five males and eight females, with a mean time between the date of the trauma and the surgery date of 8 days (range 3–24 days). The other 19 patients were treated with ORIF (12 males and 7 females), by Kocher approach and with a mean time between trauma and surgery of 7.25 days (range of 2–64 days).

Average follow-up time of all patients was 10 years (range 7–15).

Functional outcomes (as determined by performance scores) were obtained for 32 patients at the last outpatient consult (Table 3).

Table 3. Clinical and functional results of ARIF and ORIF.

	ARIF	ORIF
MEPI Score	98.07 (SD ± 4.34)	91.57 (SD ± 11.67)
BMRS Score—Variables	95.61(SD ± 5.99)	92.06(SD ± 8.66)
Duration of the procedure (minutes)	71.60 (SD ± 24.96) (range 36–135)	81.66 (SD ± 36.73) (range 29–170)
Follow-up (years) (SD; range)	10.14 (±4.32; 7–15)	10.52 (±26.46/7–15)

Independent t-test and the Chi-squared test were performed with the variables to be compared and a p value < 0.05 considered significative. The mean MEPI score for the ARIF group was 98.077 (SD ± 4.34), while ORIF group reported 91.57 (SD ± 11.67). This indicates significantly better results for the ARIF group ($p = 0.036$); mean BMRS score was 95.61 (SD ±5.99 for ARIF) and 92.06 (SD ± 8.66 for ORIF) ($p = 0.181$).

Mean duration of the procedure was 71.60 min for ARIF (SD ±24.96 and range of 36–135 min) and 81.66 min for ORIF (SD ± 36.73 and range of 29–170 min) ($p = 0.808$).

Complications

No intra operative complications were observed. A total of 15 patients reported post-operative complications, 3 for ARIF group (23.1%) and 12 for ORIF (63.5%) (Table 4).

Table 4. Post operative complications and reoperations.

	ARIF	ORIF
Complications	3 (23.1%)	12 (63.5%)
Stiffness and mild pain	2 (15.4%)	4 (21.1%)
Lateral ossification	1 (7.7%)	0
Inconstant pain	0	1 (5.3%)
Crepitation	0	1 (5.3%)
Moderate supination deficit	0	1 (5.3%)
Moderate pronation deficit	0	1 (5.3%)
Weakness in flexion	0	1 (5.3%)
Weakness in pronosupination	0	1 (5.3%)
Occasional lateral elbow pain	0	1 (5.3%)
Temporary cutaneous numbness	0	1 (5.3%)
Second surgical procedure	1 open arthrolisis and screw removal	2 arthroscopic arthrolysis with one screw removal

In the ARIF group, two patients reported elbow stiffness (15.4%). One underwent arthrolysis and screw removal; the other one had symptoms of ulnar nerve compression, with positive Tinel sign and distal dysesthesia. The third patient showed a heterotopic ossification at the lateral epicondyle margin without functional deficit (7.7%). One patient underwent a second surgery with open arthrolysis and screw removal.

In the ORIF group, the most frequent complication was persistent mild pain, followed by moderate inconstant pain, crepitation during ROM of radial head, pronosupination limitations, mild supination deficit, and weakness when complete flexion of the elbow was reached. From these patients, two underwent a second procedure: the first underwent screw removal and arthrolysis eight months after the osteosynthesis, and the second patient underwent arthroscopic arthrolysis after 15 months, with satisfactory range of motion improvement.

4. Discussion

Arthroscopic treatment of elbow pathology is increasing over time; treatments include reduction and fixation of radial head fractures that include associated injuries, such as coronoid fracture or collateral ligament avulsion [8,22,23]. This technique offers multiple advantages: a complete view of the articular surfaces of radial head and coronoid is possible [17], as well as removal of small intra-articular fragments and treatment of trochlear chondral damages or small coronoid fractures that would otherwise require extensive open medial access. There is much less tissue damage with ARIF compared to ORIF; however, ARIF still remains a technically demanding surgery that requires a long learning curve and high technical skills. Complication rate is reported with a huge variability depending on the surgeon's abilities [24].

The first arthroscopic treatment of radial head fracture was described in 2004 [25] for a fracture of the neck of the proximal radius in a child. The fracture was manually reduced and fixed by percutaneous K-wires under a direct intra-articular visualization [26].

In 2006, Rolla et al. [16] published a series of cases that included 6 fractures of the radial head (II, III and IV types according to Mason) which were reduced and fixed by percutaneous screws. The performed technique was described, with an indication to work in the anterior compartment to reduce the fracture, and then change the view position to the posterolateral portal, creating an anterolateral portal for fragment fixation.

In 2007, Michels [15] described 14 cases, all classified as Mason type II. The authors performed ARIF using only two portals (anterolateral and posterolateral) and performed a small incision to insert the screws, with good clinical and radiographic results. Wang et al. [27] reported results from 18 cases with Mason type II fractures treated with percutaneous K-wires under arthroscopy with clinical good results. In 2019, Haasters et al. [28] reported a retrospective case series of 20 patients, highlighting good results and a high capacity of arthroscopy to diagnose and treat concomitant elbow injuries that might not be visible at MRI or CT scan.

As evidenced by the literature, ARIF of radial head fracture is a procedure that is growing in popularity but is not yet widely performed. With the present study, the authors aim to report their 10 years outcome of the arthroscopic radial head osteosynthesis and describe different surgical technique using different portals, depending on the fracture pattern.

In comparison to open osteosynthesis, screw length is more difficult to assess because performing an intraoperative fluoroscopy with the tools in place is complicated. Generally, the screws range from 14 to 18 mm long and, in case of indecision, the Authors recommend choosing a shorter screw and checking at the end of fixation to avoid loss of reduction or K-wire bending while obtaining a satisfactory radiographic view. Studying a pre-operatory CT scan helps to determine appropriate screw length and avoiding excessive length.

The instruments should be chosen carefully, because drill and screwdriver might have very short results, especially when fixation is performed at the anteromedial portal. If these tools are not available, the arthroscopic cannula can be cut and shortened as necessary before being inserted into the joint.

Another important aspect of ARIF in comparison to ORIF is the surgical time. In the present study, the mean surgical time for ARIF was 74.46 min, 2.64 min faster than ORIF group; however, the independent t-test showed no statistically significant difference ($p = 0.808$) between the groups, indicating that after the proper learning curve even a technically demanding procedure can be performed with confidence and reproducibility. Obviously, considering the difficulty of this procedure, the learning curve is steep and requires high elbow arthroscopic skills.

The different position described in this paper, along with the findings in the literature that indicate how the radial head can be easily reached for screw insertion [29], aim to give elbow surgeons the tools they need to approach and improve this fixation technique. The Authors find it easier to perform the synthesis from the anteromedial portal when possible, with supination or pronation helping to reach a wider radial head surface. The AM working position gives the surgeon a wider articular space to work in without the need of an additional portal that may cause a tear (even if small) to the annular ligament. In this working position, the Authors suggest that it is more comfortable to also insert multiple screws in different directions, either parallel to the radial head surface or oblique through the radial neck. One disadvantage is the larger distance required to reach the radial head from the AM portal. Longer screwdrivers and drills may be necessary, especially in obese or highly muscular patients.

For the same reason, the Authors do not suggest the PL working position. As the capsule is very close to the radial head, it is more difficult to perform and the cartilage is easier to damage while reducing the facture. However, this position uses safer portals than anterior ones as they are far from neurovascular structures.

The AL working position can be considered a good balance between advantages and disadvantages. The space is narrow, and a small tear of the annular ligament occurs frequently, but the AL is in the same position that is used to reduce the fracture, and instrument length does not create difficulties.

In the present series, regarding the functional outcome, MEPI scores were better in the ARIF group (mean 98.07, $p = 0.036$) with statistical significance. In comparison to the previous series about arthroscopic reduction and internal fixation of radial head fractures, the presented results are comparable with results published by Rolla et al. [16], which reported three excellent and three good results for functional outcome. The present study reported 92.30% excellent and 7.69% good results (n = 13 patients, 12 excellent and 1 good). Another functional parameter used was the BMRS score, which had no statistically significative difference between the arthroscopic and the open groups ($p = 0.181$; mean score 95.615 and 92.063, respectively) and in comparison to Michel's study (mean 97.6 and range 86–100 points; 11 excellent and 3 good results) [15], the present study reported similar values for the ARIF group (mean 95.61 and range 81–100 points; 10 excellent (76.9%) and 3 good (23.1%).

Even if complications are reported in radial head ARIF, the present series included no neurological or vascular lesions other than the patient with symptoms of ulnar nerve compression. The major complication of this technique is the same as that described for elbow arthroscopy, i.e., the risk of nerve or brachial artery injury, but the frequency is not well known [5].

In the present series, the ARIF cohort had a complication rate of 23.1%. The rate of neurological complications is between 0 and 14%, according to El Hajj et al. [30], with more than half of the cases including the ulnar or median nerves. This complication can occur due to the proximity of the radial, posterior interosseous, ulnar, and median nerves to anterolateral and anteromedial portals [5]. These injuries can also be a result of laceration or be secondary to compression from a cannula, fluid extravasation, exposure to local anesthetics, or tourniquet-related problems [31]. The series by Kelly et al., a retrospective review of 473 consecutive elbow arthroscopies performed during an 18-year period, had an overall complication rate of 12%, with serious complications in less than 1% (permanent nerve lesions or infection), and minor complications (such transient nerve lesions) in 11%

of the arthroscopic procedures [32]. This matched the presented complications of this study, with exception of heterotopic ossification, which was not analyzed.

The major limitation of this study is its retrospective design. However, to our knowledge, the existing studies have not reported results and complications of radial head ARIF with this long of a follow-up. As a retrospective study, the patient selection also represents a possible source of bias, in that the Authors tried to avoid enrolling all the patients that met the inclusion criteria.

5. Conclusions

The described radial head ARIF surgical technique represents a reproducible and safe procedure. A long learning curve is necessary, but with the proper experience it represents a tool that might be beneficial for patients, allowing a radial head fracture treatment with minimal tissue damage, evaluation and treatment of the concomitant lesions, and with no limitation of screws positioning. The surgeon must perform accurate pre-operative planning and intraoperatively choose the better working position so that they can fix all fracture patterns and obtain good clinical results, comparable to the state of the art radial head ORIF.

Author Contributions: Conceptualization E.G., A.M., M.D.S.F. and M.C. methodology, E.G., A.M. and M.C.; software, A.R. and A.S.; validation, G.C. and F.T.; formal analysis, A.S.; investigation, A.M.; resources, E.G.; data curation, M.D.S.F.; writing—original draft preparation, E.G., M.C. and M.D.S.F.; writing—review and editing, F.T. and M.C.; visualization, F.T.; supervision, E.G. and M.C.; project administration, E.G. All authors have read and agreed to the published version of the manuscript.

Funding: This research received no external funding.

Institutional Review Board Statement: The study was conducted in accordance with the Declaration of Helsinki and approved by the Institutional Review Board (or Ethics Committee) of IRCCS Istituto Ortopedico Rizzoli (protocol code Artic.elb, date of approval 9 November 2016).

Informed Consent Statement: Informed consent was obtained from all subjects involved in the study.

Data Availability Statement: The data presented in this study are available on request from the corresponding author.

Conflicts of Interest: The authors declare no conflict of interest.

References

1. Kaas, L.; Van Riet, R.P.; Vroemen, J.P.A.M.; Eygendaal, D. The incidence of associated fractures of the upper limb in fractures of the radial head. *Strateg. Trauma Limb Reconstr.* **2008**, *3*, 71–74. [CrossRef] [PubMed]
2. Van Riet, R.P.; Morrey, B.F.; O'Driscoll, S.W.; Van Glabbeek, F. Associated injuries complicating radial head fractures: Ademographic study. *Clin. Orthop. Relat. Res.* **2005**, *441*, 351–355. [CrossRef] [PubMed]
3. Morrey, B.F.; An, K.N. Stability of the elbow: Osseous constraints. *J. Shoulder Elbow Surg.* **2005**, *14*, 174S–178S. [CrossRef] [PubMed]
4. Van Riet, R.; Van Glabbeek, F.; Neale, P.G.; Bimmel, R.; Bortier, H.; Morrey, B.F.; O'Driscoll, S.W.; An, K.N. Anatomical considerations of the radius. *Clin. Anat.* **2004**, *17*, 564–569. [CrossRef] [PubMed]
5. O'Driscoll, S.W.; Morrey, B.M. Arthroscopy of the Elbow: Diagnostic and Therapeutic Benefits and Hazards. *J. Bone Joint Surg.* **1992**, *74*, 84–94. [CrossRef]
6. Hotchkiss, R.N. Displaced fractures of the radial head: Internal fixation or excision? *J. Am. Acad. Orthop. Surg.* **1997**, *5*, 1–10. [CrossRef]
7. Broberg, M.A.; Morrey, B.F. Results of treatment of fracture-dislocations of the elbow. *Clin. Orthop. Relat. Res.* **1987**, *216*, 109–119. [CrossRef]
8. Van Riet, R.P.; Van den Bekerom, M.P.J. Radial head fractures. *Shoulder Elb.* **2020**, *12*, 212–223. [CrossRef]
9. Herbertsson, P.; Josefsson, P.O.; Hasserius, R.; Karlsson, C.; Besjakov, J.; Karlsson, M. Uncomplicated Mason type-II and III fractures of the radial head and neck in adults. A long-term follow-up study. *J. Bone Joint Surg. Am.* **2004**, *86*, 569–574. [CrossRef]
10. Akesson, T.; Herbertsson, P.; Josefsson, P.O.; Hasserius, R.; Besjakov, J.; Karlsson, M.K. Displaced fractures of the neck of the radius in adults. An excellent long-term outcome. *J. Bone Joint Surg. Br.* **2006**, *88*, 642–644. [CrossRef]
11. Burkhart, K.J.; Wegmann, K.; Muller, L.P.; Gohlke, F.E. Fractures of the Radial Head. *Hand Clin.* **2015**, *31*, 533–546. [CrossRef] [PubMed]
12. Lapner, M.; King, G.J.W. Radial Head Fractures. *J. Bone Joint Surg.* **2013**, *95*, 1135–1143.

13. Budge, M.D.; Armstrong, A.D. Elbow Arthroscopy: Set Up, Portals, and Tools for Success. *Oper. Tech. Orthop.* **2009**, *19*, 209–219. [CrossRef]
14. Yeoh, K.M.; King, G.J.W.; Faber, K.J.; Glazebrook, M.A.; Athwal, G.S. Evidence-Based Indications for Elbow Arthroscopy. *Arthrosc. J. Arthrosc. Relat. Surg.* **2012**, *28*, 272–282. [CrossRef] [PubMed]
15. Michels, F.; Pouliart, N.; Handelberg, F. Arthroscopic management of Mason type 2 radial head fractures. *Knee Surg. Sport Traumatol. Arthrosc.* **2007**, *15*, 1244–1250. [CrossRef]
16. Rolla, P.R.; Surace, M.F.; Bini, A.; Pilato, G. Arthroscopic treatment of fractures of the radial head. *Arthroscopy* **2006**, *22*, 233. [CrossRef]
17. Cucchi, D.; Guerra, E.; Luceri, F.; Lenich, A.; Nicoletti, S.; Randelli, P.; Wirtz, D.C.; Eygendaal, D.; Arrigoni, P.; ESSKA Elbow and Wrist Committee 2016–2018. A combination of an anteromedial, anterolateral and midlateral portals is sufficient for 360° exposure of the radial head for arthroscopic fracture fixation. *Knee Surg. Sports Traumatol. Arthrosc.* **2019**, *1*, 319–325. [CrossRef]
18. Cucchi, D.; Arrigoni, P.; Lucerim, F.; Menon, A.; Guerra, E.; Muller, L.P.; Burger, C.; Eygendaal, D.; Wegmann, K.; ESSKA Elbow and Wrist Committee 2016–2018. Modified anteromedial and anterolateral elbow arthroscopy portals show superiority to standard portals in guiding arthroscopic radial head screw fixation. *Knee Surg. Sports Traumatol. Arthrosc.* **2019**, *10*, 3276–3283. [CrossRef]
19. Longo, U.G.; Franceschi, F.; Loppini, M.; Maffulli, N.; Denaro, V. Rating systems for evaluation of the elbow. *Br. Med. Bull.* **2008**, *87*, 131–161. [CrossRef]
20. Morrey, B.F.; An, K.N. Functional evaluation of the elbow. In *The Elbow and Its Disorders*, 2nd ed.; Morrey, B.F., Ed.; W.B. Sanders: Philadelphia, PA, USA, 1993; pp. 86–89.
21. Dawson, J.; Doll, H.; Boller, I.; Fitzpatrick, R.; Little, C.; Rees, J.; Jenkinson, C.; Carr, A.J. The Development and validation of a patient reported questionnaire to assess outcomes of elbow surgery. *J. Bone Joint Surg. Br.* **2008**, *90*, 466–473. [CrossRef]
22. Conti Mica, M.; Caekebeke, P.; Van Riet, R. Lateral collateral ligament injuries of the elbow—Chronic posterolateral rotatory instability (PLRI). *EFORT Open Rev.* **2016**, *1*, 461–468. [CrossRef]
23. Savoie, F.H.; Field, L.D.; O'Brien, M.J.; Gutley, D.J. Arthroscopic and open radial ulnohumeral ligament reconstruction for posterolateral rotatory instability of the elbow. *Hand Clin.* **2009**, *25*, 323–329. [CrossRef] [PubMed]
24. Solomon, H.B.; Murthi, A.M.; Anand, M. Elbow arthroscopy: Use or abuse. *Curr. Opin. Orthop.* **2002**, *13*, 310–314. [CrossRef]
25. Pike, J.M.; Athwal, G.S.; Faber, K.J.; King, G.J.W. Radial Head Fractures-An Update. *J. Hand Surg.* **2009**, *34*, 557–565. [CrossRef] [PubMed]
26. Dawson, F.; Inostroza, F. Arthroscopic Reduction and Percutaneous Fixation of a Radial Neck Fracture in a Child. *Arthroscopy* **2004**, *20* (Suppl. S2), 90–93. [CrossRef] [PubMed]
27. Wang, J.; Qi, W.; Shen, X.; Tao, S.; Liu, Y. Results of arthroscopic fixation of Mason type II radial head fractures using Kirschner wires. *Medicine* **2018**, *97*, 0201. [CrossRef] [PubMed]
28. Haasters, F.; Helfen, T.; Bocker, W.; Mayr, H.O.; Prall, W.C.; Lenich, A. The value of elbow arthroscopy in diagnosing and treatment of radial head fractures. *BMC Musculoskelet. Disord.* **2019**, *20*, 343. [CrossRef]
29. Carroll, M.J.; Athwal, G.S.; King, G.J.W.; Faber, K.J. Capitellar and trochlear fractures. *Hand Clin.* **2015**, *31*, 615–630. [CrossRef]
30. El Hajj, F.; Hoteit, M.; Ouaknine, M. Elbow arthroscopy: An alternative to anteromedial portals. *Orthop. Traumatol. Surg. Res.* **2015**, *101*, 411–414. [CrossRef]
31. Bennett, J.M. Elbow Arthroscopy: The Basics. *J. Hand Surg.* **2013**, *38*, 164–167. [CrossRef]
32. Marti, D.; Spross, C.; Jost, B. The first 100 elbow arthroscopies of one surgeon: Analysis of complications. *J. Shoulder Elbow Surg.* **2013**, *22*, 567–573. [CrossRef] [PubMed]

Disclaimer/Publisher's Note: The statements, opinions and data contained in all publications are solely those of the individual author(s) and contributor(s) and not of MDPI and/or the editor(s). MDPI and/or the editor(s) disclaim responsibility for any injury to people or property resulting from any ideas, methods, instructions or products referred to in the content.

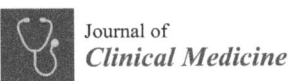

Article

Infrared Thermography in Symptomatic Knee Osteoarthritis: Joint Temperature Differs Based on Patient and Pain Characteristics

Luca De Marziani [1], Angelo Boffa [1,*], Lucia Angelelli [1], Luca Andriolo [1], Alessandro Di Martino [1], Stefano Zaffagnini [1] and Giuseppe Filardo [2]

1 Clinica Ortopedica e Traumatologica 2, IRCCS Istituto Ortopedico Rizzoli, 40136 Bologna, Italy
2 Applied and Translational Research (ATR) Center, IRCCS Istituto Ortopedico Rizzoli, 40136 Bologna, Italy
* Correspondence: angeloboffa@libero.it; Tel.: +39-0516366567

Abstract: The aim of this study was to evaluate osteoarthritis (OA) patients with infrared thermography to investigate imaging patterns as well as demographic and clinical characteristics that influence knee inflammation. Forty patients with one-sided symptomatic knee OA were included and evaluated through knee-specific PROMs and the PainDETECT Questionnaire for neuropathic pain evaluation. Thermograms were captured using a thermographic camera FLIR-T1020 and temperatures were extracted using the software ResearchIR for the overall knee and the five ROIs: medial, lateral, medial patella, lateral patella, and suprapatellar. The mean temperature of the total knee was 31.9 ± 1.6 °C. It negatively correlated with age (rho = -0.380, $p = 0.016$) and positively correlated with BMI (rho = 0.421, $p = 0.007$) and the IKDC objective score (tau = 0.294, $p = 0.016$). Men had higher temperatures in the knee medial, lateral, and suprapatellar areas ($p = 0.017$, $p = 0.019$, $p = 0.025$, respectively). Patients with neuropathic pain had a lower temperature of the medial knee area (31.5 ± 1.0 vs. 32.3 ± 1.1, $p = 0.042$), with the total knee negatively correlating with PainDETECT ($p = 0.045$). This study demonstrated that the skin temperature of OA symptomatic knees is influenced by demographic and clinical characteristics of patients, with higher joint temperatures in younger male patients with higher BMI and worst objective knee scores and lower temperatures in patients affected by neuropathic pain.

Keywords: infrared thermography; knee; osteoarthritis; joint temperature; inflammation; neuropathic pain

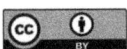

Citation: De Marziani, L.; Boffa, A.; Angelelli, L.; Andriolo, L.; Di Martino, A.; Zaffagnini, S.; Filardo, G. Infrared Thermography in Symptomatic Knee Osteoarthritis: Joint Temperature Differs Based on Patient and Pain Characteristics. *J. Clin. Med.* **2023**, *12*, 2319. https://doi.org/10.3390/jcm12062319

Academic Editor: Yves-Marie Pers

Received: 5 January 2023
Revised: 3 March 2023
Accepted: 14 March 2023
Published: 16 March 2023

Copyright: © 2023 by the authors. Licensee MDPI, Basel, Switzerland. This article is an open access article distributed under the terms and conditions of the Creative Commons Attribution (CC BY) license (https://creativecommons.org/licenses/by/4.0/).

1. Introduction

Osteoarthritis (OA) is a common form of degenerative joint disease affecting the adult population, characterized by articular cartilage loss within the synovial joints and associated with hypertrophy of the bone (osteophytes and subchondral bone sclerosis), thickening of the capsule, and synovial inflammation [1]. An important aspect of OA is the interpatient variability in clinical and structural manifestations [2,3]. This heterogeneity may be one of the major factors associated with the complexity of OA management and the difficulties in developing one-fits-all therapeutic strategies. In fact, nowadays, no conservative therapies have been proven to arrest or modify the disease progression, nor to be highly effective for symptomatic relief [4,5]. For this reason, the identification of specific OA features could help to better identify different diseases patterns and target treatments and manage each patient according to the specific disease phase and manifestation [6]. Among the key aspects investigated, lot of attention has been placed on the inflammatory process involving OA joints.

Inflammation plays a central role in the pathophysiology of OA, with the involvement of the synovial membrane and the release of pro-inflammatory cytokines. These factors induce chondrocytes to produce degradative enzymes of the extracellular matrix and inhibit both tissue repair and regeneration [7]. During the inflammatory process, there is an increase of blood flow that can manifest clinically with redness and heat, as well as with joint swelling and pain [8]. As many available treatments target the inflammatory process, the quantification of the inflammatory component in the OA process could help to better characterize patients with OA, favoring a more targeted treatment [9,10]. In this light, the temperature is a key physical property, as its values detected by infrared thermography could reflect the articular inflammatory process [11]. Therefore, infrared thermography has been proposed as a tool for OA diagnosis and monitoring of disease state, progression, and response to medical treatment, in particular in relation to the inflammatory components [12]. However, although the use of infrared thermography for the evaluation of patients with OA is growing, data are still sparse and evidence on thermographic findings in OA patients is lacking.

The aim of this study was to evaluate OA patients with infrared thermography, to investigate imaging patterns as well as demographic and clinical characteristics that could influence the skin temperature of the knee of patients affected by symptomatic OA.

2. Materials and Methods

This study was approved by the hospital ethics committee of the IRCCS Istituto Ortopedico Rizzoli, Italy (n. 0017413). Patients were enrolled by orthopedic physicians between December 2021 and April 2022 in a research outpatient clinic focused on patients with knee OA. Informed consent was obtained from each patient for study participation. Male or female patients with one-sided symptomatic knee OA (Kellgren–Lawrence grade ≥ 2) with a history of chronic pain or swelling (at least 6 months) were included in the study. The following exclusion criteria were used for selection: history of trauma or intra-articular injection therapy within 6 months before treatment or knee surgery within 12 months; presence of any concomitant knee lesion causing pain or swelling, neoplasms, dermatological and vascular conditions, systemic disorders (e.g., uncontrolled diabetes), metabolic disorders of the thyroid, severe cardiovascular diseases, rheumatoid arthritis, inflammatory arthropathy, hematological diseases, infections, immunodepression, antidepressant, anticoagulants, or antiaggregant therapy; and use of nonsteroidal anti-inflammatory drugs in the 5 days before the investigation.

Forty consecutive patients were enrolled according to the inclusion/exclusion criteria. Among them, 26 patients were men and 14 women, with a mean age of 61.3 ± 9.3 years and a mean body mass index (BMI) of 25.2 ± 3.0. All demographic and clinical patients' characteristics are reported in Table 1.

After enrollment in the study and just before the infrared thermography evaluation, patients were clinically assessed thorough knee-specific patient reported outcome measurements (PROMs) including the International Knee Documentation Committee (IKDC) subjective and objective scores, the Knee injury and Osteoarthritis Outcome Score (KOOS) sub-scales, the EuroQol Visual Analog Scale (EQ-VAS), the Tegner score, the Visual Analogue Scale (VAS) for the symptomatic knee pain, and the PainDETECT Questionnaire for the neuropathic pain evaluation. For the last score, patients with values lower than 13 were considered negative for neuropathic pain, while patients with values higher or equal to 13 were considered positive for neuropathic pain. Subjective clinical questionnaires were compiled by patients with the support of the clinician, while the IKDC objective score was evaluated by the clinician. Moreover, all participants underwent weight-bearing antero-posterior to assess the baseline OA severity according to the Kellgren–Lawrence classification. Finally, the skin temperature of the knee affected by symptomatic OA was evaluated with thermography imaging as reported below. After data collection, further analyses were performed to determine the demographic and clinical parameters that influenced the skin temperature of the OA knee.

Table 1. Included patients' characteristics.

Sex (M/W)	26/14
Age (years)	61.3 ± 9.3 [43–75]
BMI (kg/m^2)	25.2 ± 3.0 [19.9–31.1]
Side	Right: 21-Left: 19
Symptoms duration (months)	108.5 ± 91.4 [18–372]
Symptoms onset	Acute: 13-Chronic: 27
Previous knee surgery (yes/no)	22/18
Smoke (yes/no)	9/31
Kellgren–Lawrence grade	Grade 2: 19 Grade 3: 18 Grade 4: 3
VAS pain	5.0 ± 2.4 [1–9]
IKDC Subjective score	42.3 ± 15.1 [18.4–81.6]
IKDC Objective score	Grade 1: 6 Grade 2: 17 Grade 3: 9 Grade 4: 8
KOOS Pain	61.9 ± 19.1 [17–94]
KOOS Symptoms	60.5 ± 20.5 [18–100]
KOOS ADL	69.9 ± 18.6 [38–100]
KOOS QoL	34.5 ± 16.9 [0–75]
KOOS Sport/Rec	42.6 ± 17.7 [20–90]
Tegner score pre-treatment	2.3 ± 1.2 [1–5]
PainDETECT Questionnaire	8.8 ± 4.9 [2–20]
Neuropathic pain (yes/no)	8/32

Values are expressed as mean ± standard deviation and [range]. ADL, activities of daily living; BMI, body mass index; IKDC, International Knee Documentation Committee; KOOS, Knee Injury and Osteoarthritis Outcome Score; M, male; QoL, quality of life; Sport/Rec, function in sport and recreation; VAS, visual analogue scale; W, women.

2.1. Infrared Imaging Procedure and Analysis

The infrared imaging evaluation was performed in a dedicated outpatient clinic shielded from direct sunlight and with a temperature controlled and set at 23.0 °C and a mean humidity of 45 ± 3%. The image acquisition was always performed in the same time slot between 14:00 pm and 17:00 pm in order to minimize the circadian variations of the temperature. According to Marins et al. [13], participants were asked to sit for ten minutes without touching their knee before the thermal image acquisition without pants, socks, shoes, and with light clothing such as a t-shirt on the top. Participants were asked to stand on a designated floor map. The thermograms of the symptomatic knee were captured using a thermographic camera FLIR T1020 (FLIR® Systems, Täby, Sweden), which has 1024 × 768 pixels of resolution and a thermal sensitivity of 0.02 °C. The camera was positioned at 1 m of distance from the subject, adjusted to their patellar height and positioned perpendicular to the knee. An anterior view image was obtained for each patient using the autofocus modality. Then, maintaining the same knee position, an anatomical marker (a 2 cm diameter circular sticker) was placed on the center of the patella and a second anterior view image was obtained to facilitate the precise subsequent localization of the patella in infrared images. The two anterior images (one with and one without the patellar marker) were aligned side by side on the computer screen, and a template indicating the region of interests (ROIs) was centered over the patella of the unmarked image, using the marked image as a guide (Figure 1) [14]. The ROIs were defined as follows: the patellar area was a square 6 cm in width, divided in "medial patella" and "lateral patella" (6 cm high and 3 cm wide each); the "suprapatellar" area was the area 3 cm over the patella; and the "medial" and "lateral" areas were the regions 3 cm under the patella and on its medial and lateral sides, respectively.

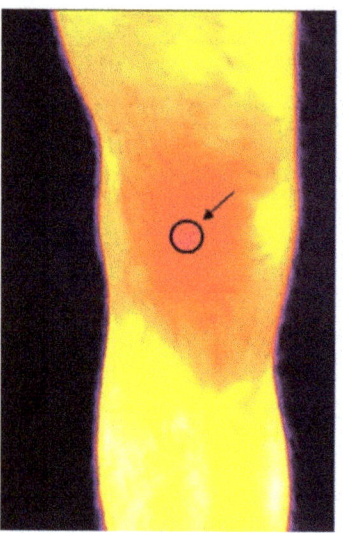 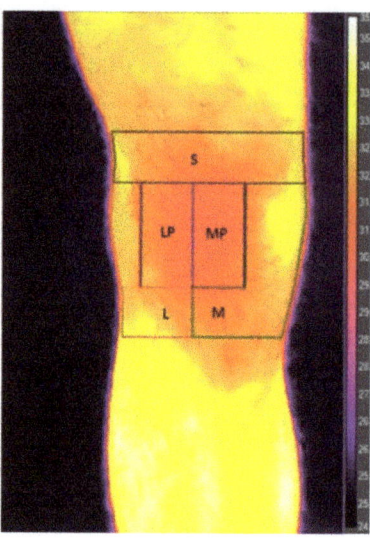

Figure 1. Infrared thermography analysis. On the left, the infrared image obtained with the patellar marker (identified with circle and arrow), while on the right, the image obtained with the considered region of interest (ROI): L, lateral; LP, lateral patella; M, medial; MP, medial patella; and S, suprapatellar.

The mean temperatures, as well as maximum and minimum temperatures, were extracted using the software ResearchIR (FLIR® Systems, Sweden) for the overall knee area and the 5 ROIs: medial, lateral, medial patella, lateral patella, and suprapatellar.

2.2. Statistical Analysis

All continuous data were expressed in terms of the mean and the standard deviation of the mean and range; the categorical data were expressed as frequency and percentages. The Shapiro–Wilk test was performed to test normality of continuous variables. The Levene test was used to assess the homoscedasticity of the data. The repeated measures general linear model (GLM) with Sidak test for multiple comparisons was performed to assess the differences in different areas. The ANOVA test was performed to assess the between groups differences of continuous, normally distributed, and homoscedastic data; the Mann–Whitney non-parametric test was used otherwise. The ANOVA test, followed by the post hoc Sidak test for pairwise comparisons, was performed to assess the among groups differences of continuous, normally distributed, and homoscedastic data; the Kruskal–Wallis non-parametric test, followed by the post hoc Mann–Whitney test with Bonferroni correction for multiple comparisons, was used otherwise. The Spearman rank correlation was used to assess correlations between temperature and continuous data; the Kendall tau rank correlation was used for ordinal data. With 40 patients, a post hoc power equal to 0.9 was obtained with the Kendall's ordinal correlation between the IKDC objective score and the total mean knee temperature. For all tests, $p < 0.05$ was considered significant. All statistical analyses were performed using SPSS v.19.0 (IBM Corp., Armonk, NY, USA).

3. Results

The mean temperatures of the evaluated OA knees are shown in Table 2. The mean temperature of the total knee was 31.9 ± 1.6 °C. Analyzing the mean temperature of the different areas, the patella (both medial and lateral areas) was found to be colder than all other areas of the knee. In particular, the mean temperature of the medial area was higher than medial patella and lateral patella areas (both $p < 0.0005$). The mean temperature of the lateral area was higher than medial patella ($p = 0.019$) and lateral patella areas ($p = 0.048$). The mean temperature of the suprapatellar area was higher than medial patella and lateral patella areas (both $p < 0.0005$). No significant differences were found among the medial, lateral, and suprapatellar areas ($p = $ n.s.).

Table 2. Temperatures of the evaluated knee areas.

Area	Mean Temperature	Minimum Temperature	Maximum Temperature
Total knee	31.9 ± 1.6	30.3 ± 1.1	33.6 ± 1.2
Medial	32.1 ± 1.0	30.7 ± 1.0	33.4 ± 1.2
Lateral	31.9 ± 1.0	30.5 ± 1.1	33.1 ± 1.1
Medial Patella	31.6 ± 1.4	30.9 ± 1.3	32.5 ± 1.4
Lateral Patella	31.6 ± 1.5	30.9 ± 1.4	32.6 ± 1.5
Suprapatellar	32.1 ± 1.2	30.7 ± 1.1	33.3 ± 1.2

The mean temperature of the total knee negatively correlated with age (rho = −0.380, $p = 0.016$) and positively with BMI (rho = 0.421, $p = 0.007$), with higher temperatures in patients younger and with higher BMI. This correlation was also confirmed for all sub-areas, except for the medial patellar area in relation to age, as shown in Table 3. Males tended to be warmer than females, with higher mean temperatures of the total knee (32.2 ± 1.2 vs. 31.4 ± 0.8, $p = 0.051$), medial area (32.4 ± 1.1 vs. 31.5 ± 0.7 $p = 0.017$), lateral area (32.2 ± 1.1 vs. 31.3 ± 0.9, $p = 0.019$), and suprapatellar area (32.4 ± 1.2 vs. 31.5 ± 0.8 $p = 0.025$), while no significant differences between sexes were found for the patella areas.

Table 3. Temperature correlates with age and BMI.

Area	Age	BMI
Total knee	Rho = −0.380, $p = 0.016$	Rho = 0.421, $p = 0.007$
Medial	Rho = −0.450, $p = 0.004$	Rho = 0.333, $p = 0.036$
Lateral	Rho = −0.387, $p = 0.014$	Rho = 0.365, $p = 0.020$
Medial Patella	Rho = −0.265, $p = 0.098$	Rho = 0.461, $p = 0.003$
Lateral Patella	Rho = −0.329, $p = 0.038$	Rho = 0.512, $p = 0.001$
Suprapatellar	Rho = −0.377, $p = 0.016$	Rho = 0.433, $p = 0.005$

Regarding clinical scores, the mean temperature of the total knee correlated with the IKDC objective score (tau = 0.294, $p = 0.016$), and this correlation was confirmed for all sub-areas (Figure 2). Patients with neuropathic pain had a lower mean temperature of the medial knee area than patients without neuropathic pain (31.5 ± 1.0 vs. 32.3 ± 1.1, $p = 0.042$), although only a tendency was found for the total knee and the remaining sub-areas. Moreover, the mean temperature of the total knee and the medial area negatively correlated with the PainDETECT Questionnaire (rho = −0.319, $p = 0.045$, rho = −0.366, $p = 0.020$, respectively), while a tendency was found for the other four sub-areas (Figure 3). The mean temperature of the medial knee area correlated with the VAS pain scale (rho = −0.361, $p = 0.022$), while a tendency was found for the mean temperature of the total knee (rho = −0.298, $p = 0.062$), the lateral area (rho = −0.291, $p = 0.068$), and the lateral area (rho = −0.301, $p = 0.060$).

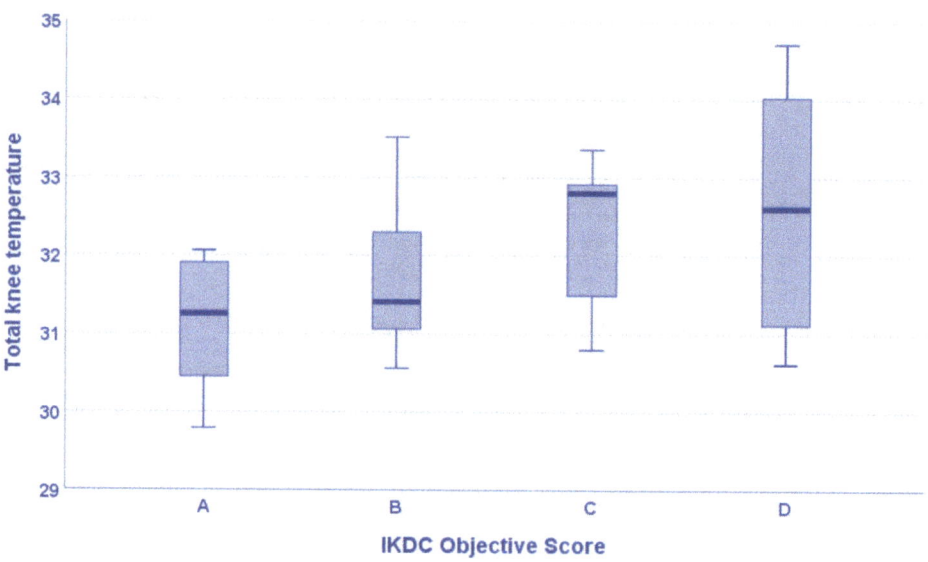

Figure 2. The mean temperature of the total knee positively correlated with the International Knee Documentation Committee (IKDC) objective score (tau = 0.294, p = 0.016). Box-and-whisker plots show median values and interquartile ranges.

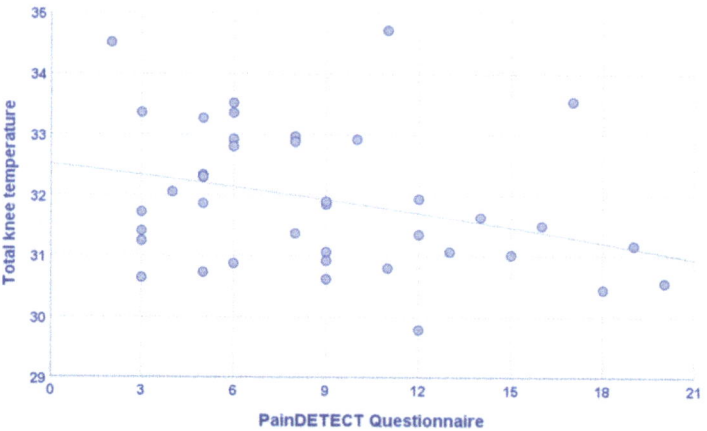

Figure 3. The mean temperature of the total knee positively correlated with the PainDETECT Questionnaire (rho = −0.319, p = 0.045).

Finally, the mean temperatures of the total knee and other sub-areas were not influenced by other factors such as side, symptom duration, Kellgren–Lawrence grade, previous surgery, and smoke.

4. Discussion

The main finding of this study is that the skin temperature of knees affected by OA is influenced by demographic and clinical characteristics of patients, including age, sex, BMI, and objective and subjective scores. In particular, higher joint temperatures were found in younger male patients with higher BMI and worst objective knee scores, while lower temperatures were found in patients affected by neuropathic pain.

The detection of knee temperature through infrared thermography can be useful for better profiling patients with different knee OA patterns. Over the years, the use of infrared thermography has gained a growing interest in the clinical research to evaluate musculoskeletal disorders, quantifying the skin temperature in order to better characterize the properties and course of a specific disease [15–17]. The study of joint temperature could potentially improve the diagnosis and therapy of orthopedic pathologies, including knee diseases such as OA [18,19]. A recent systematic review of the literature underlined the correlation between surface skin temperature and joints' inflammatory and degenerative diseases, including rheumatic pathologies and OA [20]. In particular, a correlation was shown between thermal findings and diseases' presence and stage, as well as the clinical assessment of disease activity and response to treatment, supporting infrared thermography's role in the study and management of rheumatic diseases and OA. Nevertheless, evidence on infrared thermography application for knee OA is still limited, especially on elucidating demographic and clinical characteristics that could influence the temperature of the knee in patients affected by symptomatic OA. The current study demonstrated that different factors could influence the skin temperature of symptomatic OA knees.

Age showed a negative correlation with the skin temperature of the knee, with younger patients having higher temperatures compared to older patients. The lower temperature of the knees of elderly patients is ascribable to the decrease in body temperature with aging, probably due to a reduction in basal metabolic rate and a lower muscle component compared to the younger population [21–23]. Moreover, a reduction in the overall skin temperature with aging has been justified by the reduction in core temperature in older adults due to a reduction in metabolic processes and to an alteration in the heat dissipation through the skin [22,24,25]. This was reported in healthy subjects by Ferreira et al., who found that young subjects' limbs' temperature was higher compared to the elderly subjects' limbs [26]. The current study confirmed the difference of temperature based on age also for knees affected by symptomatic OA, with lower skin temperatures in older patients considering both the overall knee temperature and most sub-areas. In fact, a further sub-analysis confirmed this correlation for all sub-regions but the region above the patellar bone.

The analysis of knee sub-regions is important when investigating knee OA thermographic patterns. Different temperatures have been detected among the different knee areas, with the area corresponding to the patella reporting the coldest temperature while the medial and suprapatellar areas reporting the highest temperatures. The patella area of the investigated knee OA patients showed a distinct thermal pattern compared to the other areas. In fact, its skin temperature was colder than all other areas of the knee, as previously reported in the literature also in healthy subjects. A description of the thermal image of the normal knee was previously given by several authors who described the thermographic image of a normal knee to be characterized by symmetry in the image of the two knees with an isothermal oval area corresponding to the patella [27,28]. The lower skin temperature of the patellar area could be explained by the fact that the skin tends to be colder above tendons and bones than above muscles [29,30]. Accordingly, the patella represents the coldest area for knee OA patients, and this could be probably linked to the fact that this area of the knee is the furthest from the intra-articular synovium due to the interposition of the patellar bone. In fact, the skin temperature of the knee could reflect the joint inflammatory process, characterized by an increased vascularization of the synovial membrane, which could be easily detected in areas without underlying bone [31].

Other aspects that influenced the skin temperature of the knee OA patients studied were sex and BMI. Neves et al. evaluated the influence of gender and body fat on temperature. They discovered that women exhibit lower values of surface temperature than man on the trunk and upper and lower limbs [32]. The literature data showed that women differ from men in thermal responses to exogenous heat load and heat loss, as well as to endogenous heat load during exercise, because they usually have a larger ratio of body surface to body mass, a greater subcutaneous fat content, and lower exercise capacity. Perhaps also a lower blood volume in women than in men may limit their heat exchange [33]. Moreover, men have a significantly higher muscle mass and lower body fat percentage than women [34]. Finally, this can be also explained by the fact that women have a lower metabolic rate than men [35]. Accordingly, the data emerged from the current study showed that men have higher knee skin temperature than women.

More controversial findings have been found regarding BMI. Higher temperatures were detected for all areas of the knee in patients with higher BMI. This finding is not in line compared to what has been reported in the literature for the overall temperature in obese subjects. In fact, subjects with increased body fat percentage showed lower temperatures of the lower limbs compared to normal-weight individuals [32]. This discrepancy could be explained by the increased inflammatory component that characterized knees of overweight or obese patients who are also affected by OA, probably resulting in an increase of the skin temperature at the OA knee level [36]. In fact, it has been demonstrated that obesity is associated with a chronic inflammatory environment at joint level, which can increase biomarkers of synovial inflammation [37–41]. The obesity-related dyslipidemia can also contribute to OA pathogenesis and increase of inflammation by an increasing matrix metalloproteinases production in joint tissues [42]. Moreover, obese patients present a higher mechanical loading on their joints, resulting in an altered activation of multiple inflammatory pathways, such as interleukin 1-beta (IL-1β) and tumor necrosis factor-alpha (TNF-α) release, chondrocyte apoptosis induction, synovial inflammation, and subchondral bone dysfunction, all contributing to OA [43]. Future studies should investigate the correlation between the skin temperature of the knee and the inflammatory biomarker profile of the affected joint and analyze these findings in relation to the clinical status of the patients.

The clinical evaluation of the knee OA joints in this series showed a significant positive correlation between the skin temperature and the IKDC objective score. This score evaluates objective features of the knee including joint effusion [44]. The current study demonstrated that OA knees with a worse objective clinical status are characterized by a higher temperature, probably related to a high inflammatory component of the joint, with consequent high functional limitations [45]. This finding was similar to a previous study which showed a correlation between higher skin temperature of the knee and worst Western Ontario and McMaster Universities Osteoarthritis (WOMAC) stiffness and function scores [46]. Conversely, the subjective scores analyzed in this case series did not correlate with the skin temperature of the evaluated knee, and the VAS pain score actually showed a negative correlation.

The controversial findings with respect to the pain perception and temperature can be explained by another result of this study, where the pain experience was investigated also in terms of another aspect, the neuropathic pain component. This was investigated with the painDETECT questionnaire, a score evaluating the contribution of neuropathic pain in the pain perceived by the patient [47,48]. A significant contribution of neuropathic pain is present in 23% of patients with knee or hip OA, with a typical symptomatologic pattern with burning pain, shooting pain or lancinating pain, tactile allodynia, and pain patterns [47,49]. Patients with a neuropathic pain showed a lower skin temperature of the knee at medial area compared with patients without neuropathic pain. A possible explanation for this result is that the pain in patients with neuropathic pain is not related to a significant inflammatory component, while it could be due to a central sensitization and an impaired pain modulation [50]. This hypothesis is confirmed by a study conducted by Ohtori S. et al., who found a tendency for negative correlation between the painDETECT score and the amount of joint fluid, with less joint fluid in patients with neuropathic pain [51]. Therefore, the evaluation of patients with symptomatic knee OA but with a "low" temperature should always be investigated for the presence of neuropathic pain, although future targeted studies are needed to better elucidate this aspect.

This study has some limitations. First of all, the sample size could limit the statistical power to better investigate correlations among sub-groups. Therefore, while this is one of the largest studies on symptomatic knee OA patients, future studies with larger populations should confirm the correlation found in the current study. Second, knees were evaluated with an anterior view alone, while further information could be obtained through lateral and posterior thermal acquisitions. Third, a control group of non-symptomatic knee OA patients or non-OA knee patients could have helped understanding the role of thermography in detecting changes of the temperature related to the severity or the presence of OA disease. Another possible weakness is that the evaluation of the neuropathic pain was performed based only on the PainDETECT questionnaire rather than on specific clinical and instrumental exams. Future studies should better investigate the influence of the neuropathic pain component on skin temperature of OA knees. Moreover, the thermographic evaluation of the knee skin temperature could be influenced by the time of the day chosen, and further studies should investigate the behavior of the knee skin temperature during the daytime. Additionally, future studies will have to better characterize the temperature differences of the knee affected by symptomatic knee OA compared to the healthy contralateral one. Finally, the method of thermographic image acquisition and analysis was based on the previous literature, but no method has been described as the gold standard in this field. It is possible that different settings, different lenses, and different devices could be more suitable for such evaluations in the clinical practice. Therefore, future studies should help standardize more the use of thermography for the evaluation of patients with knee OA in order to confirm its potential in identifying different disease patterns both in the research setting and in the clinical practice. This could have the potential to better address patients with knee OA, improving diagnosis, management, and treatment, with a possible socioeconomic and healthcare impact in the future.

5. Conclusions

This study demonstrated that the skin temperature of OA symptomatic knees evaluated with infrared thermography is influenced by demographic and clinical characteristics of patients, including age, sex, BMI, and objective and subjective scores. Higher joint temperatures were found in younger male patients with higher BMI and worst objective knee scores, while lower temperatures were found in patients affected by neuropathic pain.

Author Contributions: Conceptualization, G.F.; methodology, L.D.M., A.B. and L.A. (Lucia Angelelli); data curation, L.D.M.; writing—original draft preparation, L.D.M., A.B. and L.A. (Luca Andriolo); writing—review and editing, A.D.M. and G.F.; supervision. S.Z. and G.F. All authors have read and agreed to the published version of the manuscript.

Funding: This research was funded by the Italian Ministry of Health—5 × 1000 Anno 2019, Redditi 2018 "Termografia a infrarossi per lo studio di patologie infiammatorie e degenerative articolari".

Institutional Review Board Statement: The study was conducted in accordance with the Declaration of Helsinki and approved by the Institutional Ethics Committee of IRCCS Istituto Ortopedico Rizzoli, Bologna, Italy (Prot. n. 0017413).

Informed Consent Statement: Informed consent was obtained from all subjects involved in the study.

Data Availability Statement: Not applicable.

Acknowledgments: The authors give special thanks to Elettra Pignotti for her contribution to the statistical analysis.

Conflicts of Interest: S.Z. reports non-financial support from personal fees from I + SRL and grants from Fidia Farmaceutici SPA, Cartiheal Ltd., IGEA clinical biophysics, BIOMET, and Kensey Nash, outside the submitted work. The funders had no role in the design of the study; in the collection, analyses, or interpretation of the data; in the writing of the manuscript; or in the decision to publish the results. The other authors declare no conflict of interest.

References

1. Pereira, D.; Peleteiro, B.; Araújo, J.; Branco, J.; Santos, R.A.; Ramos, E. The effect of osteoarthritis definition on prevalence and incidence estimates: A systematic review. *Osteoarthr. Cartil.* **2011**, *19*, 1270–1285. [CrossRef] [PubMed]
2. Bierma-Zeinstra, S.M.; Verhagen, A.P. Osteoarthritis subpopulations and implications for clinical trial design. *Arthritis Res. Ther.* **2011**, *13*, 213. [CrossRef] [PubMed]
3. Felson, D.T. Identifying different osteoarthritis phenotypes through epidemiology. *Osteoarthr. Cartil.* **2010**, *18*, 601–604. [CrossRef]
4. Deveza, L.A.; Nelson, A.E.; Loeser, R.F. Phenotypes of osteoarthritis: Current state and future implications. *Clin. Exp. Rheumatol.* **2019**, *37*, 64–72.
5. De Girolamo, L.; Kon, E.; Filardo, G.; Marmotti, A.G.; Soler, F.; Peretti, G.M.; Vannini, F.; Madry, H.; Chubinskaya, S. Regenerative approaches for the treatment of early OA. *Knee Surg. Sport. Traumatol. Arthrosc.* **2016**, *24*, 1826–1835. [CrossRef] [PubMed]
6. Previtali, D.; Andriolo, L.; Frattura, G.D.L.; Boffa, A.; Candrian, C.; Zaffagnini, S.; Filardo, G. Pain Trajectories in Knee Osteoarthritis—A Systematic Review and Best Evidence Synthesis on Pain Predictors. *J. Clin. Med.* **2020**, *9*, 2828. [CrossRef] [PubMed]
7. Castrogiovanni, P.; Di Rosa, M.; Ravalli, S.; Castorina, A.; Guglielmino, C.; Imbesi, R.; Vecchio, M.; Drago, F.; Szychlinska, M.A.; Musumeci, G. Moderate Physical Activity as a Prevention Method for Knee Osteoarthritis and the Role of Synoviocytes as Biological Key. *Int. J. Mol. Sci.* **2019**, *20*, 511. [CrossRef]
8. Fokam, D.; Lehmann, C. Clinical assessment of arthritic knee pain by infrared thermography. *J. Basic Clin. Physiol. Pharmacol.* **2018**, *30*, 20170218. [CrossRef]
9. Ren, G.; Lutz, I.; Railton, P.; Wiley, J.P.; McAllister, J.; Powell, J.; Krawetz, R.J. Serum and synovial fluid cytokine profiling in hip osteoarthritis: Distinct from knee osteoarthritis and correlated with pain. *BMC Musculoskelet. Disord.* **2018**, *19*, 129. [CrossRef]
10. Siqueira, M.B.P.; Frangiamore, S.; Klika, A.K.; Gajewski, N.; Barsoum, W.K.; Higuera, C.A. Comparison of Synovial Fluid Cytokine Levels between Traumatic Knee Injury and End-Stage Osteoarthritis. *J. Knee Surg.* **2017**, *30*, 128–133. [CrossRef]
11. Salisbury, R.S.; Parr, G.; De Silva, M.; Hazleman, B.L.; Page-Thomas, D.P. Heat distribution over normal and abnormal joints: Thermal pattern and quantification. *Ann. Rheum. Dis.* **1983**, *42*, 494–499. [CrossRef] [PubMed]
12. Tattersall, G.J. Infrared thermography: A non-invasive window into thermal physiology. *Comp. Biochem. Physiol. Part A Mol. Integr. Physiol.* **2016**, *202*, 78–98. [CrossRef] [PubMed]
13. Marins, J.C.B.; Moreira, D.G.; Cano, S.P.; Quintana, M.S.; Soares, D.D.; de Andrade Fernandes, A.; Da Silva, F.S.; Costa, C.M.A.; dos Santos Amorim, P.R. Time required to stabilize thermographic images at rest. *Infrared Phys. Technol.* **2014**, *65*, 30–35. [CrossRef]
14. Denoble, A.E.; Hall, N.; Pieper, C.F.; Kraus, V.B. Patellar Skin Surface Temperature by Thermography Reflects Knee Osteoarthritis Severity. *Clin. Med. Insights Arthritis Musculoskelet. Disord.* **2010**, *3*, 69–75. [CrossRef] [PubMed]
15. Moreira, D.G.; Costello, J.T.; Brito, C.J.; Adamczyk, J.G.; Ammer, K.; Bach, A.J.; Costa, C.M.; Eglin, C.; Fernandes, A.A.; Fernández-Cuevas, I.; et al. Thermographic imaging in sports and exercise medicine: A Delphi study and consensus statement on the measurement of human skin temperature. *J. Therm. Biol.* **2017**, *69*, 155–162. [CrossRef]
16. Hildebrandt, C.; Raschner, C.; Ammer, K. An Overview of Recent Application of Medical Infrared Thermography in Sports Medicine in Austria. *Sensors* **2010**, *10*, 4700–4715. [CrossRef] [PubMed]
17. Varjú, G.; Pieper, C.F.; Renner, J.B.; Kraus, V.B. Assessment of hand osteoarthritis: Correlation between thermographic and radiographic methods. *Rheumatology* **2004**, *43*, 915–919. [CrossRef]
18. Seixas, A.; Ammer, K. Systematic Reviews and Meta-analysis about Infrared Thermography in Musculoskeletal Research: Trends and critical appraisal. *Thermol. Int.* **2022**, *32*, 65–73.
19. Ammer, K. Temperature of the human knee-a review. *Thermol. Int.* **2012**, *22*, 137–151.
20. Schiavon, G.; Capone, G.; Frize, M.; Zaffagnini, S.; Candrian, C.; Filardo, G. Infrared Thermography for the Evaluation of Inflammatory and Degenerative Joint Diseases: A Systematic Review. *Cartilage* **2021**, *13*, 1790S–1801S. [CrossRef]
21. Güneş, Ü.Y.; Zaybak, A. Does the body temperature change in older people? *J. Clin. Nurs.* **2008**, *17*, 2284–2287. [CrossRef] [PubMed]
22. Júnior, P.R.H.; Sardeli, A.V. The Effect of Aging on Body Temperature: A Systematic Review and Meta- Analysis. *Curr. Aging Sci.* **2021**, *14*, 191–200. [CrossRef] [PubMed]
23. Lu, S.-H.; Leasure, A.-R.; Dai, Y.-T. A systematic review of body temperature variations in older people. *J. Clin. Nurs.* **2010**, *19*, 4–16. [CrossRef]
24. Blatteis, C.M. Age-Dependent Changes in Temperature Regulation–A Mini Review. *Gerontology* **2012**, *58*, 289–295. [CrossRef]
25. Petrofsky, J.S.; Lohman, E., III; Suh, H.J.; Garcia, J.; Anders, A.; Sutterfield, C.; Khandge, C. The effect of aging on conductive heat exchange in the skin at two environmental temperatures. *Med. Sci. Monit.* **2006**, *12*, CR400–CR408. [PubMed]
26. Ferreira, J.J.A.; Mendonça, L.C.S.; Nunes, L.A.O.; Andrade Filho, A.C.C.; Rebelatto, J.R.; Salvini, T.F. Exercise-Associated Thermographic Changes in Young and Elderly Subjects. *Ann. Biomed. Eng.* **2008**, *36*, 1420–1427. [CrossRef] [PubMed]
27. Vujcic, M.; Nedeljkovic, R. Thermography in the detection and follow up of chondromalacia patellae. *Ann. Rheum. Dis.* **1991**, *50*, 921–925. [CrossRef]
28. Collins, A.J.; Ring, E.F.; Cosh, J.A.; Bacon, P.A. Quantitation of thermography in arthritis using multi-isothermal analysis. I. The thermographic index. *Ann. Rheum. Dis.* **1974**, *33*, 113–115. [CrossRef]
29. Ramirez-GarciaLuna, J.L.; Bartlett, R.; Arriaga-Caballero, J.E.; Fraser, R.D.J.; Saiko, G. Infrared Thermography in Wound Care, Surgery, and Sports Medicine: A Review. *Front. Physiol.* **2022**, *13*, 838528. [CrossRef]

30. Kanitakis, J. Anatomy, histology and immunohistochemistry of normal human skin. *Eur. J. Dermatol.* **2002**, *12*, 390–399.
31. Mathiessen, A.; Conaghan, P.G. Synovitis in osteoarthritis: Current understanding with therapeutic implications. *Arthritis Res. Ther.* **2017**, *19*, 18. [CrossRef] [PubMed]
32. Neves, E.B.; Salamunes, A.C.C.; de Oliveira, R.M.; Stadnik, A.M.W. Effect of body fat and gender on body temperature distribution. *J. Therm. Biol.* **2017**, *70*, 1–8. [CrossRef] [PubMed]
33. Kaciuba-Uscilko, H.; Grucza, R. Gender differences in thermoregulation. *Curr. Opin. Clin. Nutr. Metab. Care* **2001**, *4*, 533–536. [CrossRef] [PubMed]
34. Chudecka, M.; Lubkowska, A. Thermal maps of young women and men. *Infrared Phys. Technol.* **2015**, *69*, 81–87. [CrossRef]
35. Arciero, P.J.; Goran, M.I.; Poehlman, E.T. Resting metabolic rate is lower in women than in men. *J. Appl. Physiol.* **1993**, *75*, 2514–2520. [CrossRef] [PubMed]
36. Wang, C.; Zhu, Y.; Liu, Z.; Long, H.; Ruan, Z.; Zhao, S. Causal associations of obesity related anthropometric indicators and body compositions with knee and hip arthritis: A large-scale genetic correlation study. *Front. Endocrinol.* **2022**, *13*, 1011896. [CrossRef]
37. Boffa, A.; Merli, G.; Andriolo, L.; Lattermann, C.; Salzmann, G.M.; Filardo, G. Synovial Fluid Biomarkers in Knee Osteoarthritis: A Systematic Review and Quantitative Evaluation Using BIPEDs Criteria. *Cartilage* **2021**, *13*, 82S–103S. [CrossRef]
38. Kanthawang, T.; Bodden, J.; Joseph, G.B.; Lane, N.E.; Nevitt, M.; McCulloch, C.E.; Link, T.M. Obese and overweight individuals have greater knee synovial inflammation and associated structural and cartilage compositional degeneration: Data from the osteoarthritis initiative. *Skelet. Radiol.* **2021**, *50*, 217–229. [CrossRef]
39. Hung, A.; Sayre, E.C.; Guermazi, A.; Esdaile, J.M.; Kopec, J.A.; Thorne, A.; Singer, J.; Wong, H.; Nicolaou, S.; Cibere, J. Association of Body Mass Index with Incidence and Progression of Knee Effusion on Magnetic Resonance Imaging and on Knee Examination. *Arthritis Care Res.* **2016**, *68*, 511–516. [CrossRef]
40. Distel, E.; Cadoudal, T.; Durant, S.; Poignard, A.; Chevalier, X.; Benelli, C. The infrapatellar fat pad in knee osteoarthritis: An important source of interleukin-6 and its soluble receptor. *Arthritis Rheum.* **2009**, *60*, 3374–3377. [CrossRef]
41. Fujisaka, S.; Usui, I.; Ikutani, M.; Aminuddin, A.; Takikawa, A.; Tsuneyama, K.; Mahmood, A.; Goda, N.; Nagai, Y.; Takatsu, K.; et al. Adipose tissue hypoxia induces inflammatory M1 polarity of macrophages in an HIF-1α-dependent and HIF-1α-independent manner in obese mice. *Diabetologia* **2013**, *56*, 1403–1412. [CrossRef] [PubMed]
42. Thijssen, E.; van Caam, A.; Van Der Kraan, P.M. Obesity and osteoarthritis, more than just wear and tear: Pivotal roles for inflamed adipose tissue and dyslipidaemia in obesity-induced osteoarthritis. *Rheumatology* **2015**, *54*, 588–600. [CrossRef]
43. Fang, T.; Zhou, X.; Jin, M.; Nie, J.; Li, X. Molecular mechanisms of mechanical load-induced osteoarthritis. *Int. Orthop.* **2021**, *45*, 1125–1136. [CrossRef] [PubMed]
44. Irrgang, J.J.; Ho, H.; Harner, C.D.; Fu, F.H. Use of the International Knee Documentation Committee guidelines to assess outcome following anterior cruciate ligament reconstruction. *Knee Surg. Sports Traumatol. Arthrosc.* **1998**, *6*, 107–114. [CrossRef] [PubMed]
45. Mendieta, E.D.M.; Ibáñez, T.C.; Jaeger, J.U.; Hernán, G.B.; Mola, E.M. Clinical and ultrasonographic findings related to knee pain in osteoarthritis. *Osteoarthr. Cartil.* **2006**, *14*, 540–544. [CrossRef]
46. Ammer, K.; Engelbert, B.; Hamerle, S.; Kern, E.; Solar, S.; Kuchar, K. Correlation between the WOMAC index and temperature in patients with knee pain. *Eur. J. Thermol.* **1998**, *8*, 50–56.
47. Moss, P.; Benson, H.A.E.; Will, R.; Wright, A. Patients with Knee Osteoarthritis Who Score Highly on the PainDETECT Questionnaire Present with Multimodality Hyperalgesia, Increased Pain, and Impaired Physical Function. *Clin. J. Pain* **2018**, *34*, 15–21. [CrossRef]
48. Freynhagen, R.; Baron, R.; Gockel, U.; Tölle, T.R. pain*DETECT*: A new screening questionnaire to identify neuropathic components in patients with back pain. *Curr. Med. Res. Opin.* **2006**, *22*, 1911–1920. [CrossRef]
49. French, H.P.; Smart, K.M.; Doyle, F. Prevalence of neuropathic pain in knee or hip osteoarthritis: A systematic review and meta-analysis. *Semin. Arthritis Rheum.* **2017**, *47*, 1–8. [CrossRef]
50. Moreton, B.J.; Tew, V.; das Nair, R.; Wheeler, M.; Walsh, D.A.; Lincoln, N.B. Pain Phenotype in Patients with Knee Osteoarthritis: Classification and Measurement Properties of painDETECT and Self-Report Leeds Assessment of Neuropathic Symptoms and Signs Scale in a Cross-Sectional Study. *Arthritis Care Res.* **2015**, *67*, 519–528. [CrossRef]
51. Ohtori, S.; Orita, S.; Yamashita, M.; Ishikawa, T.; Ito, T.; Shigemura, T.; Nishiyama, H.; Konno, S.; Ohta, H.; Takaso, M.; et al. Existence of a Neuropathic Pain Component in Patients with Osteoarthritis of the Knee. *Yonsei Med. J.* **2012**, *53*, 801–805. [CrossRef] [PubMed]

Disclaimer/Publisher's Note: The statements, opinions and data contained in all publications are solely those of the individual author(s) and contributor(s) and not of MDPI and/or the editor(s). MDPI and/or the editor(s) disclaim responsibility for any injury to people or property resulting from any ideas, methods, instructions or products referred to in the content.

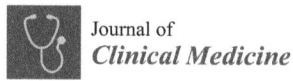

Article

Femoral Anteversion in Total Hip Arthroplasty: Retrospective Comparison of Short- and Straight-Stem Models Using CT Scans

Sebastian Martin Klim [1,†], Patrick Reinbacher [2,†], Maria Anna Smolle [1,*], Andrzej Hecker [2], Michael Maier [1], Joerg Friesenbichler [1], Andreas Leithner [1], Lukas Leitner [1], Alexander Draschl [1], Jan Lewis [1], Kevin Brunnader [1] and Werner Maurer-Ertl [1]

[1] Department of Orthopaedics & Traumatology, Medical University of Graz, Augenbruggerplatz 5, 8036 Graz, Austria
[2] Division of Plastic, Aesthetic and Reconstructive Surgery, Department of Surgery, Medical University of Graz, Auenbruggerplatz 5, 8036 Graz, Austria
* Correspondence: maria.smolle@medunigraz.at
† These authors contributed equally to this work.

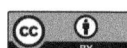

Abstract: Data on reconstruction of the femoral anteversion (FA) and the center of rotation after total hip arthroplasty (THA) are rare. We aimed to answer whether a short-stem fixation enables improved anatomical reconstruction of the FA compared to a straight-stem. Methods: One hundred and thirty patients who underwent short- (n = 89, group A, prospective) or straight-stem THA (n = 41, group B, retrospective) were included. CT scans of the hip, knee, and ankle were performed pre- and postoperatively in group A and in group B during the last follow-up. Femoral torsion was determined using three-dimensional models. Results: The mean preoperative FA was $22.4° \pm 11.0°$, and the mean postoperative FA was $23.4° \pm 10.1°$. The relative difference was $-0.8° \pm 8°$, and the absolute difference was $6.4° \pm 4.9°$. Gender analysis revealed significant differences in preoperative FA between female (f) and male (m) patients ($28.1° \pm 11.2°$ (f) vs. $18.4° \pm 8.3°$ (m); $p > 0.001$) as well as in postoperative FA ($26.7° \pm 23.5°$ (f) vs. $21.0° \pm 9.7°$ (m); $p < 0.007$) in group A. Postoperative FA was higher in group A (mean $6.8°$; $23.9° \pm 10.1°$ (f) vs. $16.6° \pm 8.6°$ (m); $p < 0.001$). Conclusions: The study's findings suggest that short-stem THA leads to improved anatomical FA reconstruction; however, a substantial postoperative gender-related FA difference was detectable, which may warrant consideration by surgeons when determining the final stem anteversion. It should be noted that the impact of the postoperative gender-related FA difference on clinical outcomes is not entirely clear, and further research is warranted to elucidate this relationship.

Keywords: CT-scan; femoral anteversion; hip geometry reconstruction; short-stem; total hip arthroplasty

1. Introduction

Total hip arthroplasty (THA) is considered to be the most successful orthopedic surgery of the 20th century, and it significantly impacts healthcare economics [1]. To achieve optimal results, the femoral stem fixation should satisfy several requirements, including ease of handling during surgery, preservation of bone stock and soft tissue, and stable long-term fixation [2–4]. Not only should the surface texture, geometric configuration, and choice of implant material be carefully considered, but the appropriate operative approach is also necessary in order to achieve the best possible results [5]. Furthermore, reconstructing the individual's hip geometry is crucial in order to achieve optimal force distribution and range of motion while minimizing the risk of aseptic loosening, component wear, and dislocation [6–8]. This is emphasized as an important consideration in the literature [9–11]. The accurate performance of a THA depends on several criteria that are not considered in a comprehensive manner in conventional THA planning. As Habor et al. suggested in their work, a patient-specific morphofunctional planning of the target zone for implants could provide a solution [12]. Another approach to reach as accurate of a result as possible in THA could be the implementation of image-based robotic assistance throughout the implantation process. Surgeons could make use of haptically controlled robotic arms to achieve more precise results in THA [13].

One of the critical goals of hip anatomy reconstruction during THA is to restore the femoral torsion (ante- or retroversion of the femoral neck) and, consecutively, the center of rotation of the femoral head [14,15]. Improper alignment of component torsion, whether excessive ante- or retrotorsion, can result in impingement and hip instability, leading to complications such as dislocation, component wear, and limited range of motion [16–18]. Moreover, failing to restore the angle of femoral anteversion (FA) to 15–20° or to adapt it to the native femoral anteversion or cup anteversion [19–21] is associated with a higher risk of dislocation, edge loading, squeaking, hip instability, and limited range of motion [14,17,22]. Therefore, correct alignment of the FA is crucial when trying to achieve an impingement-free range of motion and prevent common complications associated with THA. This can be accomplished by a patient-specific preoperative 3D simulation of range of motion (ROM), flexion, and internal rotation (IR) angle to establish the correct implantation zone of the implant components [23]. Another approach to achieve even better results with THA that are more similar to the naturally occurring physiology would be a patient-specific instrument system that can be individually manufactured for each configuration of the femur and acetabulum [24]. Furthermore, the correct choice of material and implantation site may be crucial when considering a patient's body mass index (BMI) or the implementation of intraoperational fluoroscopy for the success of THA [25,26].

Moreover, it is known that stem design plays a critical role in determining the stem's final position and, as a result, its anteversion [27]. Over the course of time, various stem and cup designs were developed to achieve precise hip joint reconstruction and to extend the lifetime of hip implants [27,28]. However, due to the continuous development of new implant designs for cementless short-stem THA as well as its increased use and related research, this method is more prominent [29–31]. Although short-stem designs gained popularity due to their ability to preserve proximal femoral bone stock and provide more natural loading in the proximal femur than straight-stems [32–36], only a limited number of studies have directly compared the two designs in terms of FA reconstruction [27,37,38], with short-stems showing higher FA restoration accuracy than straight-stems [38]. However, more data is needed to verify the superiority of short-stem designs in FA reconstruction and their clinical relevance, considering that various stem designs may affect the parameters of hip geometry reconstruction differently. Furthermore, it is important to note that, to date, no study has investigated the influence of the novel, metaphyseal-anchoring, calcar-guided, neck-sparing short-stem designs (ANA.NOVA® Alpha Schaft® Proxy, ImplanTec GmbH, Moedling, Austria) on FA restoration compared to a conventional straight-stem.

Therefore, our study aimed to (1) investigate if a novel calcar-guided short-stem design enables an improved anatomical reconstruction of FA compared to a straight-stem design and (2) whether this effect results in a difference in postoperative clinical and patient-reported outcome measures. We hypothesized that the short-stem designs would restore FA more accurately and result in better outcome measures.

2. Materials and Methods

The current study, categorized as level III evidence, involved a retrospective comparative analysis of 130 prospectively included unilateral THA patients who received either a short- or straight-stem design between 2005 and 2017 at a single institution. The anterolateral approach to the hip [39], as recently mentioned by Reinbacher et al. [40], was performed as the standard procedure in both groups, and all patients were operated on for primary hip osteoarthritis. Our research group previously described the characteristics of both stem designs [14]. The current study was approved by the Ethics Committee of the Medical University of Graz, Austria (protocol code 28-152 ex 15/16).

In group A, 89 patients underwent unilateral short-stem THA performed by a single surgeon at a single institution between 2016 to 2017. In this group, all patients were implanted with a cementless short-stem design (ANA.NOVA® Alpha Schaft® Proxy, ImplanTec GmbH, Moedling, Austria) that features epi-metaphyseal fixation combined with a press-fit cup (ANA.NOVA® Alpha Pfanne, ImplanTec GmbH, Moedling, Austria). The short-stem is available in twelve sizes, ranging from zero to eleven, and is designed for neck-shaft angles ranging from 125° to 140°. No alternative designs were provided regarding offset and collar. Pre- and postoperatively, each patient underwent low-dose rotational computed tomography (CT) imaging of the hip, knee, and ankle.

In group B, 41 THA patients received a collarless, cementless straight-stem design with a meta-diaphyseal fixation combined with a press-fit cup (Corail® stem and Pinnacle® cup DePuy Synthes, West Chester, PA, USA) at our department between 2005 and 2012. These patients were selected at random from our follow-up registry to serve as a comparison group, with the condition that postoperative CT scans would be available. The straight-stem design used in this group is available in 13 different sizes with two collar options (with and without) and neck-shaft angle variations (standard or high offset 135°, coxa vara 125°). Complete postoperative rotational CT scans of the hip, knee, and ankle were obtained in this group, but no preoperative CT scans were available. The study excluded pregnant patients, patients under custodianship, or patients with a confirmed periprosthetic joint infection from both groups (A and B).

To assess FA, 3D measurements were performed using the Hectec mediCAD hip 3D® software (mediCAD Hectec GmbH, Altdorf, Germany). The CT scan images were converted into three-dimensional digital models during this process. The FA was measured preoperatively (only in group A) and postoperatively (in both groups) using the axial oblique technique of Jarrett et al. [41]. Known for its particularly high intra- and interobserver agreement, this measurement technique uses oblique femoral slices with a slice distance and thickness of 5mm [42]. To measure femoral torsion, the angle between a proximal line (aligned with the femoral neck) and a distal femoral line (which is tangential to the posterior condyles on a single axial image with maximum anterior-posterior expansion) is used (Figure 1). Preoperative planning in terms of determining the optimal implant size and position was performed on standard anterior-posterior x-rays of the hip using the mediCAD® Classic Hip 2D software (Hectec GmbH, Altdorf, Germany) as described in a previously published study [43].

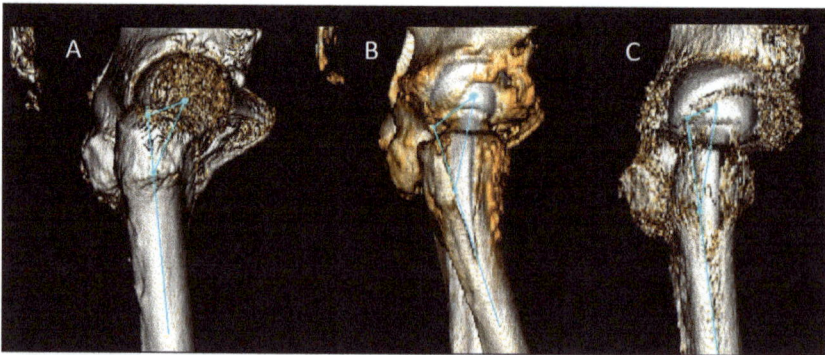

Figure 1. Preoperative and postoperative CT measurement method. 3D measurements obtained with mediCAD hip 3D software, showing the proximal femoral long axis defined by two points and the femoral anteversion angle formed between a perpendicular line through the proximal femoral long axis and the femoral head, and a line connecting the femoral condyles. (**A**): preoperative condition. (**B**): postoperative condition with short stem. (**C**): postoperative condition with straight stem.

3D measurements with mediCAD hip 3D. The femoral long axis is defined by two points in the proximal femur: (1) inferior border of the lesser trochanter; (2) at a point approximately 6 cm distal in the femoral shaft. The angle between the perpendicular line between the proximal femoral long axis and the femoral head and the line between the formal condyles is the femoral anteversion.

The surgeon aimed for a cup inclination between 30° and 50°, a cup anteversion of 10° to 20°, and a stable press-fit fixation. The femoral neck osteotomy for the two implants was performed at different resection levels according to the manufacturer's recommendations. This generally resulted in a more distal resection height of the femoral neck in group B and a more proximal, bone-preserving resection height in group A. When broaching the femur, the biggest possible stem size was used to attain secure fixation aiming for 15° of FA. In both groups, all stems were combined with cementless cups and ceramic-on-ceramic bearings. Demographic data (age at the time of surgery, gender, and body mass index (BMI)) were recorded. In addition, Western Ontario and McMaster Universities Osteoarthritis Index (WOMAC) scores as well as Harris Hip Scores (HHS) were obtained in the follow-up examinations one year postoperatively from all included patients [44,45].

To detect significant differences, paired and unpaired t-tests were used. The Mann–Whitney U test was performed if parametric distribution was not given. Regression analysis was used to detect differences in continuous variables. An alpha level <0.05 was considered significant. All evaluations were done with the statistical program Stata/MP 13.0 (StataCorp, College Station, TX, USA).

3. Results

The demographic data and results are shown in Table 1. The mean age at the time of surgery was 60.4 ± 7.5 years in group A and 63.9 ± 10.3 in group B (p = 0.03). The mean BMI was 28.5 ± 4.8 (group A) and 28.2 ± 4.5 (group B, p > 0.05). In group A, the preoperative FA was 22.4° ± 11.0°, and the postoperative FA was 23.4° ± 10.1°. The relative difference was −0.8° ± 8°, and the absolute difference was 6.4° ± 4.9°. There was no difference regarding the absolute FA change angle from pre- to postoperative phases in group A (7.6° ± 5.7° (f) vs. 5.6° ± 4.0° (m); p = 0.057). Furthermore, there was no significant correlation between the change of angle in pre- to postoperative FA and patient age (p = 0.657) or body mass index (p = 0.307) in this group. When comparing both groups, the postoperative FA was found to be higher in group A than in group B (mean 6.8°; 23.9° ± 10.1° (A) vs. 16.6° ± 8.6° (B); p < 0.001; Figure 1).

Table 1. Demographic and clinical data.

		Proxy (n = 89) N; %	Corail (n = 41) N; %	p-Value
Gender	Male	51 (57.3)	25 (61.0)	0.693
	Female	38 (42.7)	16 (39.0)	
Hip Type	Coxa vara (CCD < 125°)	47 (52.8)	0 (0.0)	**<0.001**
	Coxa norma (CCD 125–134.9°)	33 (37.1)	0 (0.0)	
	Coxa valga (CCD ≥ 135°)	9 (10.1)	41 (100.0)	
Age at Surgery (in years; mean ± standard deviation)		60.4 ± 4.5	63.9 ± 10.3	**0.030**
BMI (mean ± standard deviation)		28.5 ± 4.8	28.2 ± 4.5	0.603
Preoperative Femoral Anteversion (mean ± standard deviation)		22.4° ± 11.0°	N/A	N/A
Postoperative Femoral Anteversion (mean ± standard deviation)		23.4° ± 10.1°	16.6° ± 1.3°	**<0.001**
HHS Score after 1 year (mean ± standard deviation)		95.8 ± 8.0	93.5 ± 10.1	0.159
WOMAC Score after 1 year (mean ± standard deviation)		10.5 ± 13.6	9.7 ± 14.4	0.758

Significant p-values are in bold text.

Fifty-one (57.3%) men were included in group A, and twenty-five (60.9%) were included in group B (p = 0.693). Gender analysis in group A revealed significant differences between women (f) and men (m) in the preoperative FA phase (28.1° ± 11.2° (f) vs.

18.4° ± 8.3° (m); $p > 0.001$) as well as in the postoperative FA phase (26.7° ± 23.5° (f) vs. 21.0° ± 9.7° (m); $p < 0.007$). No such differences were found in group B when comparing the postoperative FA (17.9° ± 9.9° (f) vs. 15.7° ± 7.6° (m); $p = 0.425$), as depicted in Table 1.

The HHS in the one-year follow-up was 95.8 ± 8 for group A and 93.5 ± 10 for group B, showing no statistically significant difference between them ($p = 0.16$). The regression analysis for group A showed no significant correlation between the absolute change of angle in the femoral anteversion from the pre- to postoperative phases and the HHS ($p = 0.50$). Furthermore, the regression analysis showed a significantly lower HHS for female patients ($p > 0.01$) and a higher HHS for patients with a higher postoperative FA ($p = 0.03$). The WOMAC score in the one-year follow-up was 10.5 for group A and 9.7 for group B and showed no significant difference between them ($p = 0.75$).

4. Discussion

In this retrospective comparative analysis, we examined whether a calcar-guided short-stem design or a conventional straight-stem design would result in better FA reconstruction after THA. We also analyzed whether both stem designs differ regarding patient-reported outcome measures. The results confirmed our hypothesis that the FA was better restored with the short-stem design, but it did not confirm superior clinical outcomes (HHS) or patient-reported outcome measures (WOMAC).

The main finding of this study was the significant difference in anatomical FA reconstruction after THA when comparing a calcar-guided short-stem design with a straight-stem design. As only 17 preoperative CT scans of the contralateral native hip were available in group B, we cannot generalize these results, but in that small number, the preoperative FA was non-significantly different from that of group A (22.4° ± 11 (A) vs. 22.6° ± 8 (B); $p > 0.05$). In a similar preoperative FA situation, the implantation of the calcar-guided short-stem design led to superior FA reconstruction accuracy. This result is in accordance with the findings of Sariali and Pascal Mousselard [38], who compared an anatomic, cementless, and proximally hydroxyapatite (HA)-coated short-stem design (SPS Evolution, Symbios SA, Yverdon-les Bains, Switzerland) to a generic straight-stem design (HARMONY, Symbios SA, Yverdon-les Bains, Switzerland) similar to the straight-stem design investigated in our study. Therefore, our findings provide evidence supporting the effectiveness of short-stem designs in achieving superior FA reconstruction compared to straight-stems while also yielding comparable clinical and patient-reported outcome measures. The results of our study emphasize the effectiveness of the short-stem design, particularly the calcar-guided design that was included in our analysis. The short-stem design aims to reconstruct the hip anatomy more accurately by following the femoral neck's calcar, thereby improving proximal fit while maintaining femoral anteversion [38,46,47].

The difference in higher FA when using a short-stem design became even more distinct in the gender-based subgroup analysis, as female patients had a significantly higher FA before surgery (28.1° ± 11.2° (f) vs. 18.4° ± 8.3° (m), group A) than their male counterparts. This observation in men was previously reported by Nakahara et al. (25.2 ± 9.8° (f) vs. 20.3 ± 9.9° (m)) and others [48–50]. Similarly, a gender-related difference in postoperative FA was only significant in group A. This also lines up with the significantly lower overall postoperative FA in group B. Therefore, optimal reconstruction of the FA seems to be particularly important in women, as the FA may play a role in the significantly higher dislocation rates of women compared to male patients (4:1) after THA [51–54].

Furthermore, Yoon et al. [55] reported that using a short-stem design increased anterior femoral tilt in the sagittal plane compared to a straight-stem design, which is associated with a higher risk of posterior impingement and anterior dislocation. On the other hand, Fischer et al. [27] reported a higher frequency of postoperative retrotorsion with a collarless straight-stem design compared with a short-stem design, which bears an increased risk of posterior dislocation. Based on current knowledge, these findings suggest that surgeons may need to aim for different femoral anteversion angles for the implanted short-stem design in women and men, indicating the importance of gender-specific considerations.

However, dislocation rates were not recorded in the current study; thus, no definitive conclusions can be drawn on this matter. Future studies are needed to investigate this hypothesis further.

However, Faizan et al. [56] discovered a bimodal distribution of anteversion angles in implanted short-stem designs and a difference between pre- and post-virtual implantation anteversion angles while investigating the ABG II monolithic stem system (Stryker Orthopaedics, Mahwah, NJ, USA). Their findings suggest that THA patients may benefit from being divided into two groups, one requiring an anteverted stem and the other requiring less or no anteversion in the stem, to achieve the correct version during FA reconstruction. As the study conducted by Faizan et al. [56] does not offer sufficient information to confirm if the bimodal distribution is related to gender, we cannot determine whether it supports our hypothesis that women may have different postoperative FA requirements than men and could benefit from a stem design with little or no anteversion. Nevertheless, we did observe a significantly higher postoperative FA among women in group A, suggesting that there may be a basis for our hypothesis.

The clinical and patient-reported outcome measures evaluated in this study did not reveal any significant differences between the two groups one year after surgery. Although the HHS suggested better results in group A ($p = 0.16$) and regression analysis revealed significantly better HHS for patients with higher postoperative FA, the WOMAC score did not favor either group ($p = 0.75$). Previous studies also reported this by comparing the postoperative HHS and WOMAC scores of short- and straight-stem THA designs [57,58]. This was to be expected, as the biggest hazards of insufficiently reconstructed hip geometry mainly develop after a longer follow-up period and are usually detected radiographically (aseptic loosening, dislocation, and wear).

Overall, the results of our investigation suggest a more anatomical reconstruction of the FA after THA when using a short-stem design. However, long-term results are needed to investigate whether this improved alignment of the FA significantly impacts the rate of serious adverse events (aseptic loosening, component wear, and dislocation), patient satisfaction, and quality of life. The significant value of this work should be emphasized, as it represents one of the largest series in which the postoperative hip geometries of a short-stem and a straight-stem design were directly compared using state-of-the-art CT scans and 3D measurement techniques. Furthermore, this is the first study to provide data on FA reconstruction using a cementless short-stem design (ANA.NOVA® Alpha Schaft® Proxy, ImplanTec GmbH, Moedling, Austria) in combination with a press-fit cup (ANA.NOVA® Alpha Pfanne, ImplanTec GmbH, Moedling, Austria).

Regarding implantation breakdown in patients with a BMI categorized as obese (class I–III), Ammarullah et al. [25] suggested that material, the texture of the surface, and the use of special coatings should be considered. In addition, they said that the implant geometry and the adaption of surgical procedures to prevent the failure of implantations in obese patients should be kept in mind [25]. In terms of materials and surgical techniques, further research is necessary.

In order to improve the accuracy regarding the as-physiological-as-possible placement of the stem in total hip arthroplasty (THA), the use of patient-specific instrumentation with laser guidance to reduce the risk of femoral anteversion should be considered. Ferretti et al. [5] demonstrated that using a positioning system enables the accurate positioning of the stem and cup. When applied, operating times are not significantly prolonged and even improve in correlation with the user's learning curve [5]. Free et al. [59] were able to determine that radiological markers can be used in the specific case of the increasingly popular direct anterior approach (DAA) to predict implant malpositioning. It can be inferred that by adapting the surgical technique used, possible positioning errors can be avoided. Furthermore, in certain femur configurations, such as coxa profunda (lower femoral neck-shaft angle and higher lateral center-edge angle), a higher probability of implant malpositioning in THA was described [59]. According to Habor et al. [12], another approach to avoid an unphysiological FA outcome could be the implementation of morphofunctional planning for patient-specific THAs. In this approach, a 3D model-based calculation of the target zone of the joint head is specifically used for each individual patient to prevent poor THA outcomes [12].

Mitsutake et al. [23] showed the role that preoperative 3D imaging can have on range of motion (ROM), considering that a simulated ROM, including flexion and internal rotation angles during the preoperative planning process, can reduce the risk of posterior dislocation of the cup and, consequently, reduce the risk of non-anatomical femoral FA [23]. Another approach to increase the accuracy of THA implantation and consequently avoid unphysiological FA outcomes could be the incorporation of image-guided robotic assistance. Foissey et al. [13] demonstrated that haptically controlled robotic arms allow more precise cup implantation in patients in whom a direct anterior approach (DAA) was performed. This technique could also be helpful in the future for the implantation of stems and could be implemented throughout the whole process of THA [13].

Furthermore, intraoperative fluoroscopy was shown to have better outcomes in terms of unphysiological versions and inclinations in THA than in patients who did not undergo intraoperative fluoroscopy. Consequently, it was demonstrated that intraoperative fluoroscopy imaging enables proper abduction and version of the acetabular cup position. As a result, the desired positioning of THA components could be achieved without a significant extension of the operation time [26].

Zhang et al. [24] demonstrated that the use of a patient-specific instrumentation system promises advantages in the accuracy of implantation compared to freehand THA. Preoperatively acquired CT images are once again used, as in other procedures, and 3D models are molded afterward. These models can be applied as a guide on the femoral neck or acetabulum to ensure accurate osteotomy and, consequently, accurate implantation [24]. Due to the fact that the exact positioning of the stem and the avoidance of unphysiological FA is a matter of multimodal influences, further research in this field will be necessary.

A major limitation of this study is that group B did not undergo any preoperative CT scans of the side of the hip to be operated on. Therefore, an analysis regarding preoperative differences in FA between the two groups could not be performed. Nevertheless, CT scans of the contralateral native hip were available for 17 cases in group B, and the measurements did not show any significant difference in preoperative FA between the two groups (22.4 $\pm$ 11° (A) vs. 22.6° $\pm$ 8 (B)). Moreover, it is highly improbable that there was a significant preoperative difference in FA because patients received either a short- or straight-stem design based only on the year the surgery was performed. Another limitation is the asymmetric group size of 89 to 41 patients due to the availability of postoperative CT scans in group B bearing the risk of inaccuracies. Furthermore, owing to the short follow-up of clinical and patient-reported outcome measures, the study does not provide data on the long-term effects of different FAs between both groups. Additionally, dislocation rates and rates of ante- or retrotorsion after THA were not recorded; thus, this limits the validity of the superior FA reconstruction outcomes with short-stem designs. Lastly, only one type of short-stem design was analyzed; therefore, the results obtained may not be entirely comparable to other short-stem designs. Hence, the results of this study should be interpreted with caution and in light of its limitations.

5. Conclusions

The present study shows that, compared to a predominantly diaphyseal anchoring straight-stem design, a mainly metaphyseal anchoring short-stem design allows for improved anatomical reconstruction of the femoral anteversion in THA. This may be important in the female femoral anatomy for adequate reconstruction of the hip geometry due to their higher variability in femoral antetorsion. This study was able to confirm research from Sariali and Pascal Mousselard [38] regarding the implantation of the calcar-guided short-stem design, which led to superior FA reconstruction accuracy. Regarding materials and surgical techniques for obese THA patients (class I–III), further research is required [25].

Author Contributions: Conceptualization, J.F. and W.M.-E.; methodology, P.R., J.F. and W.M.-E.; software, S.M.K., P.R., M.A.S. and A.H.; validation, S.M.K., P.R. and M.A.S.; formal analysis, M.A.S.; investigation, S.M.K. and P.R.; data curation, S.M.K., P.R., M.M., L.L., A.D., J.L. and K.B.; writing—original draft preparation, S.M.K. and P.R.; writing—review and editing, P.R., M.A.S., A.H., A.L., A.D., J.L. and W.M.-E.; visualization, S.M.K., P.R. and M.A.S.; supervision, J.F., A.L. and W.M.-E.; project administration, W.M.-E.; S.M.K. and P.R. contributed equally to this work as first authors. All authors have read and agreed to the published version of the manuscript.

Funding: This research was partly funded by ImplanTec GmbH. Funding institution had no role in data interpretation or paper preparation.

Institutional Review Board Statement: The study was conducted in accordance with the Declaration of Helsinki and approved by the Ethics Committee of the Medical University of Graz, Austria (protocol code 28-152 ex 15/16).

Informed Consent Statement: Informed consent was obtained from all subjects involved in the study.

Data Availability Statement: The datasets generated and/or analyzed during the current study are available from the corresponding author upon reasonable request.

Conflicts of Interest: As a potential conflict of interest, we hereby state that author W.M.-E. has given paid presentations for and received a research grant from ImplanTec GmbH. Author A.L. has received institutional and educational grants from Johnson & Johnson and ImplanTec GmbH.

References

1. Kurtz, S.M.; Ong, K.L.; Lau, E.; Bozic, K.J. Impact of the Economic Downturn on Total Joint Replacement Demand in the United States: Updated Projections to 2021. *J. Bone Joint Surg. Am.* **2014**, *96*, 624–630. [CrossRef] [PubMed]
2. Sakalkale, D.P.; Sharkey, P.F.; Eng, K.; Hozack, W.J.; Rothman, R.H. Effect of Femoral Component Offset on Polyethylene Wear in Total Hip Arthroplasty. *Clin. Orthop. Relat. Res.* **2001**, *388*, 125–134. [CrossRef] [PubMed]
3. Karachalios, T.; Hartofilakidis, G.; Zacharakis, N.; Tsekoura, M. A 12- to 18-Year Radiographic Follow-up Study of Charnley Low-Friction Arthroplasty. The Role of the Center of Rotation. *Clin. Orthop. Relat. Res.* **1993**, *296*, 140–147.
4. Bunyoz, K.I.; Malchau, E.; Malchau, H.; Troelsen, A. Has the Use of Fixation Techniques in THA Changed in This Decade? The Uncemented Paradox Revisited. *Clin. Orthop. Relat. Res.* **2020**, *478*, 697–704. [CrossRef] [PubMed]
5. Ferretti, A.; Iannotti, F.; Proietti, L.; Massafra, C.; Speranza, A.; Laghi, A.; Iorio, R. The Accuracy of Patient-Specific Instrumentation with Laser Guidance in a Dynamic Total Hip Arthroplasty: A Radiological Evaluation. *Sensors* **2021**, *21*, 4232. [CrossRef]
6. Bader, R.; Scholz, R.; Steinhauser, E.; Zimmermann, S.; Busch, R.; Mittelmeier, W. The Influence of Head and Neck Geometry on Stability of Total Hip Replacement: A Mechanical Test Study. *Acta Orthop. Scand.* **2004**, *75*, 415–421. [CrossRef]
7. Stief, F.; van Drongelen, S.; Brenneis, M.; Tarhan, T.; Fey, B.; Meurer, A. Influence of Hip Geometry Reconstruction on Frontal Plane Hip and Knee Joint Moments during Walking Following Primary Total Hip Replacement. *J. Arthroplasty* **2019**, *34*, 3106–3113. [CrossRef]
8. Flecher, X.; Ollivier, M.; Argenson, J.N. Lower Limb Length and Offset in Total Hip Arthroplasty. *Orthop. Traumatol. Surg. Res.* **2016**, *102*, S9–S20. [CrossRef]
9. Archibeck, M.J.; Cummins, T.; Carothers, J.; Junick, D.W.; White, R.E. A Comparison of Two Implant Systems in Restoration of Hip Geometry in Arthroplasty. *Clin. Orthop. Relat. Res.* **2011**, *469*, 443–446. [CrossRef]
10. Berend, K.R.; Sporer, S.M.; Sierra, R.J.; Glassman, A.H.; Morris, M.J. Achieving Stability and Lower-Limb Length in Total Hip Arthroplasty. *J. Bone Jt. Surg. Am.* **2010**, *92*, 2737–2752.
11. Bourne, R.B.; Rorabeck, C.H. Soft Tissue Balancing: The Hip. *J Arthroplasty* **2002**, *17*, 17–22. [CrossRef] [PubMed]
12. Habor, J.; Fischer, M.C.M.; Tokunaga, K.; Okamoto, M.; Radermacher, K. The Patient-Specific Combined Target Zone for Morpho-Functional Planning of Total Hip Arthroplasty. *J. Pers. Med.* **2021**, *11*, 817. [CrossRef] [PubMed]
13. Foissey, C.; Batailler, C.; Coulomb, R.; Giebaly, D.E.; Coulin, B.; Lustig, S.; Kouyoumdjian, P. Image-Based Robotic-Assisted Total Hip Arthroplasty through Direct Anterior Approach Allows a Better Orientation of the Acetabular Cup and a Better Restitution of the Centre of Rotation than a Conventional Procedure. *Int. Orthop. (SICOT)* **2023**, *47*, 691–699. [CrossRef] [PubMed]
14. Maurer-Ertl, W.; Friesenbichler, J.; Pfann, M.; Maier, M.; Reinbacher, P.; Leithner, A.; Smolle, M.A. Restoration of Hip Geometry after Total Hip Arthroplasty: Retrospective Comparison of Two Short Stems and One Straight Stem. *BMC Musculoskelet. Disord.* **2022**, *23*, 1035. [CrossRef]
15. Karnezis, I.A. A Technique for Accurate Reproduction of the Femoral Anteversion during Primary Total Hip Arthroplasty. *Arch. Orthop. Trauma Surg.* **2001**, *121*, 343–345. [CrossRef]
16. Renkawitz, T.; Haimerl, M.; Dohmen, L.; Gneiting, S.; Lechler, P.; Woerner, M.; Springorum, H.-R.; Weber, M.; Sussmann, P.; Sendtner, E.; et al. The Association between Femoral Tilt and Impingement-Free Range-of-Motion in Total Hip Arthroplasty. *BMC Musculoskelet. Disord.* **2012**, *13*, 65. [CrossRef] [PubMed]

17. Zahar, A.; Rastogi, A.; Kendoff, D. Dislocation after Total Hip Arthroplasty. *Curr. Rev. Musculoskelet. Med.* **2013**, *6*, 350–356. [CrossRef] [PubMed]
18. Wines, A.P.; McNicol, D. Computed Tomography Measurement of the Accuracy of Component Version in Total Hip Arthroplasty. *J. Arthroplasty* **2006**, *21*, 696–701. [CrossRef]
19. Dessyn, E.; Flecher, X.; Parratte, S.; Ollivier, M.; Argenson, J.-N. A 20-Year Follow-up Evaluation of Total Hip Arthroplasty in Patients Younger than 50 Using a Custom Cementless Stem. *Hip Int.* **2019**, *29*, 481–488. [CrossRef]
20. Sariali, E.; Mouttet, A.; Flecher, X.; Argenson, J.N. Reproducing Proximal Femur Anatomy with Custom Stems. In *Personalized Hip and Knee Joint Replacement*; Rivière, C., Vendittoli, P.-A., Eds.; Springer: Cham, Switzerland, 2020; ISBN 978-3-030-24242-8.
21. Jolles, B.M.; Zangger, P.; Leyvraz, P.-F. Factors Predisposing to Dislocation after Primary Total Hip Arthroplasty: A Multivariate Analysis. *J. Arthroplasty* **2002**, *17*, 282–288. [CrossRef] [PubMed]
22. Sariali, E.; Klouche, S.; Mamoudy, P. Ceramic-on-Ceramic Total Hip Arthroplasty: Is Squeaking Related to an Inaccurate Three-Dimensional Hip Anatomy Reconstruction? *Orthop. Traumatol. Surg. Res.* **2014**, *100*, 437–440. [CrossRef]
23. Mitsutake, R.; Tanino, H.; Ito, H. The Effect of Range of Motion Simulated with a Patient-Specific Three-Dimensional Simulation Analysis on Dislocation after Total Hip Arthroplasty. *Hip Int.* **2023**, *33*, 313–322. [CrossRef]
24. Zhang, T.; Jia, Z.; Han, W.; Wang, J.; Li, J.; Gong, M.; Jiang, X. Effectiveness and Accuracy of a Patient-Specific Instrumentation System for Total Hip Arthroplasty. *Orthop. Surg.* **2023**, *15*, 878–887. [CrossRef]
25. Ammarullah, M.I.; Santoso, G.; Sugiharto, S.; Supriyono, T.; Kurdi, O.; Tauviqirrahman, M.; Winarni, T.I.; Jamari, J. Tresca Stress Study of CoCrMo-on-CoCrMo Bearings Based on Body Mass Index Using 2D Computational Model. *J. Tribol.* **2022**, *33*, 31–38.
26. Shah, M.; Vieira, A.; Mahajan, A.; Agrawal, L.; Shah, D.; Surme, S.; Velankar, A. Does Intra-Operative Fluoroscopy Significantly Improve Component Position in a Primary Total Hip Arthroplasty? Our Experience in a Tertiary Care Hospital. *JOIO* **2023**, *57*, 325–335. [CrossRef]
27. Fischer, T.; Stern, C.; Fritz, B.; Zingg, P.O.; Pfirrmann, C.W.A.; Sutter, R. Impact of Stem Design and Cementation on Postoperative Femoral Antetorsion in 227 Patients with Total Hip Arthroplasty (THA). *Skelet. Radiol.* **2020**, *49*, 2001–2009. [CrossRef] [PubMed]
28. Jamari, J.; Ammarullah, M.I.; Saad, A.P.M.; Syahrom, A.; Uddin, M.; van der Heide, E.; Basri, H. The Effect of Bottom Profile Dimples on the Femoral Head on Wear in Metal-on-Metal Total Hip Arthroplasty. *J. Funct. Biomater.* **2021**, *12*, 38. [CrossRef] [PubMed]
29. Migliorini, F.; Driessen, A.; Colarossi, G.; El Mansy, Y.; Gatz, M.; Tingart, M.; Eschweiler, J. Short Stems for Total Hip Replacement among Middle-Aged Patients. *Int. Orthop.* **2020**, *44*, 847–855. [CrossRef] [PubMed]
30. Ettinger, M.; Ettinger, P.; Lerch, M.; Radtke, K.; Budde, S.; Ezechieli, M.; Becher, C.; Thorey, F. The NANOS Short Stem in Total Hip Arthroplasty: A Mid Term Follow-Up. *Hip Int.* **2011**, *21*, 583–586. [CrossRef]
31. Reinbacher, P.; Smolle, M.A.; Friesenbichler, J.; Draschl, A.; Leithner, A.; Maurer-Ertl, W. Three-Year Migration Analysis of a New Metaphyseal Anchoring Short Femoral Stem in THA Using EBRA-FCA. *Sci. Rep.* **2022**, *12*, 17173. [CrossRef] [PubMed]
32. van Oldenrijk, J.; Molleman, J.; Klaver, M.; Poolman, R.W.; Haverkamp, D. Revision Rate after Short-Stem Total Hip Arthroplasty: A Systematic Review of 49 Studies. *Acta Orthop.* **2014**, *85*, 250–258. [CrossRef] [PubMed]
33. Liang, H.-D.; Yang, W.-Y.; Pan, J.-K.; Huang, H.-T.; Luo, M.-H.; Zeng, L.-F.; Liu, J. Are Short-Stem Prostheses Superior to Conventional Stem Prostheses in Primary Total Hip Arthroplasty? A Systematic Review and Meta-Analysis of Randomised Controlled Trials. *BMJ Open* **2018**, *8*, e021649. [CrossRef] [PubMed]
34. Yan, S.G.; Woiczinski, M.; Schmidutz, T.F.; Weber, P.; Paulus, A.C.; Steinbrück, A.; Jansson, V.; Schmidutz, F. Can the Metaphyseal Anchored Metha Short Stem Safely Be Revised with a Standard CLS Stem? A Biomechanical Analysis. *Int. Orthop.* **2017**, *41*, 2471–2477. [CrossRef] [PubMed]
35. Bieger, R.; Ignatius, A.; Reichel, H.; Dürselen, L. Biomechanics of a Short Stem: In Vitro Primary Stability and Stress Shielding of a Conservative Cementless Hip Stem. *J. Orthop. Res.* **2013**, *31*, 1180–1186. [CrossRef] [PubMed]
36. Salemyr, M.; Muren, O.; Ahl, T.; Bodén, H.; Eisler, T.; Stark, A.; Sköldenberg, O. Lower Periprosthetic Bone Loss and Good Fixation of an Ultra-Short Stem Compared to a Conventional Stem in Uncemented Total Hip Arthroplasty. *Acta Orthop.* **2015**, *86*, 659–666. [CrossRef]
37. Hochreiter, J.; Böhm, G.; Fierlbeck, J.; Anderl, C.; Birke, M.; Münger, P.; Ortmaier, R. Femoral Antetorsion after Calcar-Guided Short-Stem Total Hip Arthroplasty: A Cadaver Study. *J. Orthop. Res.* **2022**, *40*, 2127–2132. [CrossRef]
38. Sariali, E.; Pascal Moussellard, H. Higher Femoral Anteversion Restoration Accuracy after Total Hip Arthroplasty with a Proximally Fixed Anatomic Stem than with a Generic Straight Double-Tapered Stem. *HIP Int.* **2022**, 112070002210789. [CrossRef] [PubMed]
39. Watson-Jones, R. Fractures of the Neck of the Femur. *Br. J. Surg.* **1936**, *23*, 787–808. [CrossRef]
40. Reinbacher, P.; Hecker, A.; Friesenbichler, J.; Smolle, M.; Leitner, L.; Klim, S.; Draschl, A.; Colovic, D.; Brunnader, K.; Leithner, A.; et al. Simultaneous Bilateral Total Hip Arthroplasty with Straight-Stems and Short-Stems: Does the Short One Do a Better Job? *JCM* **2023**, *12*, 1028. [CrossRef]
41. Jarrett, D.Y.; Oliveira, A.M.; Zou, K.H.; Snyder, B.D.; Kleinman, P.K. Axial Oblique CT to Assess Femoral Anteversion. *AJR Am. J. Roentgenol.* **2010**, *194*, 1230–1233. [CrossRef] [PubMed]
42. Kaiser, P.; Attal, R.; Kammerer, M.; Thauerer, M.; Hamberger, L.; Mayr, R.; Schmoelz, W. Significant Differences in Femoral Torsion Values Depending on the CT Measurement Technique. *Arch. Orthop. Trauma Surg.* **2016**, *136*, 1259–1264. [CrossRef] [PubMed]

43. Reinbacher, P.; Smolle, M.A.; Friesenbichler, J.; Draschl, A.; Leithner, A.; Maurer-Ertl, W. Pre-Operative Templating in THA Using a Short Stem System: Precision and Accuracy of 2D versus 3D Planning Method. *J. Orthop. Traumatol.* **2022**, *23*, 16. [CrossRef] [PubMed]
44. Bellamy, N.; Buchanan, W.W.; Goldsmith, C.H.; Campbell, J.; Stitt, L.W. Validation Study of WOMAC: A Health Status Instrument for Measuring Clinically Important Patient Relevant Outcomes to Antirheumatic Drug Therapy in Patients with Osteoarthritis of the Hip or Knee. *J. Rheumatol.* **1988**, *15*, 1833–1840.
45. Harris, W.H. Traumatic Arthritis of the Hip after Dislocation and Acetabular Fractures: Treatment by Mold Arthroplasty. An End-Result Study Using a New Method of Result Evaluation. *J. Bone Jt. Surg. Am.* **1969**, *51*, 737–755. [CrossRef]
46. Kutzner, K.P. Calcar-Guided Short-Stem Total Hip Arthroplasty: Will It Be the Future Standard? Review and Perspectives. *World J. Orthop.* **2021**, *12*, 534–547. [CrossRef]
47. Kutzner, K.P.; Pfeil, J. Individualized Stem-Positioning in Calcar-Guided Short-Stem Total Hip Arthroplasty. *J. Vis. Exp. JoVE* 2018. [CrossRef]
48. Maruyama, M.; Feinberg, J.R.; Capello, W.N.; D'Antonio, J.A. The Frank Stinchfield Award: Morphologic Features of the Acetabulum and Femur: Anteversion Angle and Implant Positioning. *Clin. Orthop. Relat. Res.* **2001**, *393*, 52–65. [CrossRef]
49. Nakahara, I.; Takao, M.; Sakai, T.; Nishii, T.; Yoshikawa, H.; Sugano, N. Gender Differences in 3D Morphology and Bony Impingement of Human Hips. *J. Orthop. Res.* **2011**, *29*, 333–339. [CrossRef]
50. Noble, P.C.; Alexander, J.W.; Lindahl, L.J.; Yew, D.T.; Granberry, W.M.; Tullos, H.S. The Anatomic Basis of Femoral Component Design. *Clin. Orthop. Relat. Res.* **1988**, *235*, 148–165. [CrossRef]
51. Padgett, D.E.; Warashina, H. The Unstable Total Hip Replacement. *Clin. Orthop. Relat. Res.* **2004**, *420*, 72–79. [CrossRef]
52. Coventry, M.B. Late Dislocations in Patients with Charnley Total Hip Arthroplasty. *J. Bone Jt. Surg. Am.* **1985**, *67*, 832–841. [CrossRef]
53. Woo, R.Y.; Morrey, B.F. Dislocations after Total Hip Arthroplasty. *J. Bone Jt. Surg. Am.* **1982**, *64*, 1295–1306. [CrossRef]
54. Hartel, M.J.; Petersik, A.; Schmidt, A.; Kendoff, D.; Nüchtern, J.; Rueger, J.M.; Lehmann, W.; Grossterlinden, L.G. Determination of Femoral Neck Angle and Torsion Angle Utilizing a Novel Three-Dimensional Modeling and Analytical Technology Based on CT Datasets. *PLoS ONE* **2016**, *11*, e0149480. [CrossRef]
55. Yoon, J.Y.; Seo, W.Y.; Kim, H.J.; Yoo, J.J. The Relationship between Femoral Stem Tilt and Stem Length in Total Hip Arthroplasty: A Retrospective Case-Control Study. *Clin. Orthop. Surg.* **2022**, *14*, 184–190. [CrossRef] [PubMed]
56. Faizan, A.; Gerges, J.J.; Asencio, G.; Essig, J.; Munini, E.; Hozack, W.J. Changes in Femoral Version During Implantation of Anatomic Stems: Implications on Stem Design. *J. Arthroplast.* **2016**, *31*, 512–516. [CrossRef]
57. Yu, H.; Liu, H.; Jia, M.; Hu, Y.; Zhang, Y. A Comparison of a Short versus a Conventional Femoral Cementless Stem in Total Hip Arthroplasty in Patients 70 Years and Older. *J. Orthop. Surg. Res.* **2016**, *11*, 33. [CrossRef]
58. Huo, S.-C.; Wang, F.; Dong, L.-J.; Wei, W.; Zeng, J.-Q.; Huang, H.-X.; Han, Q.-M.; Duan, R.-Q. Short-Stem Prostheses in Primary Total Hip Arthroplasty: A Meta-Analysis of Randomized Controlled Trials. *Medicine* **2016**, *95*, e5215. [CrossRef] [PubMed]
59. Free, M.D.; Barnes, I.; Hutchinson, M.; Harvie, P. Preoperative Radiographs to Predict Component Malposition in Direct Anterior Approach Total Hip Arthroplasty. *Hip Int.* **2023**, *33*, 207–213. [CrossRef]

Disclaimer/Publisher's Note: The statements, opinions and data contained in all publications are solely those of the individual author(s) and contributor(s) and not of MDPI and/or the editor(s). MDPI and/or the editor(s) disclaim responsibility for any injury to people or property resulting from any ideas, methods, instructions or products referred to in the content.

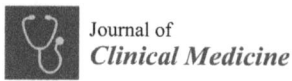

Article

Joint Response to Exercise Is Affected by Knee Osteoarthritis: An Infrared Thermography Analysis

Luca De Marziani [1], Angelo Boffa [1,*], Simone Orazi [1], Luca Andriolo [1], Alessandro Di Martino [1], Stefano Zaffagnini [1] and Giuseppe Filardo [2]

1 Clinica Ortopedica e Traumatologica 2, IRCCS Istituto Ortopedico Rizzoli, 40136 Bologna, Italy
2 Applied and Translational Research (ATR) Center, IRCCS Istituto Ortopedico Rizzoli, 40136 Bologna, Italy
* Correspondence: angeloboffa@libero.it; Tel.: +39-0516366567

Abstract: Infrared thermography can be used to evaluate the inflammation characterizing the joint environment of OA knees, but there is limited evidence on the response to physical exercise. Identifying the response to exercise of OA knees and the influencing variables could provide important information to better profile patients with different knee OA patterns. Sixty consecutive patients (38 men/22 women, 61.4 ± 9.2 years) with symptomatic knee OA were enrolled. Patients were evaluated with a standardized protocol using a thermographic camera (FLIR-T1020) positioned at 1 m with image acquisition of an anterior view at baseline, immediately after, and at 5 min after a 2-min knee flexion–extension exercise with a 2 kg anklet. Patients' demographic and clinical characteristics were documented and correlated with the thermographic changes. This study demonstrated that the temperature response to exercise in symptomatic knee OA was affected by some demographic and clinical characteristics of the assessed patients. Patients with a poor clinical knee status presented with a lower response to exercise, and women showed a greater temperature decrease than men. Not all evaluated ROIs showed the same trend, which underlines the need to specifically study the different joint subareas to identify the inflammatory component and joint response while investigating knee OA patterns.

Keywords: infrared thermography; knee; osteoarthritis; joint temperature; inflammation; response; exercise

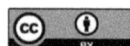

Citation: De Marziani, L.; Boffa, A.; Orazi, S.; Andriolo, L.; Di Martino, A.; Zaffagnini, S.; Filardo, G. Joint Response to Exercise Is Affected by Knee Osteoarthritis: An Infrared Thermography Analysis. *J. Clin. Med.* 2023, 12, 3399. https://doi.org/10.3390/jcm12103399

Academic Editor: Enrique Gómez-Barrena

Received: 24 January 2023
Revised: 12 April 2023
Accepted: 8 May 2023
Published: 11 May 2023

Copyright: © 2023 by the authors. Licensee MDPI, Basel, Switzerland. This article is an open access article distributed under the terms and conditions of the Creative Commons Attribution (CC BY) license (https://creativecommons.org/licenses/by/4.0/).

1. Introduction

Infrared thermography is an established method that is able to detect the infrared radiation emitted by the human body, which correlates with the temperature distribution of a defined region [1]. This technology, used for the first time in the 1960s [2], allows us to identify and locate thermal abnormalities characterized by an increase or decrease in temperature at the skin surface, which can reflect the status of a specific pathology [3]. In particular, infrared thermography has been proposed as a method to evaluate conditions with an inflammatory component, which plays a central role in the pathophysiology of several diseases [4]. The awareness of the role of inflammation within a wide range of diseases as well as the technological advancements in cameras and improvements in software used for image analysis has led to increased use of infrared thermography in different scientific fields, from dermatology to oncology [5,6]. Recently, the use of infrared thermography has been proposed in the orthopedic field as a potential method for evaluating patients with knee osteoarthritis (OA) to better characterize the pathology and guide personalized treatment [4].

Knee OA is one of the most common musculoskeletal diseases. It is characterized by the deterioration and loss of articular cartilage with concomitant structural and functional changes across the entire joint [7]. Inflammation plays a key role in the pathophysiology of knee OA, with the involvement of the synovial membrane and the release of several proinflammatory cytokines [8–10]. The inflammatory component leads to an increase in blood flow that can manifest clinically as redness and heat as well as joint swelling and pain [4]. Infrared thermography has been proven, through the evaluation of the skin temperature of the knee, to be able to evaluate the inflammation component that characterizes the joint environment of OA knees [11–14]. However, although the use of infrared thermography in this setting is growing, there is limited evidence on its use for the evaluation of the inflammatory response to physical exercise in OA knees. While a few reports suggest that there are activity-related changes in OA knees, despite documenting temperature-induced changes after exercise, no studies have evaluated possible factors influencing the temperature response [15,16]. Identifying the response to exercise of OA knees and the variables that influence this response could provide important information to better profile patients with different knee OA patterns.

The aim of this study was to evaluate, through infrared thermography, the response to a knee flexion–extension exercise and identify the clinical and demographic variables able to influence this response in patients with symptomatic knee OA.

2. Materials and Methods

This study was approved by the hospital ethics committee of the IRCCS Istituto Ortopedico Rizzoli, Italy (n. 0017413). Patient screening was performed by orthopedic physicians in a research outpatient department of a highly specialized referral center for orthopedics focused on patients with knee OA. The evaluation was performed from December 2021 to December 2022. Informed consent was obtained from each patient prior to study participation. Patients were clinically evaluated for their eligibility for study inclusion according to the following criteria: patients with monolateral symptomatic knee OA (Kellgren–Lawrence grade ≥ 2) with a history of chronic pain or swelling (for at least 6 months) were included in the study. The exclusion criteria were as follows: previous total knee arthroplasty; history of trauma or intra-articular injections within 6 months before treatment or knee surgery within 12 months; the presence of concomitant lesions causing knee pain or swelling, including radiculopathy; clinical signs of dermatological and vascular conditions; neoplasms; systemic disorders (i.e., uncontrolled diabetes); uncontrolled metabolic disorders of the thyroid; severe cardiovascular diseases; rheumatoid arthritis and other inflammatory arthropathies; hematological diseases; infections; immunodepression; anticoagulant or antiaggregant therapy; the use of nonsteroidal anti-inflammatories or other analgesic drugs in the 5 days before the evaluation. According to the Thermographic Imaging in Sports and Exercise Medicine (TISEM) guidelines [17] as well as considering the guidelines of the American Academy of Thermology [18], patients were asked to respect some instructions: avoidance of exercise and physical activity within 48 h; avoidance of alcohol beverages, smoking, caffeine, large meals, any type of ointment, cosmetics, and showering within 4 h; avoidance of ice or lotion applications within 48 h; and avoidance of knee exposure to the sun for long periods during the week prior to the examination.

A total of 60 consecutive patients with symptomatic knee OA were enrolled in accordance with the inclusion/exclusion criteria. Among them, 38 patients were men and 22 were women, aged 61.4 ± 9.2 years, and with a body mass index (BMI) of 25.4 ± 3.0. All demographic and clinical characteristics are reported in Table 1.

After enrollment, patients were evaluated clinically thorough knee-specific patient reported outcome measurements (PROMs), including the International Knee Documentation Committee (IKDC) subjective score, the Knee Injury and Osteoarthritis Outcome Score (KOOS) subscales, the Tegner score for activity level, the Visual Analogue Scale (VAS) for pain, and the PainDETECT questionnaire for the evaluation of the neuropathic pain component. Clinical questionnaires were administered via paper questionnaires during clinical visits in the research outpatient clinic. Patients completed the questionnaires, and doctors were available in case of questions. Moreover, the IKDC objective scores were evaluated by the clinician. All participants underwent weight-bearing antero-posterior radiographs to assess the baseline OA severity according to the Kellgren–Lawrence classification. Finally, the skin temperature of the knee affected by symptomatic OA was evaluated with thermographic imaging.

Table 1. Included patients' characteristics.

Sex, M/W	38/22
Age, years	61.4 ± 9.2 (43–75)
BMI, kg/m^2	25.4 ± 3.0 (19.5–33.8)
Side	Right: 33—Left: 27
Symptom duration, months	108.3 ± 99.3 (18–372)
Symptom onset	Acute: 14—Chronic: 46
Previous knee surgery, yes/no	31/29
Smoker, yes/no	13/47
Kellgren–Lawrence grade	Grade 2: 30
	Grade 3: 21
	Grade 4: 9
VAS pain	5.6 ± 2.3 (1–9)
IKDC subjective score	41.3 ± 14.2 (9.2–81.6)
IKDC objective score	Grade 1: 8
	Grade 2: 29
	Grade 3: 10
	Grade 4: 13
KOOS pain	59.8 ± 18.9 (2–94)
KOOS symptoms	60.4 ± 19.7 (18–100)
KOOS ADL	69.5 ± 18.4 (6–100)
KOOS QoL	34.5 ± 16.2 (0–75)
KOOS Sport/Rec	43.8 ± 17.7 (20–90)
Tegner score pre-treatment	2.2 ± 1.2 (1–5)
PainDETECT questionnaire	8.7 ± 5.5 (0–25)

Values are expressed as mean ± standard deviation and range (). ADL, Activities of daily living; BMI, body mass index; IKDC, International Knee Documentation Committee; KOOS, Knee Injury and Osteoarthritis Outcome Score; M, men; QoL, Quality of Life; Sport/Rec, Function in Sport and Recreation; VAS, visual analogue scale; W, women.

2.1. Infrared Thermography Procedure, Exercise, and Analysis

The infrared imaging evaluation was performed in a dedicated outpatient clinic shielded from direct sunlight and with the temperature controlled at 23.0 °C [19,20] and a mean humidity of 45 ± 3%. Image acquisition was performed between 14:00 and 17:00 to minimize the circadian temperature variations. According to Marins et al. [21], the thermalization period was 10 min. To speed up thermalization, patients were asked to remove trousers, shoes, and socks, remain seated and undressed on the lower limbs with light clothing (such as a t-shirt) on the top, and not touch their knees. The patient only rested the buttocks region on the medical bed, while the remaining parts of the lower limbs had no contact with other objects or body parts; only feet without socks touched a paper towel, thus separating them from direct contact with the floor. Thermograms were acquired using a FLIR T1020 thermographic camera (FLIR® Systems, Stockholm, Sweden) with a resolution of 1024 × 768 pixels and a thermal sensitivity of 0.02 °C. The camera was positioned at a distance of 1 m, perpendicular to the knee and adjusted to the patellar height [22]. After the patient was acclimatized, he was positioned on a designated floor map, and image acquisition (T0) of an anterior view was performed using the autofocus mode.

Then, one 2 kg anklet was positioned on the ankle of the symptomatic lower limb of the patient. At this point, with the patient seated, a knee flexion–extension exercise was performed for 2 min at the rate of one extension every 2 s (1 s flexion phase and 1 s extension phase). A metronome was used to standardize pacing. Immediately after performing this exercise, the anklet was removed, and the patient was positioned again on the floor map and a second anterior view image was acquired (T1). Afterwards, the patient waited in the room for 5 min in a sitting position without touching or moving the lower limbs. At the end of this resting period, the patient was positioned on the floor map and a third anterior view image was acquired (T2). Finally, maintaining the same position of the knee, an anatomical marker (circular adhesive of 2 cm in diameter) was placed at the center of the patella to obtain a further image in the anterior view in order to facilitate the precise subsequent location of the patella in the analysis of the previous infrared images (Figure 1).

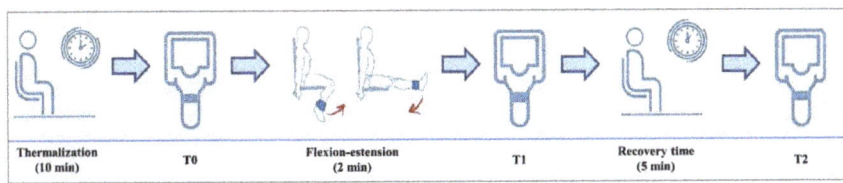

Figure 1. Timeline of the study.

During the image analysis process, the three anterior images acquired at T0, T1, and T2 were aligned side by side with the image with the patellar marker on the computer screen, and a template indicating the region of interests (ROIs) was centered over the patella of each unmarked image, using the marked image as a guide [23,24]. The ROIs were defined as follows: the patellar area was a square, 6 cm in diameter, divided into the medial patella and lateral patella (each area 6 cm high and 3 cm wide); the suprapatellar area was the area 3 cm over the patella; the medial and lateral areas were the regions 3 cm below the patella on its medial and lateral sides, respectively. The mean temperatures were extracted using ResearchIR software (FLIR® Systems, Stockholm, Sweden) to determine the overall knee area and the 5 ROIs: medial patella, lateral patella, suprapatellar, and medial and lateral knees.

2.2. Statistical Analysis

All continuous data are expressed in terms of the mean and the standard deviation of the mean and range, and the categorical data are expressed as frequencies and percentages. The Shapiro–Wilk test was performed to test normality of continuous variables. The Levene test was used to assess the homoscedasticity of the data. The Repeated Measures General Linear Model (GLM) with the Sidak test for multiple comparisons was performed to assess the differences in different areas. The ANOVA test was performed to assess the between-group differences of continuous, normally distributed, and homoscedastic data; the Mann–Whitney nonparametric test was used otherwise. The ANOVA test, followed by the post-hoc Sidak test for pairwise comparisons, was performed to assess the among-group differences of continuous, normally distributed, and homoscedastic data, the Kruskal–Wallis nonparametric test, followed by the post-hoc Mann–Whitney test with Bonferroni correction for multiple comparisons, was used otherwise. The Spearman rank correlation was used to assess correlations between temperature and continuous data; the Kendall tau rank correlation was used for ordinal data. For all tests, $p < 0.05$ was considered significant. All statistical analyses were performed using SPSS v.19.0 (IBM Corp., Armonk, NY, USA).

3. Results
3.1. Temperature Changes

The mean temperature of the total knee significantly changed after exercise, ranging from the baseline (T0) value of 32.13 ± 1.07 °C to 31.86 ± 1.12 °C at T1 and 31.94 ± 1.10 °C at T2 ($p = 0.002$). In detail, the mean temperature of the total knee detected at T0 was higher compared to that at T1 ($p = 0.001$) with a mean difference T0-T1 (ΔT0 T1) of 0.27 °C and compared to that at T2 ($p = 0.036$) with a mean difference T0-T2 (ΔT0 T2) of 0.20 °C. No significant differences in the mean temperature of the total knee were found between T1 and T2 (Figure 2).

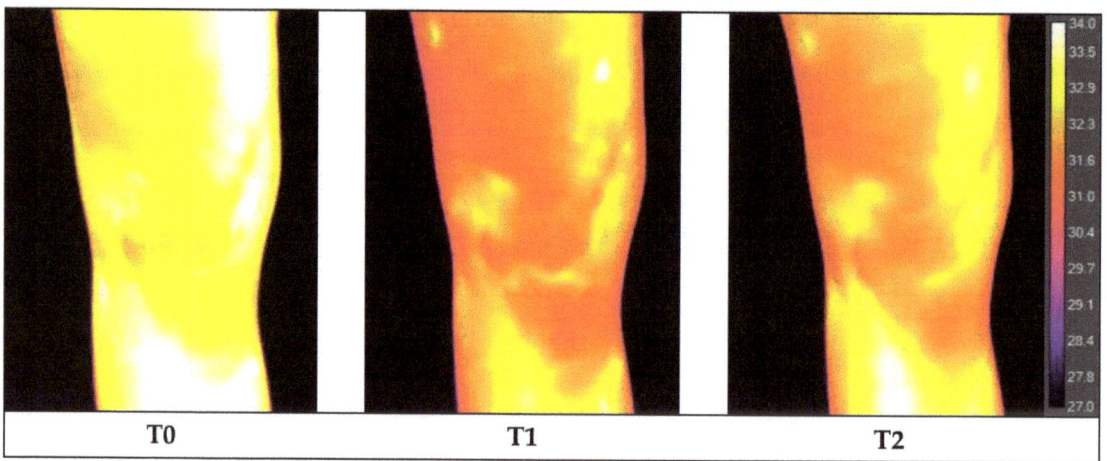

Figure 2. Thermographic basal image (**T0**), at the end of the 2-min flexion–extension exercise (**T1**) and after the 5-min rest period (**T2**).

Similar changes in the mean temperature after exercise were observed for all knee subareas (Figure 3). In particular, statistically significant changes (ANOVA test) were detected for the lateral ($p = 0.001$), medial ($p = 0.002$), suprapatellar ($p < 0.0005$), and medial patella subareas ($p = 0.011$), while no significant changes were observed for the lateral patella subarea. A higher change in temperature from T0 to T1 (ΔT0-T1) was found for the suprapatellar area ($p < 0.0005$) with a mean ΔT0-T1 of 0.33 °C, while a smaller change was detected for the lateral patella area ($p = $ n.s) with a mean ΔT0 T1 of 0.19 °C. A higher change in temperature from T0 to T2 (ΔT0 T2) was found for the medial area with a mean ΔT0-T2 of 0.25 °C, while a smaller change was detected for the suprapatellar area (n.s) with a mean ΔT0-T2 of 0.15 °C. Analyzing the changes in temperature between T1 and T2 (ΔT1-T2) showed a significant increase in the suprapatellar area (+0.18, $p = 0.030$), while no differences were found in any other areas.

3.2. Influences of Demographic Variables

Sex influenced the temperature changes after the exercise (Figure 4). Women had a greater decrease in temperature than men after exercise (ΔT0-T1) in the total knee (-0.47 ± 0.64 vs. -0.16 ± 0.49, $p = 0.021$) and the medial (-0.48 ± 0.73 vs. -0.17 ± 0.50, $p = 0.042$) and suprapatellar (-0.56 ± 0.70 vs. -0.19 ± 0.55, $p = 0.022$) areas. Similarly, women had a greater decrease in temperature between T0 and T2 (ΔT0-T2) in the total knee (-0.46 ± 0.49 vs. -0.05 ± 0.59, $p = 0.009$) and the medial (-0.52 ± 0.50 vs. -0.10 ± 0.60, $p = 0.007$), medial patella (-0.48 ± 0.62 vs. -0.03 ± 0.60, $p = 0.018$), and suprapatellar (-0.50 ± 0.51 vs. -0.06 ± 0.66, $p = 0.001$) areas. No significative differences were found in ΔT1T2 between women and men. The other demographic characteristics, including age, BMI, OA grade, sport activity level, smoking status, previous surgery, and symptom onset did not influence the thermic response after exercise.

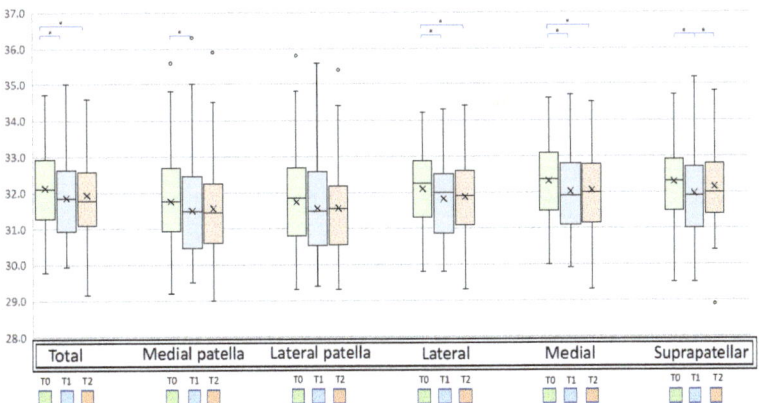

Figure 3. Mean temperatures of the total knee and subareas at T0, T1, and T2 (* $p < 0.05$, post-hoc Sidak test). Box-and-whisker plots showing median values and interquartile ranges. The "x" represents the mean temperature. T0: baseline; T1: immediately after performing this exercise; T2: 5 min after performing this exercise.

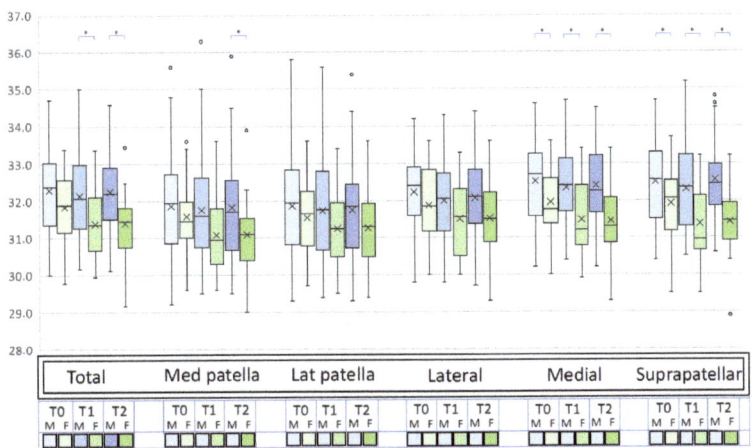

Figure 4. Differences in the total mean knee temperature and subareas at T0, T1, and T2 in men and women (* $p < 0.05$). Box-and-whisker plots showing median values and interquartile ranges. "x" represents the mean temperature. F: females; M: males; T0: baseline; T1: immediately after performing this exercise; T2: 5 min after performing this exercise.

3.3. Influence of Clinical Variables

The ΔT0-T1 of the total knee was negatively correlated with the VAS score (rho = −0.296, $p = 0.022$), with a higher temperature change occurring in patients with lower VAS scores (Figure 5a). This correlation was confirmed for the medial area (rho = −0.320, $p = 0.013$) and medial patella area (rho = −0.294, $p = 0.023$). The medial area was also positively correlated with the IKDC subjective score (rho = 0.363, $p = 0.004$) and the KOOS ADL subscale (rho = 0.259, $p = 0.045$), with higher temperature changes occurring in patients with better clinical values.

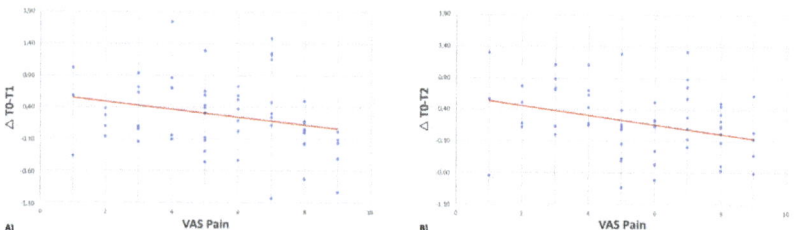

Figure 5. VAS pain is negatively correlated with ΔT0-T1 (**A**, rho = −0.296, p = 0.022) and ΔT0-T2 (**B**, rho = −0.318, p = 0.013).

The ΔT0-T2 of the total knee was negatively correlated with the VAS score (rho = −0.318, p = 0.013), with a higher temperature change occurring in patients with lower VAS scores (Figure 5b). Similar trends were observed for all subareas: lateral (rho = −0.256, p = 0.049), medial (rho = −0.365, p = 0.004), suprapatellar (rho = −0.270, p = 0.037), medial patellar (rho = −0.310, p = 0.016), and lateral patellar areas (rho = −0.271, p = 0.036). The IKDC subjective score was positively correlated with the ΔT0-T2 of the total knee (rho = 0.299, p = 0.020) and the medial area (rho = 0.371, p = 0.004), with higher temperature changes occurring in patients with higher IKDC subjective scores. The ΔT0-T2 of the total knee and the medial area were also positive correlated with the KOOS ADL subscale (rho = 0.256, p = 0.048 and rho = 0.298, p = 0.021, respectively) and the KOOS Sport/Rec subscale (rho = 0.307, p = 0.017 and rho = 0.369, p = 0.004, respectively), with higher temperature changes occurring in patients with higher activity levels. The PainDETECT questionnaire scores were negatively correlated with the ΔT0-T2 of the total knee (rho = −0.270 and p = 0.037) and the medial area (rho = −0.281, p = 0.030), with lower temperature variations occurring in patients with higher PainDETECT scores.

No correlations were found between ΔT1T2 temperatures of all areas and the clinical variables analyzed.

4. Discussion

This study demonstrated that the temperature response to exercise in symptomatic knee OA is affected by the different demographic and clinical characteristics of the assessed patients. Patients with a poor clinical knee status presented with a lower response to exercise, and women showed a greater temperature decrease compared to men.

The use of infrared thermography for the evaluation of musculoskeletal diseases has gaining increased interest in recent years, thanks to its simple method of evaluating the temperature of a body region, for example, for the study of tendinopathies and rheumatic diseases [4,25–27]. Recently, infrared thermography was proposed as a method for the evaluation of patients with knee OA to better characterize this pathology and possibly guide the treatment [4]. Although preliminary studies investigated the use of infrared thermography as a method for diagnosing and monitoring knee OA, its actual potential for use in clinical practice is still unclear, and its application remains limited [24,27,28]. In this scenario, defining how the OA knees respond to physical exercise and identifying which variables can influence this response could be useful to optimize its potential to detect OA patterns.

Previous studies evaluated the response to physical exercise in different body areas of healthy volunteers, reporting different temperature patterns [19,29,30]. In particular, significant heterogeneity among the different studies was found in terms of the response to exercise in relation to the intensity and duration of exercise [31]. Studies evaluating the skin temperature after brief exercise reported an initial temperature decrease and a subsequent temperature increase, while other studies analyzing skin temperature directly after a long bout of exercise directly detected a temperature increase compared to baseline conditions, probably hiding the initial temperature decrease [15,16]. In detail, Arfaoui et al. performed a 5-min running exercise at a speed of 8 km/h with thermalization for 30 min, a room temperature of 18 ± 0.5 °C, and a humidity of 60%, while Brito et al. performed a 50-min training session with thermalization for 10–15 min, a room temperature of 28.2 ± 0.5 °C, and a humidity of $48.1 \pm 1.2\%$. The initial temperature decrease appeared to be due to vasoconstriction of the skin circulation and a redistribution of blood flow from the skin to the muscles involved in the exercise [29,30,32]. The following increase in temperature above the baseline values appeared to be due to the activation of cutaneous mechanisms of heat dissipation [31].

The current study, focusing on older patients (mean age 61 years) with knee OA, demonstrated that the temperature of symptomatic OA knees changes in response to two minutes of physical exercise with a temperature decrease immediately after exercise. This temperature change two minutes after exercise is similar to that reported in a previous study conducted by Formenti et al. [33]. Through infrared thermography, these authors analyzed the response to exercise in 13 young healthy volunteers (mean age 25 years), showing a peak temperature reduction of between two and three minutes from the beginning of exercise. However, in this study, the authors documented a subsequent increase in the temperature which was not confirmed in the different population used in the current study. The temperature of OA knees seven minutes after the beginning of exercise remained unchanged compared with that at two minutes, and it was lower than the baseline temperature. On one hand, this difference could be justified by the different participant ages between the two studies, with possible differences in the vascular response to exercise [34,35]. On the other hand, the differences could be explained by the detection of temperature in the different skin areas in the two studies. In fact, Formenti et al. analyzed the skin temperature above the quadriceps muscles, while in the current study, the temperature was evaluated above the knee joint. Interestingly, the subdivision of the knee into subareas allowed us to highlight different behaviors in different subareas following exercise. For example, the region of the patella is cooler due to the underlying bone, and other areas may respond differently. The suprapatellar area showed a response to the exercise similar to that found in the study of Formenti et al., with a temperature decrease occurring two minutes after the beginning of exercise, followed by a significant temperature increase. Perhaps this is due to the proximity of the suprapatellar area to the distal part of the quadriceps muscle, thus showing a behavior similar to that of the skin over the muscles. On the other hand, all other subareas and the total knee temperatures demonstrated an initial decrease that was not followed by a return to baseline values after this short exercise bout and at the last studied timepoint.

This study also detected a correlation between the clinical status of the patients and the thermal response of their knees to exercise. A positive correlation was found between the evaluated clinical scores and the changes in temperature after physical exercise. Patients with a better clinical status showed a greater change in temperature compared to patients with a worse clinical status. Therefore, patients with fewer symptoms demonstrated a temperature decrease comparable with that of healthy subjects, as analyzed in previous studies [30,33,36]. This trend was confirmed by subjective scores evaluating pain, such as the VAS, or more complex functional scales, such as the IKDC subjective score and the KOOS subscales. On the other hand, patients with a worse clinical status had a lower response to exercise with a reduced temperature variation. This could be explained by the fact that patients with a worse clinical status could have performed the exercise at a lower intensity, activating the muscles less. Moreover, the higher association of a worse clinical status with a higher inflammatory component in knee OA [8,37,38] could also partly explain the altered response to physical exercise.

The response to exercise in this population also correlated with the results of the PainDETECT questionnaire, which evaluates the contribution of neuropathic pain to pain perception by the patient [39,40]. This score has not only been associated with impaired pain modulation but also with neuropathy, which may contribute to OA knee pain through damage to nerve fibers in the joint [41–43]. Considering that nerve fibers have a fundamental role in regulating skin circulation by releasing catecholamines, their alteration could lead to an impaired response to external stimuli, such as exercise [41,44,45]. In fact, patients in the current study with high PainDETECT questionnaire scores showed less temperature variation after exercise. This result could be explained by altered cutaneous vasoconstriction due to neuropathy, resulting in an alteration of the peripheral neuromodulation mechanisms. While the clinical relevance of this finding remains to be established, this finding confirms the presence of different factors influencing OA joints and the need to better study knee OA patterns.

The thermal response to exercise in patients with knee OA was also affected by sex. Women had a greater decrease in skin temperature than men immediately after exercise and at five minutes after its end. This could be related to differences in the metabolic, contractile, and hemodynamic properties of skeletal muscle between women and men, as well as the different cutaneous adipose tissue distribution [46,47]. Women have greater capillarization of the muscle than men and also a greater vasodilatory response of the arteries supplying the skeletal muscles, which leads to a greater increase in blood flow [48–50]. Moreover, women usually have a reduced exercise capacity and a lower blood volume than men; therefore, the same physical exercise could require a major effort and thus a relatively high level of blood transfer from the skin to the muscles compared to men. [51]. In previous work, it has been shown that the same type of exercise with the same number of repetitions can provide a greater training stress in women than in men [52]. In the current study, both sexes performed the same exercise for the same amount of time and at the same frequency. From this perspective, the greater activation of compensatory mechanisms aimed at redistributing the flow to the muscles involved in the exercise could explain the greater cutaneous vasoconstriction detected by the infrared thermography in women. Further studies on a larger numbers of patients should explore whether, besides the overall higher temperature changes, women present similar or different response patterns to men based on demographic, clinical, or other influencing factors.

This study presents some limitations. Although this is the largest study evaluating the thermal response to exercise in symptomatic patients with knee OA, future studies with larger populations are needed to confirm the identified correlations. Second, a control group of nonsymptomatic knee OA patients or non-OA knee patients could be used to better characterize the response of the knee to the exercise stimulus and to better evaluate temperature changes related to the presence and severity of OA disease. Third, the performed exercise may not have been optimal to generate the largest thermal response of the evaluated knee, and it could require different stresses among different patients. Therefore, future studies should investigate other possible exercises tailored to patients in terms of the type, time, and effort. It was not possible to perform evaluations using tests, such as Doppler vascular examination to exclude varicose veins or electrodiagnostic testing to better characterize the neuropathic component of the patients' pain, and future studies should better characterize the neuropathic component of pain in these patients. Although the results obtained are statistically significant, the large interindividual variability and the many variables influencing temperature may have reduced the power of the study, so the results need future confirmation. Finally, the method of thermographic image acquisition and analysis was based on previous literature, but no method has been described as the gold standard in this field. For example, we adopted a 10-min protocol for patient thermalization, while other authors prefer a 15-min window of thermalization before the thermographic evaluation. It is possible that different settings, different lenses, and different devices could be more suitable for such evaluations in clinical practice. The standardization of thermography use for the evaluation of knee OA could improve its potential for identifying different disease patterns both in research and in clinical practice. In this regard, this study provides new input on how the thermographic findings can be influenced by simple exercise testing, which could be useful for studying patients and knees with different OA patterns so that they can be targeted by specific and more effective treatment approaches in the future.

5. Conclusions

This study demonstrated that the temperature response to knee flexion–extension exercise in symptomatic knee OA is affected by the demographic and clinical characteristics of the assessed patients. Patients with a poor clinical knee status presented a lower response to exercise, and women showed a greater temperature decrease compared to men. Not all evaluated ROIs showed the same trend, which underlines the need to specifically study the different joint subareas to identify the inflammatory component and joint response while investigating knee OA patterns.

Author Contributions: Conceptualization, G.F.; methodology, L.D.M., A.B. and S.O.; data curation, L.D.M.; writing—original draft preparation, L.D.M., A.B. and L.A.; writing—review and editing, A.D.M. and G.F.; supervision. S.Z. and G.F. All authors have read and agreed to the published version of the manuscript.

Funding: This research and APC were funded by the Italian Ministry of Health—5 × 1000 Anno 2019, Redditi 2018 "Termografia a infrarossi per lo studio di patologie infiammatorie e degenerative articolari".

Institutional Review Board Statement: The study was conducted in accordance with the Declaration of Helsinki and approved by the Institutional Ethics Committee of IRCCS Istituto Ortopedico Rizzoli, Bologna, Italy (Prot. n. 0017413).

Informed Consent Statement: Informed consent was obtained from all subjects involved in the study.

Data Availability Statement: Not applicable.

Acknowledgments: Special thanks are given to Elettra Pignotti for her contribution to the statistical analysis.

Conflicts of Interest: S.Z. reports nonfinancial support through personal fees from I + SRL and grants from Fidia Farmaceutici SPA, Cartiheal ltd, IGEA clinical biophysics, BIOMET, and Kensey Nash, outside the submitted work. The funders had no role in the design of the study, in the collection, analyses, or interpretation of data, in the writing of the manuscript, or in the decision to publish the results. The other authors declare no conflict of interest.

References

1. Hildebrandt, C.; Raschner, C.; Ammer, K. An Overview of Recent Application of Medical Infrared Thermography in Sports Medicine in Austria. *Sensors* **2010**, *10*, 4700–4715. [CrossRef] [PubMed]
2. Ring, F. Thermal Imaging Today and Its Relevance to Diabetes. *J. Diabetes Sci. Technol.* **2010**, *4*, 857–862. [CrossRef] [PubMed]
3. Tattersall, G.J. Infrared Thermography: A Non-Invasive Window into Thermal Physiology. *Comp. Biochem. Physiol. A Mol. Integr. Physiol.* **2016**, *202*, 78–98. [CrossRef] [PubMed]
4. Schiavon, G.; Capone, G.; Frize, M.; Zaffagnini, S.; Candrian, C.; Filardo, G. Infrared Thermography for the Evaluation of Inflammatory and Degenerative Joint Diseases: A Systematic Review. *Cartilage* **2021**, *13*, 1790S–1801S. [CrossRef]
5. Khan, A.A.; Arora, A.S. Thermography as an Economical Alternative Modality to Mammography for Early Detection of Breast Cancer. *J. Healthc. Eng.* **2021**, *2021*, 5543101. [CrossRef]
6. Nakagami, G.; Sanada, H.; Iizaka, S.; Kadono, T.; Higashino, T.; Koyanagi, H.; Haga, N. Predicting Delayed Pressure Ulcer Healing Using Thermography: A Prospective Cohort Study. *J. Wound Care* **2010**, *19*, 465–466, 468, 470. [CrossRef]
7. Wallace, I.J.; Worthington, S.; Felson, D.T.; Jurmain, R.D.; Wren, K.T.; Maijanen, H.; Woods, R.J.; Lieberman, D.E. Knee Osteoarthritis Has Doubled in Prevalence since the Mid-20th Century. *Proc. Natl. Acad. Sci. USA* **2017**, *114*, 9332–9336. [CrossRef]
8. Sanchez-Lopez, E.; Coras, R.; Torres, A.; Lane, N.E.; Guma, M. Synovial Inflammation in Osteoarthritis Progression. *Nat. Rev. Rheumatol.* **2022**, *18*, 258–275. [CrossRef]
9. Boffa, A.; Merli, G.; Andriolo, L.; Lattermann, C.; Salzmann, G.M.; Filardo, G. Synovial Fluid Biomarkers in Knee Osteoarthritis: A Systematic Review and Quantitative Evaluation Using BIPEDs Criteria. *Cartilage* **2021**, *13*, 82S–103S. [CrossRef]
10. Nanus, D.E.; Badoume, A.; Wijesinghe, S.N.; Halsey, A.M.; Hurley, P.; Ahmed, Z.; Botchu, R.; Davis, E.T.; Lindsay, M.A.; Jones, S.W. Synovial Tissue from Sites of Joint Pain in Knee Osteoarthritis Patients Exhibits a Differential Phenotype with Distinct Fibroblast Subsets. *EBioMedicine* **2021**, *72*, 103618. [CrossRef]
11. de Silva, M.; Kyle, V.; Hazleman, B.; Salisbury, R.; Page Thomas, P.; Wraight, P. Assessment of Inflammation in the Rheumatoid Knee Joint: Correlation between Clinical, Radioisotopic, and Thermographic Methods. *Ann. Rheum. Dis.* **1986**, *45*, 277–280. [CrossRef] [PubMed]
12. Varjú, G.; Pieper, C.F.; Renner, J.B.; Kraus, V.B. Assessment of Hand Osteoarthritis: Correlation between Thermographic and Radiographic Methods. *Rheumatology* **2004**, *43*, 915–919. [CrossRef] [PubMed]

13. Ahn, S.M.; Chun, J.H.; Hong, S.; Lee, C.-K.; Yoo, B.; Oh, J.S.; Kim, Y.-G. The Value of Thermal Imaging for Knee Arthritis: A Single-Center Observational Study. *Yonsei Med. J.* **2022**, *63*, 141–147. [CrossRef] [PubMed]
14. Romanò, C.L.; Logoluso, N.; Dell'Oro, F.; Elia, A.; Drago, L. Telethermographic Findings after Uncomplicated and Septic Total Knee Replacement. *Knee* **2012**, *19*, 193–197. [CrossRef]
15. Brito, C.J.; Miarka, B.; García-Pastor, T.; Pérez, D.I.V.; Marins, J.C.B.; Sillero-Quintana, M. Osteoarthritis Subjects Have Differentiated Lower Extremity Thermal Skin Response after the Concurrent Acute Training Session. *J. Therm. Anal. Calorim.* **2021**, *145*, 2467–2475. [CrossRef]
16. Arfaoui, A.; Bouzid, M.A.; Pron, H.; Taiar, R.; Polidori, G. Application of Infrared Thermography as a Diagnostic Tool of Knee Osteoarthritis. *J. Therm. Sci. Technol.* **2012**, *7*, 227–235. [CrossRef]
17. Moreira, D.G.; Costello, J.T.; Brito, C.J.; Adamczyk, J.G.; Ammer, K.; Bach, A.J.E.; Costa, C.M.A.; Eglin, C.; Fernandes, A.A.; Fernández-Cuevas, I.; et al. Thermographic Imaging in Sports and Exercise Medicine: A Delphi Study and Consensus Statement on the Measurement of Human Skin Temperature. *J. Therm. Biol.* **2017**, *69*, 155–162. [CrossRef]
18. Schwartz, R.G.; Getson, P.; O'Young, B.; Bernton, T.; Brioschi, M.; Schakaraschwilli, G.; Terzella, M.; Habibi, B.; Zhang, H.-Y. Guidelines for Neuro-Musculoskeletal Infrared Medical Thermology & Sympathetic Skin Response (SSR) Studies. *Pan Am. J. Med. Thermol.* **2021**, 1–13. Available online: https://aathermology.org/wp-content/uploads/2018/04/AAT-NMSK-Guidelines-2021.pdf (accessed on 23 January 2023).
19. Merla, A.; Mattei, P.A.; Di Donato, L.; Romani, G.L. Thermal Imaging of Cutaneous Temperature Modifications in Runners during Graded Exercise. *Ann. Biomed. Eng.* **2010**, *38*, 158–163. [CrossRef]
20. Ring, E.F.J.; Ammer, K. The Technique of Infrared Imaging in Medicine. In *Infrared Imaging: A Casebook in Clinical Medicin*; IoP Publishing: Bristol, UK, 2015; pp. 1-1–1-10.
21. Marins, J.C.B.; Moreira, D.G.; Cano, S.P.; Quintana, M.S.; Soares, D.D.; de Andrade Fernandes, A.; da Silva, F.S.; Costa, C.M.A.; dos Santos Amorim, P.R. Time Required to Stabilize Thermographic Images at Rest. *Infrared Phys. Technol.* **2014**, *65*, 30–35. [CrossRef]
22. Danko, M.; Hudak, R.; Foffová, P.; Zivcak, J. An Importance of Camera—Subject Distance and Angle in Musculoskeletal Application of Medical Thermography. *Acta Electrotech. Inf.* **2010**, *10*, 57–59.
23. De Marziani, L.; Boffa, A.; Angelelli, L.; Andriolo, L.; Di Martino, A.; Zaffagnini, S.; Filardo, G. Infrared Thermography in Symptomatic Knee Osteoarthritis: Joint Temperature Differs Based on Patient and Pain Characteristics. *J. Clin. Med.* **2023**, *12*, 2319. [CrossRef] [PubMed]
24. Denoble, A.E.; Hall, N.; Pieper, C.F.; Kraus, V.B. Patellar Skin Surface Temperature by Thermography Reflects Knee Osteoarthritis Severity. *Clin. Med. Insights Arthritis Musculoskelet. Disord.* **2010**, *3*, 69–75. [CrossRef] [PubMed]
25. de Lacerda, A.P.D.; de Andrade, P.R.; Kamonseki, D.H.; Parizotto, N.A.; da Silva, A.S.A.; de Medeiros, L.B.; de Almeida Ferreira, J.J. Accuracy of Infrared Thermography in Detecting Tendinopathy: A Systematic Review with Meta-Analysis. *Phys. Ther. Sport Off. J. Assoc. Chart. Physiother. Sports Med.* **2022**, *58*, 117–125. [CrossRef]
26. Kumar, P.; Gaurav, A.; Rajnish, R.K.; Sharma, S.; Kumar, V.; Aggarwal, S.; Patel, S. Applications of Thermal Imaging with Infrared Thermography in Orthopaedics. *J. Clin. Orthop. Trauma* **2022**, *24*, 101722. [CrossRef]
27. Calin, M.A.; Mologhianu, G.; Savastru, R.; Calin, M.R.; Brailescu, C.M. A Review of the Effectiveness of Thermal Infrared Imaging in the Diagnosis and Monitoring of Knee Diseases. *Infrared Phys. Technol.* **2015**, *69*, 19–25. [CrossRef]
28. Lohchab, V.; Rathod, P.; Mahapatra, P.K.; Bachhal, V.; Hooda, A. Non-invasive Assessment of Knee Osteoarthritis Patients Using Thermal Imaging. *IET Sci. Meas. Technol.* **2022**, *16*, 242–249. [CrossRef]
29. Formenti, D.; Ludwig, N.; Gargano, M.; Gondola, M.; Dellerma, N.; Caumo, A.; Alberti, G. Thermal Imaging of Exercise-Associated Skin Temperature Changes in Trained and Untrained Female Subjects. *Ann. Biomed. Eng.* **2013**, *41*, 863–871. [CrossRef]
30. Merla, A.; Iodice, P.; Tangherlini, A.; De Michele, G.; Di Romualdo, S.; Saggini, R.; Romani, G. Monitoring Skin Temperature in Trained and Untrained Subjects throughout Thermal Video. In Proceedings of the 2005 IEEE Engineering in Medicine and Biology 27th Annual Conference, Shanghai, China, 17–18 January 2006; pp. 1684–1686. [CrossRef]
31. Hillen, B.; Pfirrmann, D.; Nägele, M.; Simon, P. Infrared Thermography in Exercise Physiology: The Dawning of Exercise Radiomics. *Sport. Med. Auckl. NZ* **2020**, *50*, 263–282. [CrossRef]
32. Vainer, B.G. FPA-Based Infrared Thermography as Applied to the Study of Cutaneous Perspiration and Stimulated Vascular Response in Humans. *Phys. Med. Biol.* **2005**, *50*, R63–R94. [CrossRef]
33. Formenti, D.; Ludwig, N.; Trecroci, A.; Gargano, M.; Michelon, G.; Caumo, A.; Alberti, G. Dynamics of Thermographic Skin Temperature Response during Squat Exercise at Two Different Speeds. *J. Therm. Biol.* **2016**, *59*, 58–63. [CrossRef]
34. Kenney, W.L.; Armstrong, C.G. Reflex Peripheral Vasoconstriction Is Diminished in Older Men. *J. Appl. Physiol.* **1996**, *80*, 512–515. [CrossRef] [PubMed]
35. Holowatz, L.A.; Kenney, W.L. Peripheral Mechanisms of Thermoregulatory Control of Skin Blood Flow in Aged Humans. *J. Appl. Physiol.* **2010**, *109*, 1538–1544. [CrossRef] [PubMed]
36. Kalliokoski, K.K.; Knuuti, J.; Nuutila, P. Relationship between Muscle Blood Flow and Oxygen Uptake during Exercise in Endurance-Trained and Untrained Men. *J. Appl. Physiol.* **2005**, *98*, 380–383. [CrossRef] [PubMed]
37. Collins, J.E.; Losina, E.; Nevitt, M.C.; Roemer, F.W.; Guermazi, A.; Lynch, J.A.; Katz, J.N.; Kent Kwoh, C.; Kraus, V.B.; Hunter, D.J. Semiquantitative Imaging Biomarkers of Knee Osteoarthritis Progression: Data from the Foundation for the National Institutes of Health Osteoarthritis Biomarkers Consortium. *Arthritis Rheumatol.* **2016**, *68*, 2422–2431. [CrossRef]

38. Riis, R.G.C.; Gudbergsen, H.; Henriksen, M.; Ballegaard, C.; Bandak, E.; Röttger, D.; Bliddal, H.; Hansen, B.B.; Hangaard, S.; Boesen, M. Synovitis Assessed on Static and Dynamic Contrast-Enhanced Magnetic Resonance Imaging and Its Association with Pain in Knee Osteoarthritis: A Cross-Sectional Study. *Eur. J. Radiol.* **2016**, *85*, 1099–1108. [CrossRef]
39. Moss, P.; Benson, H.A.E.; Will, R.; Wright, A. Patients with Knee Osteoarthritis Who Score Highly on the PainDETECT Questionnaire Present with Multimodality Hyperalgesia, Increased Pain, and Impaired Physical Function. *Clin. J. Pain* **2018**, *34*, 15–21. [CrossRef] [PubMed]
40. Freynhagen, R.; Baron, R.; Gockel, U.; Tölle, T.R. PainDETECT: A New Screening Questionnaire to Identify Neuropathic Components in Patients with Back Pain. *Curr. Med. Res. Opin.* **2006**, *22*, 1911–1920. [CrossRef]
41. Moreton, B.J.; Tew, V.; das Nair, R.; Wheeler, M.; Walsh, D.A.; Lincoln, N.B. Pain Phenotype in Patients with Knee Osteoarthritis: Classification and Measurement Properties of PainDETECT and Self-Report Leeds Assessment of Neuropathic Symptoms and Signs Scale in a Cross-Sectional Study. *Arthritis Care Res.* **2015**, *67*, 519–528. [CrossRef]
42. Bonnet, C.S.; Walsh, D.A. Osteoarthritis, Angiogenesis and Inflammation. *Rheumatology* **2005**, *44*, 7–16. [CrossRef]
43. French, H.P.; Smart, K.M.; Doyle, F. Prevalence of Neuropathic Pain in Knee or Hip Osteoarthritis: A Systematic Review and Meta-Analysis. *Semin. Arthritis Rheum.* **2017**, *47*, 1–8. [CrossRef] [PubMed]
44. Cracowski, J.-L.; Roustit, M. Human Skin Microcirculation. *Compr. Physiol.* **2020**, *10*, 1105–1154. [CrossRef] [PubMed]
45. Minson, C.T.; Berry, L.T.; Joyner, M.J. Nitric Oxide and Neurally Mediated Regulation of Skin Blood Flow during Local Heating. *J. Appl. Physiol.* **2001**, *91*, 1619–1626. [CrossRef]
46. Blaak, E. Gender Differences in Fat Metabolism. *Curr. Opin. Clin. Nutr. Metab. Care* **2001**, *4*, 499–502. [CrossRef] [PubMed]
47. Ansdell, P.; Thomas, K.; Hicks, K.M.; Hunter, S.K.; Howatson, G.; Goodall, S. Physiological Sex Differences Affect the Integrative Response to Exercise: Acute and Chronic Implications. *Exp. Physiol.* **2020**, *105*, 2007–2021. [CrossRef]
48. Roepstorff, C.; Thiele, M.; Hillig, T.; Pilegaard, H.; Richter, E.A.; Wojtaszewski, J.F.P.; Kiens, B. Higher Skeletal Muscle Alpha2AMPK Activation and Lower Energy Charge and Fat Oxidation in Men than in Women during Submaximal Exercise. *J. Physiol.* **2006**, *574*, 125–138. [CrossRef]
49. Hill, E.C.; Housh, T.J.; Smith, C.M.; Schmidt, R.J.; Johnson, G.O. Gender- and Muscle-Specific Responses During Fatiguing Exercise. *J. Strength Cond. Res.* **2018**, *32*, 1471–1478. [CrossRef]
50. Parker, B.A.; Smithmyer, S.L.; Pelberg, J.A.; Mishkin, A.D.; Herr, M.D.; Proctor, D.N. Sex Differences in Leg Vasodilation during Graded Knee Extensor Exercise in Young Adults. *J. Appl. Physiol.* **2007**, *103*, 1583–1591. [CrossRef]
51. Kaciuba-Uscilko, H.; Grucza, R. Gender Differences in Thermoregulation. *Curr. Opin. Clin. Nutr. Metab. Care* **2001**, *4*, 533–536. [CrossRef]
52. Alizadeh, S.; Rayner, M.; Mahmoud, M.M.I.; Behm, D.G. Push-Ups vs. Bench Press Differences in Repetitions and Muscle Activation between Sexes. *J. Sport. Sci. Med.* **2020**, *19*, 289–297.

Disclaimer/Publisher's Note: The statements, opinions and data contained in all publications are solely those of the individual author(s) and contributor(s) and not of MDPI and/or the editor(s). MDPI and/or the editor(s) disclaim responsibility for any injury to people or property resulting from any ideas, methods, instructions or products referred to in the content.

MDPI
St. Alban-Anlage 66
4052 Basel
Switzerland
www.mdpi.com

Journal of Clinical Medicine Editorial Office
E-mail: jcm@mdpi.com
www.mdpi.com/journal/jcm

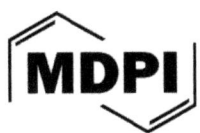

Disclaimer/Publisher's Note: The statements, opinions and data contained in all publications are solely those of the individual author(s) and contributor(s) and not of MDPI and/or the editor(s). MDPI and/or the editor(s) disclaim responsibility for any injury to people or property resulting from any ideas, methods, instructions or products referred to in the content.